FELINE BEHAVIOR:

A Guide for Veterinarians

FELINE BEHAVIOR:

A Guide for Veterinarians

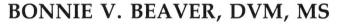

BONNIE V. BEAVER, DVM, MS

Department of Small Animal Medicine and Surgery
College of Veterinary Medicine
Texas A&M University
College Station, Texas

W. B. SAUNDERS COMPANY

Harcourt Brace Jovanovich, Inc.

Philadelphia   London   Toronto   Montreal   Sydney   Tokyo

W. B. SAUNDERS COMPANY
Harcourt Brace Jovanovich, Inc.

The Curtis Center
Independence Square West
Philadelphia, Pennsylvania 19106

Library of Congress Cataloging-in-Publication Data

Beaver, Bonnie V.

Feline behavior: a guide for veterinarians / Bonnie V. Beaver—1st ed.

    p.   cm.

1. Cats—Behavior.   I. Title.

SF446.5.B38 1992

ISBN 0–7216–3992–5

636.8—dc20   92–4228

Last digit is the print number: 9   8   7   6   5   4   3   2   1

Dedication

I have been blessed by being able to interact with and gain from a large number of outstanding individuals: my parents, relatives, friends, teachers, students, and colleagues. It is these wonderful people who have enriched and encouraged me throughout my life.

There is one person I hold especially dear and to him I dedicate this book, my husband, Larry J. Beaver.

Preface

Very little research has been done on the ethological approach to domestic animal behavior because, in the past, the human-animal relationship did not need a deep understanding. Times have changed and pets now share a close relationship with their owners, an affinity that is causing clients to ask "why" about a number of different observations. Little has been written about the cat's general behaviors because the animal was simply considered to be a farm-variety mobile mousetrap. The cat is unique among pets because of its historical influence and asocial nature, which are the same elements that make understanding cats difficult for humans.

Veterinary practice is changing, with the amount of time spent on pets becoming significantly greater than in years past. Most veterinarians have not formally learned the answers to the "why" questions their clients are asking and have had to rely on experience, common sense, and guesses.

For persons with a special interest in feline behavior, information has been particularly hard to find, as it is widely scattered and difficult to locate even with access to a large library. In addition, much information on the domestic felid is scattered throughout the literature on humans. Researchers have also had difficulty determining exactly what work has been done.

Working with feline behavior problems is an art and science that is still in its infancy. Information about specific problems is particularly difficult to obtain, much less explain to a client. Veterinarians with an interest in this area have not had a reference of origin from which they can agree and build or disagree and determine new approaches.

It was with these things in mind that I wrote the original version of this book, *Veterinary Aspects of Feline Behavior:* (1) to describe the cat's behavior and its changing role for humans, (2) to provide the practicing veterinarian with important information on how to deal with feline behavior problems, (3) to collect a bibliography for those interested in pursuing specific areas of interest, (4) to bring together scattered information to portray the complete felid, and (5) to provide a reference of origin from which feline behaviorists may build. Since that publication, additional information has been gained about cat behavior and new treatments have been developed for feline behavior problems. These changes have been incorporated into this newer version of the book, *Feline Behavior: A Guide For Veterinarians.*

I would like to thank the personnel of the Medical Sciences Library and the secretarial staff of the Department of Small Animal Medicine and Surgery at Texas A&M University for their assistance in the preparation of this book. Drs. George Shelton and John August are to be thanked too for their support, each in a unique way. Special appreciation is expressed to Sharon Ashby, Kelly Chaffin, Margaret Fisher, Kelly Helmick, and Linda Mills for their extra efforts toward the success of this endeavor and to the veterinarians throughout the country for their referrals and valuable input.

BONNIE V. BEAVER

Contents

5

Male Feline Sexual Behavior 121

6

Female Feline Sexual Behavior 141

7

Feline Ingestive Behavior 171

8

Eliminative Behavior Development 203

9
Feline Locomotive Behavior 225

10
Feline Grooming Behavior 255

Appendix

Introduction to Feline Behavior

HISTORY OF FELINE DEVELOPMENT

Earliest Origins of the Cat

Down through the ages we have had a curious relationship with the cat. More inconsistent than our relationship with any other domestic animal, it has nurtured the behavior of the modern cat.

The earliest known ancestors of the Felidae date back between 10 million and 45 million years. Carnivores are believed to have shared at that time a common forest-dwelling ancestor: the Miacidae. The cat was derived from a later subdivision, the *Dinictis*. We do not know when the cat was first considered domesticated or which of the wild cats are its ancestors. What is recorded is that by 1600 B.C., cats were domesticated in Egypt. Most authorities agree that the modern cat, *Felis catus*, is derived from *Felis libyca*, the Kaffir cat (also known as the small African bush cat, the African wild cat, or the Caffre cat), which was numerous in Egypt at that time.

The role played by the European wild cat *Felis silvestris* in the development of the modern cat is uncertain. Some contend that *F. silvestris* (formerly called *F. catus*) was crossed with the Egyptian cat to produce the modern *F. catus* (formerly called *F. domestica*), whereas others give behavioral, cultural, and physical reasons to refute this theory. A recent theory is that the two wild types are actually subspecies (*F. silvestris silvestris* and *F. silvestris libyca*), since domestic and wild have identical karyotypes.[12, 50] Molecular studies show a close lineage between the domestic cat and four wild cats, including *F. libyca*.[62]

1

Spread of the Cat from Ancient Egypt

In ancient Egypt the cat initially was kept to control the rodent population on farms and in granaries. Later the cat also was used to fish and to hunt and retrieve wild birds. As time passed, the cat became associated with religion. Bastet (also called Bast, Bassett), the cat goddess, daughter of the sun god Re, represented the fertility of plants and women as well as good health (Fig. 1–1). As Bastet became the primary goddess, the cat became a prized animal—legally protected; mourned at death by its owner, who showed his grief by shaving off his eyebrows; and mummified for burial in special cemeteries.

The range of the domesticated cat expanded slowly, possibly because of tight export restrictions, which limited emigration to the cat's own ingenuity.[3, 50, 54, 66] Merchants and soldiers eventually introduced *F. catus* to Asia and Europe, so that between A.D. 300 and 500, the cat reached Britain. The correlation between water trade routes and the existence of feline populations shows that water posed no problem to migration; the cats probably traveled by ship, coming and going as they pleased.[58]

Because Muhammad's favorite animal was the cat, it has always enjoyed favor in Islamic countries. Islamic teachings include specific references to punishment for the harsh treatment of cats and other animals.[16] The treatment this animal received from Christians, however, has had a more profound effect on its behavioral development. When

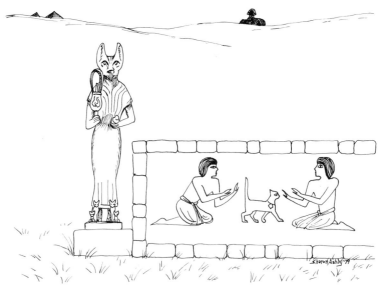

FIGURE 1–1. The Egyptian cat goddess Bastet.

introduced into Europe, the cat was believed to have protected the Christ child in the stable from the Devil's mouse.[3] As time passed, the independent nature of the cat and its prominent eyes led to its association with Diana, the moon goddess (Fig. 1–2).[29] Legend has it that she created the cat to mock the sun god Apollo.[3] This association of the cat with the moon led to the connection of the cat with the Devil and witchcraft.[19, 53] During the Middle Ages, not only were vast numbers of cats exterminated, but the same fate was met by people who showed compassion for them. When the European Crusaders returned around A.D. 1600, they brought with them an invasion of the brown rat, the bubonic plague, and a gradual reacceptance of the only effective rat control method—the cat. Introduction into America came in the seventeenth century, probably because the cat served as the principal method of rodent control on British vessels bound for the New World. Along with the cat, however, came the witchcraft cult.[19]

When Pasteur discovered in the 1800s that bacteria spread diseases, people became extremely conscious of cleanliness. By another twist of

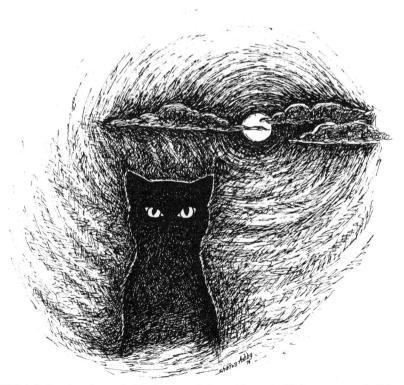

FIGURE 1–2. Prominent eyes led to the association of the cat with the moon and witchcraft.

fate, the cat came to be considered the only clean animal and was allowed in food markets, acquiring a position of favor by merchants.[19, 49]

Domestication of the Cat

Domestication requires several generations of selective breeding to produce physiological, morphological, and behavioral changes. For *F. catus* this process has been unique. Except for the cat, breeding during domestication of most animals had been done by selection of behavioral characteristics, primarily to increase gentleness. The cat, however, was first brought into the home for religious reasons, not utilitarian ones.[35, 63] Because cats followed the urbanization of human populations, mating was a matter of proximity rather than of human selection.[53, 59] Not only was it difficult to control mating in cats, but the religious connotation prohibited selective breeding. The actual date of domestication varies from 100 B.C. to as early as 7000 B.C., and several authorities imply that even now the cat is not fully domesticated because it can revert to total self-sufficiency.[50] The first recorded planned feline breeding did not occur until A.D. 999, at the Japanese Imperial Palace. It soon became fashionable in that country to control cat matings and environments. But mice subsequently devastated the silkworm industry, so that by 1602, Japanese cats were released from these controls.[49]

During the time the cat fell from favor and met with mass extermination in Europe, selective breeding was not practiced. Even with the Crusaders helping the cat return to favor, the prevailing attitude was one of tolerance rather than of full acceptance. Historically, then, it took many years before the cat achieved a position whereby the behavioral characteristics desired in a domesticated animal could be developed by selective breeding.

CURRENT STATUS OF THE FELID

Cat Population Statistics

The recent increase in the number of cats—especially registered cats—in the United States has been dramatic. This may be due in part to their adaptability to living in apartments and small homes. Figures vary greatly and are inaccurate because of the number of stray cats, but the pet cat population is between 23.1 and 56 million.[1, 24, 44, 47, 60, 64] Associated figures estimate 1.6 to 2.2 cats for each house that has cats, or one cat in every 3.2 single-family dwelling units.[15, 46, 52, 60, 64] Of this cat population, only between 3 and 13 million are seen by veterinarians.[24, 30, 44, 60] Stray cats represent between 2 per cent and 28 per cent of the known population.[23, 42, 46] Each year as many as 20 per cent of a city's pet population pass through its animal shelter.[47] This large stray feline population may be reflected in another statistic: Only 38 per cent of male cats are castrated and 31 per cent of females are spayed[64]; however, local differences have been reported.[45]

Cat ownership is increasing worldwide, often in parallel to trends in the United States. In several European countries cat numbers now exceed those for dogs, as does the percentage of households owning cats.[41]

Cat Owner Categorization

In addition to surviving a varied history, the cat has withstood many types of owners. Cat owners have been classified in several ways by researchers, but they tend to fall in one of two categories: those who have a weak attachment and those who have a strong one.[30, 64] The classification "low-involvement owner" is applied to 59 per cent of the 14,645,000 cat-owning households in one study of pet owners.[64] These people devote little time to the care or company of the cat, and seem to enjoy having a cat around more than interacting with it. This lack of involvement with the pet is reflected in trauma statistics. Of 126 cats (89 males, 37 females) reported injured during a period of slightly more than a year, 16.3 per cent had been hit by a car, 14.7 per cent had been involved in animal interaction, and 39.5 per cent received injuries from causes unknown to the owner.[31] The average life span for a cat is 12 years, but ages of 20 or more years are not uncommon.[13, 56] The current longevity record is 36 years.[65] Although the average age for the general population is 3 years, that of the neutered cat is 3 to 5 years longer and that of the traumatized cat is only 1.3 years.[8, 31, 64] One study of road kills indicated that most were kittens or young adults.[10] Because of the low-involvement owners, cat populations, for the most part, still fulfill the criteria of random mating.[51]

The second classification of cat owners, those with a strong attachment, has been subdivided. "Quality- or status-conscious owners" compose 21 per cent of all cat owners. The pet is an expression of how this owner views himself or herself and reflects his or her good taste, as would other material possessions. These owners believe that the cat depends on them for love, affection, and care, and as a result, the animal is well groomed and only reluctantly left alone.[18, 64]

"High-involvement owners," the second subdivision, constitute the remaining 20 per cent of the cat-owning population.[64] Unlike owners in the other two categories, these people rely on the cat to supply love and affection or to serve as an emotional crutch, such as a child substitute. Attachments to the cat frequently are described as those to a human family member, friend, or child.[1, 22] The person believes that the cat enjoys humans, feeds it specially prepared foods, has photographs of the pet, and may celebrate the cat's birthday.[22] Owners from this group are most likely to bury a deceased pet in a pet cemetery or mausoleum or to leave an estate to their cats. This kind of owner was responsible for bequeathing $415,000 to two cats in 1965, making them the richest cats in history.[18, 64]

Quality- or status-conscious owners and high-involvement owners, many of whom are in the middle or upper socioeconomic level, spend billions of dollars each year on their pets. Such people have a higher percentage of neutered cats than do low-involvement owners and a preference for lighter-colored cats.[11]

Modern Roles for the Cat

Pets take on many roles in society, and these roles change as the needs of civilization change. Whereas individuals can be shown to be unique, all cats are products of species-specific characteristics.[17] People's reasons for having cats vary, but most owners indicate that personality and appearance are important features.[48] The cat still controls rodents, but closer contact with humans is adding new dimensions of purpose. As a research animal, the cat has become invaluable for studies of aggression, neurology, anatomy, ecology, and aging.

Developing children derive significant benefits from having a pet, and the cat has long been important in this regard. The animal can assume different roles during a child's maturation. A child may relate better to a pet than to adults, and with this friend, she or he may be better able to work out many of the normal problems of childhood. Caring for a cat teaches the child to assume responsibility, and watching the cat's normal body functions results in self-understanding and a respect for life. The cat also provides companionship. Motivation for learning and creativity also is stimulated by a cat's presence.[18, 36, 39, 57] Even the painful experience of the death of a beloved pet can help to prepare a child for the future loss of loved ones. Interest in pets sharply decreases in boys and, to a lesser extent, in girls when adolescence is reached.[32, 35, 36]

Cats and other pets are assuming an increasingly important role in maintaining the mental health of our society. The fast pace of modern civilization isolates humans from one another, and the animal may be the only constant factor in a person's environment to help maintain psychological equilibrium. The role a pet plays within a family varies with individuals. For a wife, petting the cat may represent affection for a child substitute or a safe expression of desire for sexual sensations, whereas for the husband, the pet may represent an object of ego expression.[20, 36]

Serving as a catalyst and facilitator of human relations, the cat has been especially helpful to the elderly and the young. A person in either age group may find it difficult to accept a dependent role, and the cat, as a subordinate, can boost that person's self-esteem.[14, 33, 37] To the aged individual, a pet also may serve as a living memory of a deceased spouse. Widows are more likely to tend to preserve this memory at all costs, whereas widowers tend to destroy guilt-laden reminders of the past.[35, 37] Although most authorities believe that relationships such as loving a cat promote good mental health, a minority opinion has been expressed that attachment to a pet is a symptom of alienation from other humans.[9]

The cat has been used increasingly in psychotherapy sessions to stimulate communication, provide an object for affection, and allow the patient's mastery of a situation. Cats also have been prescribed for home therapy, working 24 hours a day to draw individuals into an awareness of their surroundings or to provide affection and emotional security where they might be lacking. Therapy in institutional settings for the emotionally disturbed and the mentally retarded also has received a big boost when cats are part of the settings because the animals increase the effect of the professional staff and provide continuity during staff turn-overs.[34]

Pets often reflect the psychological state of their families, even to the point of taking on the same neuroses as the family.[55] The animal may receive the abuse that a parent would have otherwise directed toward the child or the abuse from a child mimicking his or her parents.[26, 28] Even the cat's name may indicate its role to the family. "Ugly" or "Shorty" may represent the low regard the owner has for the animal, and human names may be indicative of a peer ranking.

The veterinarian is in a unique position as a result of the owner-pet relationship. The increased use of the cat as a mental health tool forces such patients to become more dependent on the veterinarian. This dependency requires the veterinarian to become more aware of human behavior and more familiar with methods of communicating with affected individuals. In this regard, a special facility has been established to study the human-animal interrelationship.[40] Because the veterinarian also may be called on to help select pets for therapy, he or she must be knowledgeable about the characteristics that make an animal desirable or undesirable for a particular emotional or physical need.[4, 5, 33]

If the trend toward pet dependence continues even to the point that "in the year 2000 pets will become a very important safety valve in a sick society,"[38] if civilization continues to gather in suburban areas, and if pets take on neuroses from family members, then the veterinarian will have to be prepared to treat more abnormal behavior in the cat.

Each animal species has certain behavior patterns that are stereotyped among the individuals of that species. These are the behaviors that are discussed here, behaviors that have resulted in F. catus through years of evolution. Individual variations caused by environmental alterations are so inconsistent as to be essentially meaningless. To evaluate any behavioral problem, one must decide whether the behavior pattern is objectionable to the owner but normal for the cat, or whether it is both objectionable to the owner and abnormal for the cat.[25] Fortunately euthanasia is no longer the only alternative for dealing with a cat that shows abnormal behavior.

INTRODUCTION TO EVALUATING BEHAVIOR PROBLEMS

Several methods can be used to classify feline behavior problems, with the simplest being to determine whether the behavior is normal or abnormal.[7, 61] Normal behaviors are those that are species-specific but not appreciated by the owner. Clawing wood, including furniture, and urination, anywhere in a house, are examples. Abnormal behaviors are those that result from learning or from pathophysiologic processes. Psychogenic grooming and hypothyroid aggression are included in this category.

Classification of behavior problems by the signs shown by the cat is another method. This scheme is most often used because problems generally fall into one of several categories. Descriptive classification does not account for multiple causes of the same sign, such as distinguishing between fear-induced, intermale, and epileptic aggression.

Functional classifications are the most specific because they take environmental and physiological factors into consideration. The list of specific problems becomes very long, however, and difficult to keep in mind.[7] From a clinical approach, it may be useful to minimize the number of major categories by putting functional diagnoses under them.

Major Classifications of Behavior Problems

Feline behavior problems can be broadly divided into four categories.[6] Although the same four categories could be applied to any animal, the frequency of each category varies among the species.

Frustration. The most frequent cause of primary problems for the cat is stress, or "frustration." This can be expressed in many forms for many reasons.[2, 43] All animals are creatures of habit, and unless a change is gradual, a break in routine can be upsetting. The introduction of a new pet or family member, inconsistent punishment, a change in litter brands, or the lack of proper exercise increases tension. Reactions vary between individuals and within individuals at different times. Unfortunately for the cat, as for other animals, there is no normal innate pattern for releasing these frustrations. Because the animal cannot reason away this stress, the resulting behavior is a normal pattern expressed in an inappropriate situation. Examples include housesoiling, aggression, and a psychosomatic condition. Fortunately the cat is still relatively independent of humans; however, as society asks that *F. catus* change, the number of behavior problems will rise.

Improper Socialization. Socialization is the process by which an animal learns to accept certain animal species—including its own—in proximity. It occurs only during a limited time span. Improper or inadequate socialization of a cat during its first few months of life can result in an individual that does not relate socially to other cats, the family dog, or people. The animal is handicapped in a social situation that is normal for most families and undergoes a great deal of stress if forced into such a situation.

Genetics. An animal's genetic makeup can affect behavioral inheritance, but the cat's history has been good in one respect: Genetic behavioral problems are minimal. For this species, the minimal use of selective breeding has allowed it to maintain a diverse gene pool. Even today, only 7 per cent of cats are pedigreed, compared with 51 per cent of dogs, indicating that human intervention is minimal.[21, 64] As cats undergo an increasing amount of selective breeding, chances are that the primary consideration will be for physical characteristics, not behavioral ones.

Medical Conditions. Abnormal behavior in a domestic animal usually is due to an organic state of neurologic or systemic origin. An owner takes his cat to a veterinarian because of an observed change in the animal's behavior, such as sneezing, lameness, or depression. A physical examination and some laboratory data usually provide a diagnosis. Just as frequent urinations may indicate urinary calculi or renal problems, aggression may indicate thyroid dysfunction or central nervous system abnormalities. Although much is still unknown about abnormal behaviors related to medical conditions, there have been significant advances.

Diagnostic History Taking

When one is presented with a case of abnormal behavior, the value of obtaining an accurate, complete history cannot be overemphasized. The initial history-taking session will be longer than for most medical problems, but it is crucial to the ultimate understanding of the behavioral complaint. One format that is used to take a behavioral history utilizes a list of specific questions. Although this may seem convenient, owners prefer to give a more rambling history, and it becomes necessary to organize the information somehow.[27] In addition, a specific list of questions has to be long to include items relative to all the various possibilities. Four questions help to classify the condition into one of the major categories of initiating factors.

1. *What specifically happens?* This question should be the first, and may determine if the cat is clawing the furniture, spraying the house, or refusing to eat. The history also may reveal other maladaptations of which the owner is unaware or to which he or she has already adjusted.

2. *Where does the behavior occur?* Events restricted to one area may indicate a frustration located somewhere nearby. The cat that sprays near a window may be taunted by a neighbor cat that walks on the window ledge. The cat's defecating next to the litter pan may indicate that a new type of litter is unacceptable to the cat.

3. *When did the problem start?* This question is designed to determine how longstanding the problem is. It also might help to tie the start of a problem to another event that occurred shortly before it. For example, the acquisition of a new pet may initiate marking behavior by the resident cat. The duration of the problem may affect how long it takes to eliminate the undesirable behavior.

4. *When does the behavior happen?* Many behavioral patterns have a precipitating event, such as aggression that occurs when the neighbor child pulls the cat's tail. In this case, the problem is associated only with the child's presence. If an event occurs only while the owner is away, perhaps a friend or neighbor could be asked to see if the event is occurring just after the owner leaves, throughout the owner's absence, or immediately before the owner's return.

From the answers supplied to these questions and to others that are generated during the interview, offending behaviors can be classified according to the major behavioral categories previously described.

REFERENCES

1. America is going to the cats. D.V.M. 18:59, Aug. 1987.
2. Astrup, C.: Pavlovian concepts of abnormal behavior in man and animal. In Fox, M. W., ed.: Abnormal Behavior in Animals. Philadelphia: W. B. Saunders Co., 1968.
3. Beadle, M.: The Cat: History, Biology, and Behavior. New York: Simon & Schuster, 1977.
4. Beaver, B. G.: The veterinarian's role in prescribing pets. Vet. Med. Small Anim. Clin. 69:1506, 1974.
5. Beaver, B. V.: Animal Behavior: Pets and People. American Humane Assoc. Proceedings of the National Conference on Dog and Cat Control, Denver, 1976.
6. Beaver, B. V.: Disorders of behavior. In Sherding, R. G., ed.: The Cat: Diseases and Clinical Management. New York: Churchill Livingstone, 1989.
7. Borchelt, P. L., and Voith, V. L.: Classification of animal behavior problems. Vet. Clin. North Am. [Small Anim. Pract.] 12:571, 1982.
8. Bronson, R. T.: Age at death of necropsied intact and neutered cats. Am. J. Vet. Res. 42:1606, 1981.
9. Cameron, P., and Pope, C.: Are pets harmful to the mental and physical health of our society? Good Morning America Faceoff, Dec. 22, 1977.

10. Childs, J. E., and Ross, L.: Urban cats: Characteristics and estimation of mortality due to motor vehicles. Am. J. Vet. Res. 47:1643, 1986.
11. Clark, J. M.: The effects of selection and human preference on coat colour gene frequencies in urban cats. Heredity [Lond.] 35:195, 1975.
12. Clutton-Brock, J.: Domesticated Animals from Early Times. Austin: University of Texas Press, 1981.
13. Comfort, A.: Maximum ages reached by domestic cats. J. Mammal. 37:118, 1956.
14. Corson, S. A., Corson, E. O., Gwynne, P. H., and Arnold, L. E.: Pet-facilitated psychotherapy in a hospital setting. In Masserman, J. H., ed.: Current Psychiatric Therapies. New York: Grune & Stratton, 1975.
15. Dorn, C.: Veterinary medical services: Utilization by dog and cat owners. J. Am. Vet. Med. Assoc. 156:321, 1970.
16. Excerpts from the Islamic teachings on animal welfare. Latham Letter 10:14, Summer 1989.
17. Feaver, J., Mendl, M., and Bateson, P.: A method for rating the individual distinctiveness of domestic cats. Anim. Behav. 34:1016, 1986.
18. Feldmann, B. M.: Why people own pets: Pet owner psychology and the delinquent owner. Gaines Dog Res. Prog. 1:6, Summer 1977.
19. Fox, M. W.: Understanding Your Cat. New York: Coward, McCann, Geoghegan, 1974.
20. Fox, M. W.: The veterinarian: Mercenary, Saint Francis—or humanist? J. Am. Vet. Med. Assoc. 166:276, 1975.
21. Franti, C. E., and Kraus, J. F.: Aspects of pet ownership in Yolo County, California. J. Am. Vet. Med. Assoc. 164:166, 1974.
22. Ganster, D., and Voith, V. L.: Attitudes of cat owners toward their cats. Fel. Pract. 13:21, Mar.-Apr. 1983.
23. Griffiths, A. O., and Silberberg, A.: Stray animals: Their impact on a community. Mod. Vet. Pract. 56:255, 1975.
24. Hanson, R. L., and Clark, A. P.: Number of cat owners. Fel. Pract. 7:52, Sept. 1977.
25. Hart, B. L.: Social interactions between cats and their owners. Fel. Pract. 6:6, Jan. 1976.
26. Hart, B. L.: Children and pets: An interview with a child psychiatrist. Fel. Pract. 8:8, Jan. 1978.
27. Hart, B. L., and Hart, L. A.: Canine and Feline Behavioral Therapy. Philadelphia: Lea & Febiger, 1985.
28. Heiman, M.: Man and his pet. In Slovenko, R., and Knight, J. A., eds.: Motivations in Play, Games and Sports. Springfield, IL: Charles C Thomas, 1967.
29. Huidekopper, R. S.: The Cat. New York: D. Appleton & Co., 1895.
30. Karsh, E. B., and Turner, D. C.: The human-cat relationship. In Turner, D. C., and Bateson, P., eds.: The Domestic Cat: The Biology of its Behaviour. New York: Cambridge University Press, 1988.
31. Kolata, R. J., Kraut, N. H., and Johnston, D. E.: Patterns of trauma in urban dogs and cats: A study of 1,000 cases. J. Am. Vet. Med. Assoc. 164:499, 1974.
32. Lehman, H. C.: The child's attitude toward the dog versus the cat. J. Genet. Psychol. 35:62, 1928.
33. Levinson, B. M.: Pets: A special technique in child psychotherapy. Ment. Hygiene 48:243, 1964.
34. Levinson, B. M.: Household pets in residential schools: Their therapeutic potential. Ment. Hygiene 52:411, 1968.
35. Levinson, B. M.: Interpersonal relationships between pet and human being. In Fox, M. W., ed.: Abnormal Behavior in Animals. Philadelphia: W. B. Saunders Co., 1968.
36. Levinson, B. M.: Pet-Oriented Child Psychotherapy. Springfield, IL: Charles C Thomas, 1969.
37. Levinson, B. M.: Pets and old age. Ment. Hygiene 53:364, 1969.
38. Levinson, B. M.: Forecast for the year 2000. In Anderson, R. S., ed.: Pet Animals and Society. London: Bailliere Tindall, 1974.
39. Levinson, B. M.: Pets and environment. In Anderson, R. S., ed.: Pet Animals and Society. London: Bailliere Tindall, 1974.
40. Major research set on man-animal role. D.V.M. 9:1, Feb. 1978.
41. Marchand, C., and Moore, A.: Pet populations and ownership around the world. Waltham Internat. Focus 1:14, 1991.

42. Matheson, C.: The domestic cat as a factor in urban ecology. J. Anim. Ecol. 13:130, 1944.
43. Mosier, J. E.: Personal communication, 1970.
44. MVP Staff Report: Outlook for the 70's. Mod. Vet. Pract. 51:39, Oct. 1970.
45. Nassar, R., and Mosier, J. E.: Feline population dynamics: A study of the Manhattan, Kansas, feline population. Am. J. Vet. Res. 43:167, 1982.
46. Nassar, R., Mosier, J. E., and Williams, L. W.: Study of the feline and canine populations in the greater Las Vegas area. Am. J. Vet. Res. 45:282, 1984.
47. Pet estimates vary. NACA News 6:1, June/July 1984.
48. Podberscek, A. L., and Blackshaw, J. K.: Reasons for liking and choosing a cat as a pet. Aust. Vet. J. 65:332, 1988.
49. Pond, G.: The Complete Cat Encyclopedia. New York: Crown Publishers, 1972.
50. Robinson, R.: Cat. In Mason, I. L., ed.: Evolution of Domesticated Animals. New York: Longman, 1984.
51. Searle, A. G.: Gene frequencies in London's cats. J. Genet. 49:214, 1949.
52. Selby, L. A.: Family life cycle as related to cat, dog ownership. D.V.M. 9:20, Feb. 1978.
53. Serpell, J. A.: The domestication and history of the cat. In Turner, D. C., and Bateson, P., eds.: The Domestic Cat: The Biology of its Behaviour. New York: Cambridge University Press, 1988.
54. Smith, R. C.: The Complete Cat Book. New York: Walker & Co., 1963.
55. Speck, R. V.: Mental health problems involving the family, the pet, and the veterinarian. J. Am. Vet. Med. Assoc. 145:150, 1964.
56. Suehsdorf, A.: The cats in our lives. National Geographic 125:508, 1964.
57. Swingler, R. C.: Educational value of classroom pets. Educ. Dig. 31:50, Feb. 1966.
58. Todd, N. B.: Cats and commerce. Sci. Am. 237:100, Nov. 1977.
59. Todd, N. B.: An ecological, behavioural genetic model for the domestication of the cat. Carnivore 1:52, 1978.
60. Veterinary health care market for cats. J. Am. Vet. Med. Assoc. 184:481, 1984.
61. Voith, V. L., and Marder, A. R.: Introduction to behavior disorders. In Morgan, R. V., ed.: Handbook of Small Animal Practice. New York: Churchill Livingstone, 1988.
62. Wayne, R. K., Benveniste, R. E., Janczewski, D. N., and O'Brien, S. J.: Molecular and biochemical evolution of the carnivora. In Gittleman, J. L., ed.: Carnivore Behavior, Ecology, and Evolution. Ithaca, NY: Cornell University Press, 1989.
63. Weigel, I.: Small cats and clouded leopards. In Grzimek, H. C. B., ed.: Grzimek's Animal Life Encyclopedia. Vol. 12. New York: Van Nostrand Reinhold Co., 1975.
64. Wilbur, R. H.: Pets, pet ownership and animal control: Social and psychological attitudes, 1975. In American Humane Assoc., Proceedings of the National Conference on Dog and Cat Control, Denver, 1976.
65. Wood, G. L.: Animal Facts and Feats. Garden City, NY: Doubleday, 1972.
66. Zeuner, F. E.: A History of Domesticated Animals. New York: Harper & Row, 1963.

ADDITIONAL READINGS

Anderson, R. K., Fenderson, D. A., Schuman, L. M., et al. A description of the responsibilities of veterinarians as they relate directly to human health. Report for Bureau of Health Manpower. Washington, D.C.: U.S. Department of Health, Education, and Welfare, 1976.
Antelyes, J. Pets and mental health—but whose? Mod. Vet. Pract. 54:69, Aug. 1973.
Arendt, J., Minors, D. S., and Waterhouse, J. M. Biological Rhythms in Clinical Practice. Boston: Wright, 1989.
Beaver, B. V. G. Feline behavioral problems. Vet. Clin. North Am. 6:333, 1976.
Bierma, N. H. Prescription pet. Cats 34:10, Mar. 1977.
Biologist sees link of pets with health. D.V.M. 10:30, Jan.1979.
Boudreau, J. C., and Tsuchitani, C. The cat *Felis catus*. In Boudreau, J. C., and Tsuchitani, C., eds. Sensory Neurophysiology. New York: Van Nostrand Reinhold Co., 1973.
Brunner, F. The application of behavior studies in small animal practice. In Fox, M. W., ed. Abnormal Behavior in Animals. Philadelphia: W. B. Saunders Co., 1968.

Bryant, D. The Care and Handling of Cats. New York: Ives Washburn, 1944.

Bustad, L. K., Gorham, J. R., Hegreberg, G. A., and Padgett, G. A. Comparative medicine: Progress and prospects. J. Am. Vet. Med. Assoc. 169:90, 1976.

Colbert, E. H.: Evolution of the Vertebrates. 2nd ed. New York: John Wiley & Sons, 1969.

Corson, S. A., Corson, E. O., and Gwynne, P. H.: Pet facilitated psychotherapy. In Anderson, R. S., ed. Pet Animals and Society. Baltimore: Williams & Wilkins Co., 1975.

Council for Science and Society. Companion Animals in Society. New York: Oxford University Press, 1988.

Drewitt, M. St.G. N. Cats at war: A letter to the editor. Vet. Rec. 93:351, 1973.

Eleftheriou, B. E., and Scott, J. P. The Physiology of Aggression and Defeat. New York: Plenum Publishing Corp., 1971.

Ewer, R. F. The Carnivores. Ithaca, NY: Cornell University Press, 1973.

Fox, M. W. Influence of domestication upon behavior of animals. Vet. Rec. 80:696, 1967.

Fox, M. W. The place and future of animal behavior studies in veterinary medicine. J. Am. Vet. Med. Assoc. 151:609, 1967.

Fox, M. W. Ethology: An overview. In Fox, M. W., ed., Abnormal Behavior in Animals. Philadelphia: W. B. Saunders Co., 1968.

Fox, M. W. The influence of domestication upon behavior of animals. In Fox, M. W., ed., Abnormal Behavior in Animals. Philadelphia: W. B. Saunders Co., 1968.

Fox, M. W. Psychomotor disturbances. In Fox, M. W., ed., Abnormal Behavior in Animals. Philadelphia: W. B. Saunders Co., 1968.

Fox, M. W. The behavior of cats. In Hafez, E.S.E., ed., The Behavior of Domestic Animals. 3rd ed. Baltimore: Williams & Wilkins Co., 1975.

Fraser, A. F. Behavior disorders in domestic animals. In Fox, M. W., ed., Abnormal Behavior in Animals. Philadelphia: W. B. Saunders Co., 1968.

Hart, B. L. Genetics and behavior. Fel. Pract. 3:5, Feb. 1973.

Hart, B. L. The medical interview and clinical evaluation of behavioral problems. Fel. Pract. 5:6, Dec. 1975.

Hatcher, M. G. In defense of the cat. J. Am. Vet. Med. Assoc. 160:802, 1972.

Kleiman, D. G., and Eisenberg, J. F. Comparisons of canid and felid social systems from an evolutionary perspective. Anim. Behav. 21:637, 1973.

Kling, A., Kovach, J. K., and Tucker, T. J.: The behavior of cats. In Hafez, E.S.E., ed., The Behavior of Domestic Animals. 2nd ed. Baltimore: Williams & Wilkins Co., 1969.

Levinson, B. M. Influence of pets on families. J. Am. Vet. Med. Assoc. 156:639, 1970.

Levinson, B. M. Pets, child development, and mental illness. J. Am. Vet. Med. Assoc. 157:1759, 1970.

Levinson, B. M. Man and his feline pet. Mod. Vet. Pract. 53:35, 1972.

Levinson, B. M. Pets and Human Development. Springfield, IL: Charles C Thomas, 1972.

Levoy, R. P. Important things to learn about new clients. Vet. Med. Small Anim. Clin. 73:224, 1978.

Littlejohn, A. An approach to clinical veterinary ethology. Br. Vet. J. 125:46, 1969.

Moss, L. C. Psychoneurosis—a veterinary problem. J. Am. Vet. Med. Assoc. 114:1, 1949.

MVP Staff Report. Euthanasia: An act of compassion or one of expediency? Mod. Vet. Pract. 56:395, 1975.

Pet day at the Falls Nursing Home. Shoptalk 24:4, May 1976.

Pond, G., and Calder, M. The Longhaired Cat. New York: Arco Publishing Co., 1974.

Schmidt, J. P. Psychosomatics in veterinary medicine. In Fox, M. W., ed., Abnormal Behavior in Animals. Philadelphia: W. B. Saunders Co., 1968.

Seal, U. S. Carnivora systematics: A study of hemoglobins. Comp. Biochem. Physiol. 31:799, 1969.

Shebar, S., and Schoder, J. The pet burial business. Dog Fancy 7:22, Apr. 1977.

Szasz, K. Petishism: Pets and their People in the Western World. New York: Holt, Rinehart & Winston, 1969.

Top cats: Good medicine for emotionally handicapped. Vet. Econ. 15:14, Aug. 1974.

Voith, V., and Borchelt, P. History taking and interviewing. Compendium on Continuing Education 7:432, May 1985.

Wolpe, J. Parallels between animal and human neuroses. Proceedings of the Annual Psychopathological Association 55:305, 1967.

Worden, A. N.: Abnormal behavior in the dog and cat. Vet. Rec. 71:966, 1959.

2

Feline Behavior of Sensory and Neural Origin

In studying the senses of an animal, humans often are limited by the capacities of their own senses. It is difficult to understand that which cannot be experienced. Mammalian senses differ greatly, developing primarily to meet biologic need. Thus the importance of each sense varies among the species.

THE SENSES

The comparative development of the senses is shown in Appendix B.

Sense of Vision

External Visual System Development. Like the young of several other species, the newborn kitten is care-dependent at birth and for several weeks thereafter. This immature state is reflected in the visual system, which needs postnatal time for development. At birth the kitten's ocular development is about equivalent to that of a 5-month human fetus. Anatomic changes in vascularization occur in about 3 weeks, and result in a sudden improvement in the kitten's visual optics.[157] Although visual electric potentials can be recorded from the cortex of the brain as early as 4 days of age and the first electroretinogram can be recorded at day 6, the eyes are sealed until 5 to 14 days after birth (mean is 8 days).[61, 135] At first, the eye opens only slightly, but by 17 days (mean is 9 days), both eyes are completely open (Fig. 2–1). Early handling can accelerate this process by about 24 hours.[56, 74]

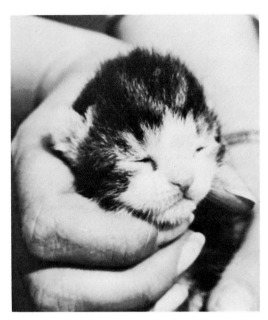

FIGURE 2–1. A 7-day-old kitten with eyes beginning to open.

A few reflexes associated with vision appear before the opening of the eyes. The palpebral reflex starts as a slow-blink response during the first 3 days of life, becoming adultlike by the 9th day. The light-blink reflex develops as early as day 50 of gestation or as late as day 13 of postnatal life (mean is 6 days after birth). Although the palpebral reflex continues, the light-blink reflex disappears around 21 days, probably because of the development of acute pupil control. Pupillary response normally appears within 24 hours after the eyes open and takes 2 to 3 days to develop normal speed. Until this time, the kitten usually tries to turn its head away from the light source.

Visual acuity develops independently of the opening of the eyes.[168] Visual pursuit first occurs as an eye- and head-turning action at about 11 days, when kittens first visually follow people and moving objects. Visual acuity, measured in terms of visual angles, gradually improves from a 180-minute arc around 16 days, to a 43-minute arc about 21 days, and then to an 11-minute arc around 25 days.[168] Between 22 and 28 days (mean is 25 days), visual placing reactions of the forelimbs first occur, and are significantly related to good visual acuity.[38, 168]

Depth perception initially appears a few days after the eyes open (mean is 13 days) and is well developed by 4 weeks of age. With continued maturation of the visual system, the kitten gradually increases the use of its eyes for behaviors such as avoiding objects and finding food, with good binocular vision by 47 days.[162] By about 2 months of age, the kitten has adult sight capacities, although the visual system continues to develop for another 2 months.[61, 106] There is an accompanying sudden onset of light-seeking behavior at 2 months of age.[43]

Eye color starts changing around 23 days of age, although early handling can speed this up slightly.[74]

External Visual System Characteristics. Because adult visual characteristics in the cat are closely related to behavioral characteristics of this species, it is important to note the anatomic adaptations that make night hunting possible. The size of the cat's pupil can change rapidly from being extremely large to being a mere slit. Because of eye shape and pupil extremes, both the lens and the cornea are larger and more highly curved than their counterparts in the human.[23, 50] As a result, a relatively large portion of the retina is activated. The tapetum lucidum reflects light within the eye for maximal stimulation of the rods in the retina. In addition to the many low-threshold rods (the rod-cone ratio is 25:1, compared with 20:1 in humans), the cat eye has more layers of sensitive cells in this area.[50, 76] These retinal differences allow cats the use of up to 50 per cent more of the available light than humans are able to use and to see in one-sixth the illumination needed by humans. The cat has an absolute brightness threshold of 1.32×10^{-7} millilamberts.[115]

The retinal fovea (macula, area centralis), the area of most acute vision, is located a mean distance of 3.42 mm dorsolateral from the center of the optic disc.[19, 39] In the cat, this area is relatively large and indefinite because both cones and rods are present, although the cones are most concentrated here.[13, 37, 89, 92, 179] In the human, there are only cones in the area of the optic disc. Although visual acuity is most accurate at 75 cm, it is compromised for night-hunting abilities.[89, 150] The visual acuity of the cat matures from slightly more than 1 cycle per degree at 35 days of age, to 5 to 6 cycles per degree at 4 months, to 8 to 9 cycles per degree as an adult.[50, 93, 118, 174] These figures are 10 per cent of those of humans.[20, 50] The low level of visual acuity is due to three internal factors: (1) reflection by the tapetum lucidum blurs the image; (2) the increased number of rods decreases the resolution of the image by lowering the visual stimulus threshold; and (3) the lens loses one-half to one-third of its capacity for accommodation. Accommodation does, however, relate to the significance of the viewed subject.[48] Although some retinal ganglion cells are comparable to those in humans, the brain is apparently unable to make use of incoming information to the same degree.[145] Despite its slight myopia, the cat shows a marked ability to notice movement, a necessity in hunting behaviors.[13, 48] Thresholds to recognize real movement are as little as 0.4 cm/sec movement.[101] Each feline eye has a blind spot on the dorsolateral retina at 13 degrees lateral.[19, 161]

The iris has a prominent bulging and changes colors during sympathetic stimulation.[90, 152]

The cat is considered color blind, but the presence of cones in the retina has been puzzling. Experimental evidence shows that cats can perceive limited color. Data as to specific color vision are contradictory, but it is agreed that color vision, although possible, is of little natural importance to the cat. Further evidence of this is suggested by the relatively low number of cones compared with rods in the retina as a whole.[179] Brightness is of much greater significance in visual discrimination, allowing the cat to detect luminance differences of only 10 per cent to 12 per cent.[174] It can perceive illumination at one-fifth the threshold of humans.[87]

Binocular vision contributes much toward the hunting success of this predator. Because of eye position and head shape, each eye has a visual field between 155 and 208.5 degrees, of which 90 to 130 degrees overlap the visual field of the opposite eye to produce binocular vision (Fig. 2–2).[13, 37, 50, 146] The remaining 73- to 173-degree field behind the head is a blind area. To provide this much binocular vision, the median plane of the eye is at an angle of only 4 to 9 degrees from that of the body.[37, 50] About 40 per cent of the cats studied show no convergence of both eyes while examining close objects, although with certain life-styles, such as hunting insects, this percentage may decrease (Fig. 2–3).[89]

Internal Visual System Characteristics. The optic nerve of the cat has a 65 per cent decussation of fibers at the optic chiasm.[13, 39] Those fibers from areas medial to the retinal fovea cross to the opposite cerebral hemisphere, whereas those lateral to it do not decussate.[39] Once they reach the brain, the impulses are received by ordered sections of the visual cortex (Fig. 2–4).[151] The cortical area is apparently important in integration of bilateral stimuli. Depth discrimination of prey is governed by this integration, the corpus callosum, and by the possibility that different cortical units are optically excited by objects on different sides and at different distances.[9, 47, 51]

Form discrimination by cats is based primarily on size differences, orientation of shapes, and general form. These general forms are basically open or closed, such as an O shape as opposed to a V shape, or a slot in contrast to a post. Neurons in the visual cortex appear selectively sensitive to orientation, length, width, and movement, and their reaction to these stimuli is based on early visual orientation.[59, 140] Four-fifths of these cells are influenced independently by both eyes, although not necessarily in equal amounts.[88] There is evidence that the central nervous system has physiologic mechanisms to differentiate newness of a stimulus, which is an extremely valuable feature for a predator.[155]

Visual acuity develops gradually as the nervous system of the neonate matures, and its development requires light stimulation during the first

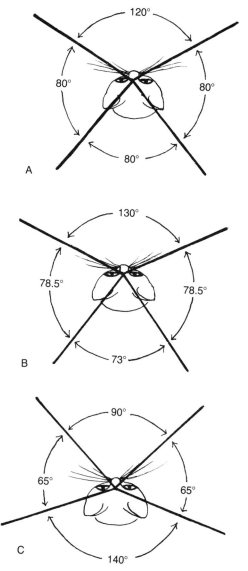

FIGURE 2–2. Visual fields of binocular, uniocular, and blind vision. (*A,* Data from Beadle, M.: The Cat: History, Biology, and Behavior. New York: Simon & Schuster, 1977. *B,* Data from Ewer, R. F.: The Carnivores. Ithaca, NY: Cornell University Press, 1973. *C,* Data from Sherman, S. M.: Visual field defects in monocularly and binocularly deprived cats. Brain Res. 49:25, 1973.)

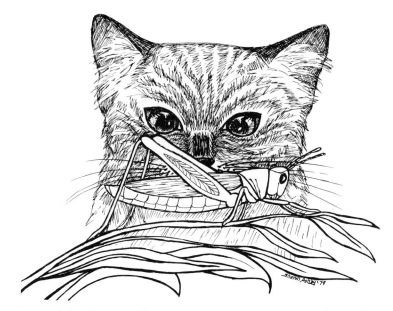

FIGURE 2–3. Small-prey hunting may require convergence of the lines of sight.

3 months, peaking between 28 and 35 days.[43, 122, 180] Deprivation of these stimuli, achieved experimentally by suturing the eyelids closed or by dark-rearing, results in a loss of visual acuity, even to the point of behavioral blindness. Concurrently, varying histologic changes occur in the cells of the visual cortex. Eye movements also are thought to be important for development of visual-motor skills.[84]

As a model for neurologic investigations, the visual cortex of the cat

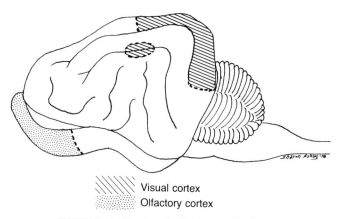

//// Visual cortex
∷∷∷ Olfactory cortex

FIGURE 2–4. Visual and olfactory cortical areas.

brain has been extensively studied. This area has been removed and the animal evaluated with regard to visual deficits. Studies showed that despite major ablations of the cortex, impairment of visual performance is minimal.

Although color vision is not well developed, certain parts of the brain have been identified as being related to this function. The ventral lateral geniculate nucleus has areas within it that respond differently to colors, particularly blue.[91]

The Siamese Visual System. External appearances are not the only variations from normal that accompany Siamese eyes. The characteristic crossing of the eyes does not appear until 6 to 8 weeks of age and is not present in all Siamese cats. Abnormal retinocerebral connections are typical of all albino animals, whether cross-eyed or not, and are associated with albino, Himalayan (Siamese), and, occasionally, chinchilla (Burmese) feline color genes.[13, 62] The visual field is normal, but the cats react to visual stimuli as if each eye does not see past the median plane.[62, 113, 147] As a result, these cats have difficulty locating objects in space. In the normal animal, visual input from the left eye goes to the top layer of the left lateral geniculate nucleus and to the second layer of the right lateral geniculate nucleus, whereas right eye input goes to the top of the right lateral geniculate nucleus and to the second layer of the left lateral geniculate nucleus. In the Siamese cat, hemispheric vision is such that fibers at the optic chiasm are misdirected: Each eye has fibers going to the appropriate position on the top layer but on the contralateral side. In addition, each eye lacks some fibers going to the top layer of the ipsilateral lateral geniculate nucleus.[13, 62, 147] Non–cross-eyed Siamese and heterozygous albino cats show abnormal optic fiber decussation to a lesser degree.[62, 109]

Sense of Audition

Auditory Development. Development of hearing in the kitten is not complete at birth. This is evidenced by the fact that the external auditory canal only begins to open between 6 and 14 days of age (mean is 9 days) and is completed by day 17 (Fig. 2–5). Electronically, the earliest evoked potential of the auditory system can be recorded at 2 to 3 days of age, and kittens initially hear sound of 100 dB SPL in the range of 500 to 2000 cycles per second (cps).[131] By day 6, the range has expanded to cover 200 to 6000 cps.[131] The development of the auditory startle response to sharp noise is highly variable, and appears within a few days of the ear canal's opening. Kittens begin orienting toward a sound as early as the 7th day, and they use this orientation for investigation by 13 to 16 days.[162] Sound recognition of littermates or people follows during the 3rd to 4th week and is coordinated with the appearance of the condi-

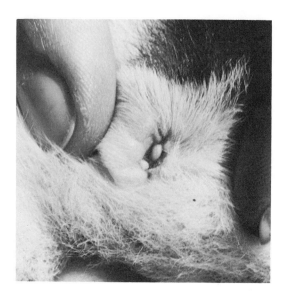

FIGURE 2–5. A 6-day-old kitten with the external auditory canals beginning to open.

tioned defense response: an arched-back, hissing response, which stabilizes during the 5th week.[56, 162, 166]

Auditory Characteristics. The auditory capabilities of the cat are not completely known. The lower audible frequencies are probably between 20 and 55 cps. From that up to 4000 cps, the cat's hearing ability is about the same as the human's. Maximal sensitivity is between 1,000 and 20,000 cps. Although the upper limit of audition is about 78,000 cps at 60 db SPL, the actual limit may be closer to 100,000 cps.[50, 83, 131, 177] The use of different instrumentation has shown that cochlear activity is present at these high frequencies, but whether the cat can hear these sounds is unknown.[177] This acute perception may be significant because social interactions between a rodent female and its young use frequencies of 17,000 to 148,000 cps, but mainly below 80,000 cps.[131] Inexperienced kittens will attack baby mice if stimulated by the squeak of the female mouse.[58, 76]

The cat can accurately hear one-tenth to one-fifth of a tone difference at higher pitches, but only about half of a tone change at lower frequencies.[13, 50, 152] With age, this ability decreases, especially in higher ranges.[13, 50]

Sound Reception and Interpretation. As a nocturnal hunter, the cat must rely on its sense of hearing to locate prey. Sound localization and maximal reception are primarily functions of the cup-shaped pinna, particularly at high frequencies.[53] Because the pinna can rotate approximately 180 degrees and acts as a funnel, it may introduce, or at least amplify, complex variations in sound quality with relation to the source, which is an important factor in localization.[23, 50]

Within the ear, the tympanic bulla is large, thus increasing acoustic resonance.

Carrying impulses to the brain are about 40,000 cochlear nerve fibers—10,000 more than in the human.[13, 40, 50, 87] These sound impulses travel a well-defined neural pathway to the auditory cortex, being analyzed there as well as along the way.[153, 155] Although the auditory fibers are the only sensory fibers completely myelinated at birth, the auditory system continues to undergo maturation, evidenced by decreasing peak latencies of cortical evoked potentials, until the minimal adult refractory interval of about 1 millisecond between discharges is reached.[40, 96, 125, 159] The rate of development of the central nervous system is faster than that of the visual system.[61] Studies in conscious cats indicate that other areas of the brain also may be involved with electric potentials from sound.[95]

In addition to the movable pinna, auditory neurons play a significant role in sound localization, which is 75 per cent accurate to an angle of about 5 degrees, only 2 degrees less accurate than for the human.[13, 50, 126] Certain neurons respond to contralateral stimuli but are inhibited by stimuli of the same frequency presented biaurally.[22, 28, 136] Other neurons respond to different latencies of the stimuli between the ears, and still others may be affected by differences in stimuli intensity between the two sides.[28, 114, 127, 136]

As with the visual system, the effects of ablation of the cortical portions of the auditory system have been studied (Fig. 2–6). Although amplitude and frequency discrimination in the adult can be affected to varying degrees, localization of sound is the most severely impaired by this procedure.

Hearing losses in cats also have been attributed to certain drugs. Kanamycin affects hair cells at the basal end of the cochlea and results

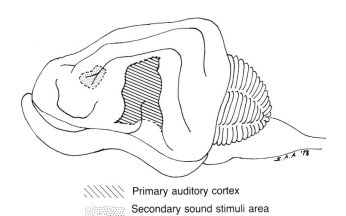

\\\\\\ Primary auditory cortex

Secondary sound stimuli area

FIGURE 2–6. Auditory cortical areas.

in loss of high-frequency perception; neomycin can damage the auditory function of the eighth cranial nerve.[16, 23] Deafness also can result from prolonged administration of streptomycin.[16]

Sense of Gustation

The sense of taste has been studied less than the other senses, perhaps because it has proved more difficult to evaluate. Taste buds are found on the vallate, fungiform, and, occasionally, foliate papillae of the tongue, as well as on the epiglottis, soft palate, lips, buccal walls, and pharynx.[23, 39] By stimulating these taste buds with chemicals known to produce certain tastes in humans and recording from afferent nerves or the presylvian gyrus, the primary center for taste reception, researchers have arrived at a few probabilities concerning the sense of taste in the cat.[39, 108] Within the 1st day of life, the kitten can distinguish sodium chloride in milk and by 10 days shows definite responses to salt and bitter, with possible responses to sweet and sour.[38, 132] The adult cat responds to chemicals associated with salt, sour, and bitter, but response to sweet is minimal at best. Considering foods eaten naturally by cats, one is not surprised that sweetness is not a major part of the cat's taste spectrum, although some cats develop a strong liking for foods with high sugar content. Maximal sensitivity to the three taste stimuli occurs at 30° C, the normal temperature of the tongue.[124]

Water fibers, maximally receptive to water, have been described in the chorda tympani. They are proposed to extend taste sensitivity to salt solutions.[35]

Neurologic studies indicate that the limbus of the brain is concerned with the memory of past gustatory experiences.[39]

Sense of Olfaction

Olfactory Development. The sense of smell is highly developed at birth, and within the first 2 days, the kitten shows a strong avoidance reaction to offensive odors.[14, 38, 106] Olfaction is well developed at this early age because of its importance in guiding the young animal to the mammary gland for nursing. By 3 days of age each kitten establishes a preferred nipple position and primarily uses odor to identify and follow previous paths to the specific nipple.[137, 138] Distress caused by removing the young kitten from its home area can be quieted by providing the smell of the area, even without physical contact. If placed near the home area, a kitten will crawl to it, guided by smell, and then fall asleep.[138] It is the gradual building of olfactory cues from the home area that provides odor orientation when the kitten begins to explore outside areas.[139] As vision develops, especially after 3 weeks of age, olfactory cues become less important but may have already influenced later stimulus prefer-ences.[55]

Olfactory Characteristics. In the adult, scent is used for identification during the typical behavioral approach of familiar cats—first face to face and then face to anus. Epithelia of the anal sacs in felids contain sebaceous tissue that can give off oils unique to that of other carnivores, which only have apocrine glands.[4] Scents also are used to explore and habituate to new environments.[1] Certain odors cause an immediate response and are said to be releasers. Moth balls, for example, cause avoidance. Primers, such as the cat's own urine, are odors that have a delayed effect or one that is not behaviorally obvious.[46]

In regard to size, the nasal olfactory area of the cat is larger than its corresponding area in the human.[13] In addition, the olfactory bulb is relatively larger and contains about 67 million cells, around 15 million more cells than in the human but far fewer than in the dog (Fig. 2–4).[13, 75] Because cats use smell behaviorally but not for tracking prey, these findings are not surprising.

Vomeronasal Olfactory System. Central olfactory pathways eventually connect to the amygdala area of the brain, a factor of significance when considering the second olfactory system of the cat.[5, 44] Immediately caudal to the incisor teeth is a papilla onto which open two nasopalatine canals. These canals allow slow passage of odors from the mouth to the vomero-nasal organ located within the hard palate. The vomeronasal organ (organ of Jacobson) is lined with olfactory cells, and has central pathways different from those of olfactory epithelium. Impulses first travel to the accessory olfactory bulb and then to areas of the hypothalamus associated with sexual behavior, feeding behavior, and, possibly, social interactions.

Flehmen is the behavior associated with the inhalation of odors into the nasopalatine canals. Beginning as early as 6 weeks, a cat will sniff a particular odor source, such as urine, often touching it with its nose and perhaps its tongue.[106] The head is then raised with the lips drawn back, nose wrinkled, and mouth partially open for inhalation (Fig. 2–7). This behavior is similar to that seen in ruminants and horses; however, the philtrum of the feline upper lip prevents its complete elevation. Flehmen, also called lip curl or gape, is most frequently displayed by tomcats.

Plant-induced Olfactory Behavior. Fourteen chemicals of diverse bio-logic origin, including certain plants, are known to affect the behavior of the cat when their fragrances are inhaled. The three chemical groups from these compounds include the 7-methylcyclopentapyranones, 7-methyl-2-pyridines, and 4-methylbenzofuranones.[160] A few of the more common plants include matatabi (*Actinidia polygama*, oriental vine, silvervine), valerian (*Valeriana officinalis*), cat thyme (*Teucrium manum*), buckbean (*Menyanthes triboliata*, bog myrtle), and, the most famous, catnip (*Nepeta cataria*, catmint). Reactions to catnip are specu-

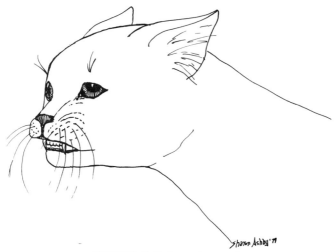

FIGURE 2–7. Flehmen by a cat.

lated to be hallucinogenic because humans who have smoked it report effects similar to those produced by marijuana. The active ingredient, cis-trans-nepetalactone, is a monoterpene that can be detected at levels as low as one part in 10^9 to 10^{11}.[4] After approaching the catnip plant, the cat will smell it and may lick, chew, or eat it. After head shaking, gazing, and salivating, the cat may rub its head on the catnip, usually while holding it in the forepaws. The skin over its back frequently twitches. As the intensity of the response increases, the cat will roll on its side, holding the catnip in its paws. There also may be animated leaping. The response usually lasts for 5 to 15 minutes, with the mean intensity lasting for 2.7 minutes.[15, 69, 82] Satiation lasts for at least an hour. It also has been speculated but is not widely accepted that catnip's odor activates central areas associated with estrous behavior because the behavioral response of the cat is similar to that during certain phases of female estrus.[69]

Individual reactions to catnip vary widely, and 30 per cent to 50 per cent of the cats studied do not respond.[23, 73, 75] Although the response is inherited by means of an autosomal dominant gene, it is modified by age and experience.[13, 23, 69, 82] Cats that show a decreased reaction to napetalactone include kittens less than 2 months old, fearful animals, and those under stress. Estrus can extend the response, and prolonged use of the drug has led to a chronic state of partial unawareness of surroundings.[15]

Sense of Touch

External Tactile Development. Like olfaction, the sense of touch is fairly well developed at birth, probably because it, too, plays a role in orientation of the neonate. Developing fetuses are responsive to tactile sensations by 24 days of gestation and exhibit flexor withdrawal to the toe pinch by 37 days.[61, 182] It is not surprising, therefore, that tactile response is present at birth and cutaneous pain reaction appears within the first 4 days after birth.[14, 38] Because their homeostatic mechanisms are not functioning completely immediately after birth, kittens also are responsive to temperature influences, and huddling is necessary for survival. For this reason, rooting behavior, the pushing of the head into warm objects, is present up to 16 days of age (mean day of ending is 8 days) (Fig. 2–8). The auriculonasocephalic reflex, a turning of the head when the side of the face is touched (Fig. 2–9), and Galant's reflex, a turning of the head and trunk when the flank region is touched (Fig. 2–10), occur in kittens but not consistently between individuals. Physical contact with the dam has a calming effect on young kittens, which, after being reunited with the queen, bury their heads in her hair. This behavior may be carried over to the adult cat that can be calmed by having its face covered with a pair of hands.[10] Odor may be slightly more important at this older age because the technique usually works better if the cat's owner covers its face.

Tactile placing of forelimb appears during the first 5 days, almost 3 weeks before visual placing occurs (Fig. 2–11). Then, as late as 6 weeks, kittens still show a preference for tactile determination of depth, using vision only secondarily.[141] The difference between dependence on the two senses represents the difference in time required for completion of connections with the motor cortex.[168]

External Tactile Characteristics. In adults, areas of tactile dermatomes have been well mapped, and Pinkus' plates, specialized tactile pads or

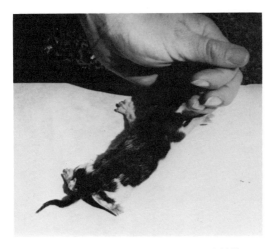

FIGURE 2–8. The rooting reflex in a day-old kitten.

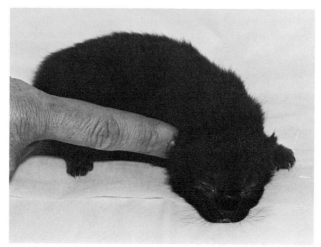

FIGURE 2–9. The auriculonasocephalic reflex is directed toward the cervical touch stimulus by a day-old kitten.

touch areas, have been found covering the skin at a rate of 7 per centimeter to 25 per centimeter by the 7th week of age.[13, 29, 99] Skin sensitivity varies. The cat's face is about a third as sensitive to radiant heat as a human face, although the nasal area can respond to minute changes, as little as 0.2° C rise or 0.5° C decrease.[13, 103, 104–105] Response in the remainder of the body requires a level of heat change that would be

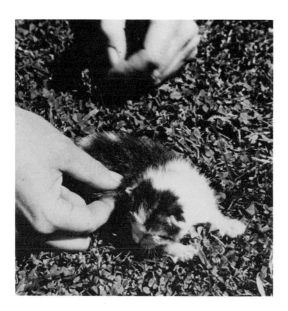

FIGURE 2–10. Galant's reflex is directed toward the abdominal touch stimulus by a 7-day-old kitten.

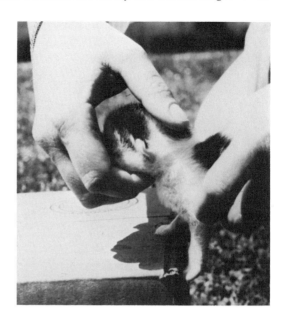

FIGURE 2–11. Tactile placing of the forelimbs in a 7-day-old kitten.

painful to humans, from 6° to 9° C.[25, 102, 104, 105] Humans report pain at 44° C, whereas cats react between 51° and 54° C.[103] This lack of sensitivity on the trunk accounts for the cat's ability to sit on a stove or radiator, apparently comfortable, even though its hair may singe. Prolonged exposure to high environmental temperatures (25° to 30° C) results in hypoexcitability, and at temperatures over 30° C, the cat exhibits panting, hyperexcitability, and circling. Cold exposure increases somatic rage (bared teeth) as well as circling.[60]

Response to touch varies among breeds and individuals. Most cats prefer to be held firmly but not tightly, so as to be sure of their support, and usually prefer gentle stroking to patting. Some cats resent being handled near the base of the tail and will turn to confront the source of stimulation or twitch the tail and skin of the lumbar region. Also, cats usually do better with minimal restraint, so that giving an intramuscular injection often is possible while holding only the cat's pelvic limb.

Tactile Vibrissae. As a nocturnal hunter, the cat may use touch for stalking or, at least, measuring areas of location. In this regard, the special vibrissae transmit sensory information only.[128] Impulses have been demonstrated with as little as a 2-mg weight or 5-nm directional movement when the direction of movement of these sinus hairs is opposite the natural slant.[36, 52] By this means an animal can detect wind currents and air currents reflected from nearby objects. Loss of these hairs makes the cat more dependent on vision. Facial vibrissae, or whiskers, are located in specific areas (Fig. 2–12). A large area of mystacial tufts is present on

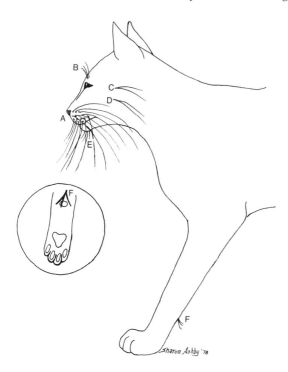

FIGURE 2–12. Location of facial and carpal vibrissae. A, Mystacial tufts; B, superciliary tuft; C, genal tuft one; D, genal tuft two; E, mandibular tuft; F, carpal vibrissae.

each upper lip; a large superciliary tuft is above each eye; a genal tuft one is ventral to the base of each ear; a genal tuft two is ventral to each genal tuft one near the angle of the mandible; and a poorly developed mandibular tuft is on the chin.[13, 50] The dorsal two rows of mystacial vibrissae move independently of the ventral two rows, and their positions vary with movement and behavior.[13] When the cat is walking the whiskers project far forward as well as laterally to scan a wide angle. When at rest the cat moves them laterally for a much narrower area. During a greeting, defense, or sniff, these tactile hairs are folded back along the side of the head.[29, 175]

Carpal vibrissae, structurally identical to cranial vibrissae, are found on the caudal surface of the forearm immediately proximocaudal to the carpus. Because the associated nerves are sensitive to a proximal displacement of the tactile hair, it has been speculated that their presence is related to the use of the forelimbs for functions other than ambulation, such as capturing prey.[17, 128, 129]

Internal Tactile Characteristics. Cerebral studies have mapped cortical locations of touch-sensitive areas, with few differences found between the young and the adult cat (Fig. 2–13).

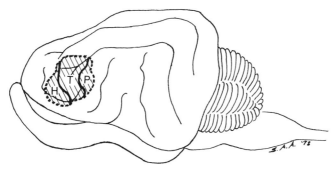

FIGURE 2–13. Somatic sensory cortical areas. *H,* Somatic sensory cortex for the head; *T,* somatic sensory cortex for the thoracic limb; *P,* somatic sensory cortex for the pelvic limb.

Unexplained Senses

Certain behaviors are probably related to neurologic capabilities, although the exact relation has not been defined.

Earthquake Prediction. Before some earthquakes, cats have been reported to undergo behavioral changes. Behavior typical of extreme fear or excitement, including restlessness and piloerection, may be seen in the cats even though electrical instruments do not perceive environmental changes.[7, 76] What the cat detects is unknown, but speculations include variations in electromagnetic fields, atmospheric electrostatic charges, air pressure, ultrasonic or subsonic emissions, the earth's level, water levels, and gaseous emissions.[76]

Homing Behavior. Many cats go back to a previous home after a move, especially if the old location is nearby. This behavior demonstrates the importance of a territory to a cat. Individuals are said to "run away" during this search, especially if they become lost. Some cats reportedly can travel great distances returning to an old home, and many such trips have been documented. Care must be exercised in studying such travels to be sure that the same cat arrives as the one that left. Great similarities in behaviors as well as physical characteristics can be misleading and are not positive proof of identification. This homing ability is apparently independent of memory because cats often do not retrace paths, but take a direct route instead. In addition, this directional orientation is not blocked by anesthesia.[173] Careful investigations have documented extended trips by cats to meet owners at new locations as far as 1,500 miles from the original home.[133]

FELINE PLAY BEHAVIOR

Of all developmental behaviors associated with kittens, play is probably the most familiar. Play assumes a wide variety of patterns, so a broad definition is: behaviors of specific patterns performed in disconnected and varying groupings, during which each action develops its own spontaneous, exuberant, action-specific energy and is not directly useful.

Play Behavior Development. At about 2 weeks self-play begins with attempts to bat moving objects. This play progresses with muscle coordination, so that at about 3 weeks of age, social play appears as oriented pawing and occasional biting. Within another few weeks interactions with littermates and specific patterns appear. By day 35 stalking, chasing, and arching of the back are seen, and wrestling appears at day 43.[56, 162] Climbing and balancing on frames starts around day 48.[111] Leaping is more variable in time of development, ranging from day 17 to day 43.[56]

Play serves many purposes. Each of the numerous types of play can result in several things. Physical fitness is the most obvious benefit derived. When the kitten becomes independent, certain species-specific behaviors, such as hunting, must be mature enough to allow its survival. Play permits the acquisition of endogenous pattern coordination, timing, physical coordination, and central nervous system maturation. In addition, play behaviors provide a method for kittens to explore their environment and make social contacts that decrease the probability of serious fighting later.

Social Play. Social play involves two or more cats, and it has eight associated categories of behaviors. These are most prevalent during weeks 4 through 16, and the decline of social play is related to the decreased preference for social contact and the need for dispersal.[32, 86, 167, 176] Early weaning and all-male groups have been associated with a higher frequency of social play by kittens.[32, 112]

"Belly-up" describes a posture of dorsal recumbency, with the thoracic limbs making a pawing motion while the pelvic limbs tread air (Fig. 2–14). The mouth often is open, exposing the teeth. Belly-up, first seen between days 21 and 23, is specific for social play but may be seen during mating.[56] At 6 weeks of age, this behavior occurs during 13 per cent of the social play, and at 12 weeks, it occupies 16 per cent of this play.[176]

"Stand-up" involves one kitten standing over a second kitten that is in a belly-up posture (Fig. 2–15). These two social play patterns appear together 67 per cent of the time. With heads oriented in the same direction, the kittens may paw and bite each other. Stand-up play first appears at about 23 days of age and obtains a frequency of about 15 per cent of social play.[176]

A third social play, "side step," develops at about 32 days of age and occupies 20 per cent of play time by 6 weeks of age. It involves one kitten showing a lateral body position, including a slight body arch and an upward curve in the tail, to a second kitten (Fig. 2–16). The posturing kitten then walks laterally toward the second kitten or circles around

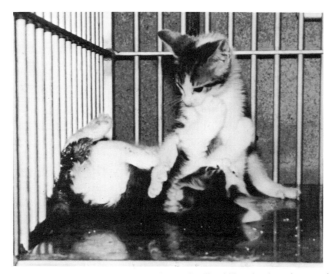

FIGURE 2–14. "Belly-up" play posture shown by the kitten in dorsal recumbency.

it.[176] This lateral posturing contains many of the same positions later used in distance-increasing silent communication.

In the "pounce" the kitten crouches low, with the pelvic limbs underneath its body and its tail straight back (Fig. 2–17). The weight initially is shifted forward and back by the pelvic limbs, which then

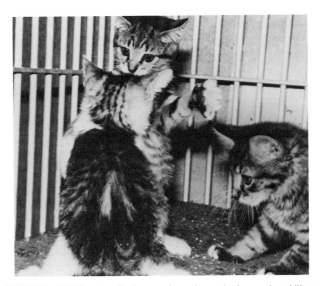

FIGURE 2–15. "Stand-up" play posture shown between two kittens.

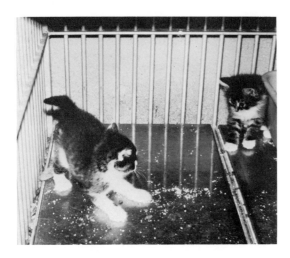

FIGURE 2–16. The lateral body position of "side step."

provide a sudden forward thrust toward the other kitten. This particular social play begins between days 33 and 35 and occupies 42 per cent of a 6-week-old kitten's play behavior. By 12 weeks 5 per cent less time is devoted to it.[176]

From a sitting position the kitten shifts its weight to its hindquarters, thereby raising its forelimbs perpendicular to the body. By extending the pelvic limb joints into a stationary bipedal position, the kitten assumes "vertical stance" (Fig. 2–18). Appearing at about 35 days of age, this posture does not occupy a large portion of play until about 12 weeks of age, when it occurs during about 25 per cent of the play time.[176]

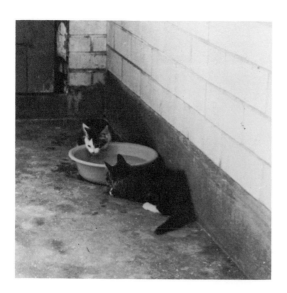

FIGURE 2–17. The crouched play posture of "pounce."

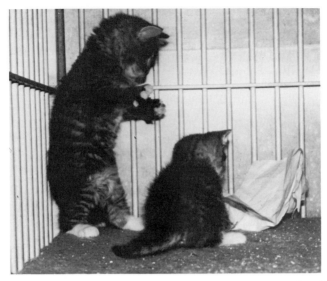

FIGURE 2–18. The "vertical stance" play posture directed toward another kitten and a paper.

"Chase" is the social play of pursuit and flight, which develops between 38 and 41 days of age (Fig. 2–19).[176] Kittens eventually spend a considerable amount of a play period in pursuit of one another, although at times, one kitten runs but the second fails to follow.

About 5 days after the appearance of chase, the "horizontal leap" develops. With body postures like those associated with side-step play, the kitten suddenly leaps off the ground.[176]

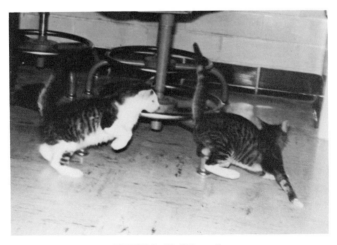

FIGURE 2–19. "Chase."

The eighth of the social play categories to develop is "face-off." By 48 days, two kittens sit looking at each other, intensely leaning forward. They simultaneously direct paw movements at each other's face. Frequently only one of the kittens participates, in a solitary version of the game (Fig. 2–20).[176]

Individual Play. Play behaviors associated with predatory behavior take different forms and may be self-rewarding, since kittens will perform them for long periods, even to the point of exhaustion. Isolated kittens play more individually and play more with their mothers than do those raised with littermates, and object play occurs more often in kittens if the mother was on a rationed diet.[11, 12, 63, 116]

Games of prey perfect some hunting skills as well as provide exercise. The game "mouse" involves leaping on a small movable object, such as a ball, and securing it with the forepaws while doing body acrobatics (Fig. 2–21). In other versions, the paw is used to bat the object. Two kittens occasionally join in this game, so that one holds the "mouse" as the other bats at it, alternating paws. "Bird" involves intercepting flying objects and bringing them into the mouth (Fig. 2–22). Intense interest is directed toward the interception of objects that take off from the ground or that fly from one point to another. As skills progress kittens undertake the game of "rabbit," in which they ambush large moving objects, such as another cat (Fig. 2–23). To succeed is to bring the object to the ground and use the neck bite. Two cats often will alternate between stalking and being chased, but with age, the game can become rough, so that the cat prefers a younger or less animated playmate.[23, 56]

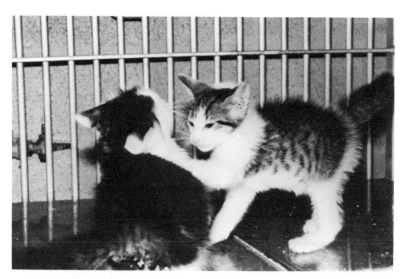

FIGURE 2–20. Unilateral "face-off" from a standing position.

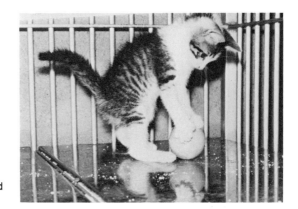

FIGURE 2–21. "Mouse" played with a ball.

In addition to living and inanimate things, play behavior can be directed toward imaginary objects. During "hallucinatory" play the kitten leaps at a wall to catch an imaginary object or bats and chases imaginary objects along the ground (Fig. 2–24).[56] A kitten may express another form of this behavior, usually in the early evening, by suddenly jumping up with dilated pupils and running wildly around the house as if chasing an invisible kitten.

FELINE LEARNING

Learning Development. Learning is a change in behavior as the result of an individual's experience.[158] It contrasts with instinctive behavior,

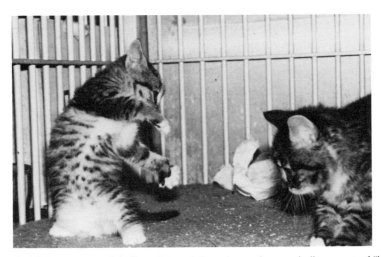

FIGURE 2–22. An unsuccessful attempt to catch a piece of paper in the game of "bird."

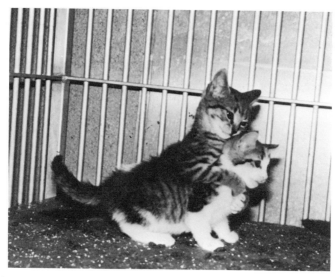

FIGURE 2–23. The top kitten is using the lower one as the target in a game of "rabbit."

which involves inherited, species-specific patterns. Learning behavior in cats, as in other animals, does involve certain genetically determined characteristics of the nervous and musculoskeletal systems. Kittens can learn immediately after birth, an important capability for the future development of the individual. By at least 10 days of age kittens learn to locate a preferred teat for nursing, primarily through trial and error. It

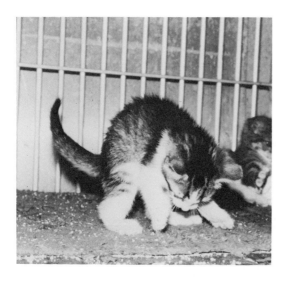

FIGURE 2–24. "Hallucinatory" play.

has been experimentally shown that at this age, they are capable of learning to avoid or escape offensive situations.[8, 49]

In certain situations the cat demonstrates a behavior somewhat unique to the species—observational learning. The queen is responsible for much of this stimulus-controlled response by her kittens. One extreme example of this early induced response is the orphaned kitten, raised with dogs, that learned to lift its leg to a tree by observing its male dog companion doing so (Fig. 2–25). Kittens frequently do not exhibit an observed behavior immediately after observing the queen perform it, but by 9 to 10 weeks of age, they will suddenly perform the act with the same directness as an individual that has performed it many times.[34, 134] The importance of imitation is probably variable, depending on the particular action involved.[3, 18, 85] Instinctive imitation, such as the learning of hunting behaviors, is important to mental development as well as to self-preservation. In contrast, the imitation of many voluntary acts requires several observations to learn and a reward to perform. To retain the connection between a previous learning experience and its external stimuli, a cat may imitate the act even though the stimulus is no longer

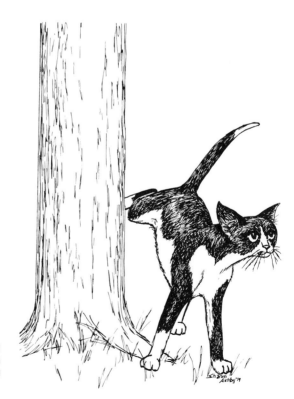

FIGURE 2–25. Observational learning by an orphaned kitten that learned from a male dog companion.

present.[18] For example, a cat trained to pull a string for a food reward would continue pulling at a nonexistent string.

At 8 weeks of age the kitten still lacks a stable attention span; thus learning is difficult to evaluate. Kittens, however, are capable of working certain specific types of problems.[24, 170] Individuals of this age can solve oddity sets by choosing the different shape from a group with several similar figures. The kitten also can learn to select choices that had previously been incorrect and leave previously correct responses alone. Probability problems have been solved by kittens 8 weeks of age. Motivation at this age is probably a limiting factor in experimental studies. Food and play behaviors are effective incentives for early learning. Prey species are in fact learned.[31] Pain also has been an effective motivator, but success depends on the difficulty of the problem's discrimination.[42, 117]

Certain types of early experiences allow for latent learning, that is, learning that is not immediately obvious. Between 5 and 6½ weeks of age human handling is effective in developing an individual that shows much less fear of strangers later in life, and early activity-encouraging environments produce less active kittens, which are affected by novel stimuli.[56, 63, 107, 181] Discipline begun before 6 weeks results in a generalized learned response that lasts into adulthood, whereas that which is started later is effective on the cat only in the specific incident.[56]

Learning Characteristics. Adult cats have been used as experimental models of learning, with vision the primary modality studied. Discrimination between patterns of different shapes can be learned whether or not the shape differences are paired with other cues, such as brightness.[149, 171] Even for the adult, the learning of oddity sets is possible though difficult.[71, 169] Teaching cats to stay out of or off certain places is exceedingly difficult unless people are present to serve as negative cues. Search techniques in strange areas are random, although each area is searched only once.[64] This indicates a high degree of trial-and-error learning. Transfer learning also occurs in cats.[172] For this learning the animal uses information from one problem to solve a second problem. For example, a circular form selected from square figures in one oddity set is generalized to a dull object placed among illuminated objects in a second problem.

Motivational factors play an important part in adult learning and behavioral choice.[143] Avoidance learning is widely used with adults as well as kittens. It can be taught by yelling and throwing things at the cat or by picking it up on the dorsum of its neck or by its chest and shaking the cat. These latter two have the advantage of discomfort without pain. Affection and attention or their lack, food, and stimulus strength have been successful motivational factors. With proper motivation and a great deal of patience a cat can be taught several tricks such as sitting up and rolling over. Training sessions must be short, not more than 5 minutes a session, for two or three sessions a day. It is easiest to start with a task that uses a natural behavior, such as jumping up on something or getting something from under a cover; shaping, placing the cat in the desired position, also can be successful. Through successive approximation from an initial behavior that is gradually increased for the reward, a cat can be taught such behaviors as using a cat door and a toilet. Once the given task has been performed correctly, it should be repeated for reinforcement. The latency period between performance and reward can affect the learning. Reinforcement is optimally given within a half second of initiation; with a 30-second delay cats are still 68 per cent correct.[163, 173] Thus, discipline must be applied immediately and in a form understood by the cat. Intrinsic motivational factors certainly exist, such as itch reduction from scratching, but they are difficult to evaluate.[140]

Intelligence. The intelligence of *Felis catus* frequently is discussed and compared with that of other animals, with these comparisons usually based on certain learned behaviors. For perspective, one should note that there is much controversy regarding the definition of intelligence and how to measure it, even in humans. Not until this controversy is settled can intelligence in animals be measured. Considering motivational differences between individuals and species, inherent differences in natural behavioral patterns, and various physical limitations of individuals and species makes the task especially difficult.

The Brain and Learning. Studies of the central nervous system's involvement in learning have been variable. The hippocampus is probably most important because of its control over attention spans and its relation to learning habits that require discrimination.[2, 6] It has been theorized that maturation of this brain area transforms an exuberant juvenile into a placid adult.[6] Other brain areas also have been studied for learning, with experimental results often related to the sensory areas.

NEUROLOGIC ORIGINS OF BEHAVIOR

The incompletely developed neonatal brain is extremely resistant to hypoxia (Fig. 2–26). Because their brain cells use anaerobic glycolysis when deprived of oxygen, individuals tested have survived for more than 20 minutes with no ill effects. This is probably why young kittens are said to be so difficult to drown.[13, 178]

Although the brain has been extensively studied with respect to the specific senses, numerous studies also have been conducted to show the interrelations between the neural areas and the behavioral functions of each. Stimulation of one sense can stimulate cortical neurons associated

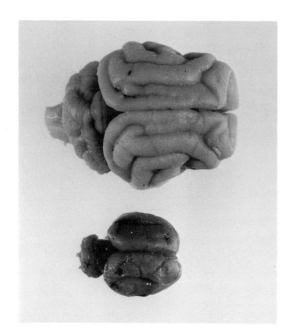

FIGURE 2–26. The brain of a newborn kitten is physically and functionally less developed than that of an adult cat.

with other senses. Peripheral stimuli have been hypothesized to activate a common central association system that projects equally to all sensory cortical fields.[156] This explains why sharp noise or sudden pain also can be perceived as a flash of light.

In considering the role of the brain in behavior, one invariably discusses the limbic system. Although some authors are more inclusive, most agree that the limbic system is composed of the limbic lobe and associated subcortical nuclei. The limbic lobe comprises the following: parahippocampal gyri, cingulate gyri, subcallosal gyri, hippocampus, and dentate gyri. The associated subcortical nuclei include the amygdaloid complex, hypothalamus, epithalamus, septal nuclei, and rostral thalamic nuclear areas. Several complicated tracts with specific behavioral functions have been defined within the limbic system. An example of such a tract is the Papez circuit (hippocampus to fornix, to mammillary body, to rostral thalamic nucleus, to cingulate gyrus, to cerebral cortex), which deals with emotion.[94]

Specific areas of the limbic system have particular functions. The cingulate gyri are thought to be involved in the functional organization of associated behaviors because they have been shown to maintain lack of aggression and to have a role in psychomotor seizures.[39, 110, 120] More thoroughly studied and complex, the hippocampus functions in broad behavioral contexts, including emotion, attention mechanisms, personality, recent memory, internal physiologic changes, submissive behavior patterns without response to social threat, and psychomotor seizures.[39, 94, 100, 130] The amygdaloid complex mainly modulates the activity of the hypothalamus and is particularly involved with regulation of agonistic behavior. Agonistic behavior is divided into four aggression components: flight, defense, predatory attack, and offensive attack, which includes a ragelike response. In addition, the amygdaloid complex regulates hypothalamic output with respect to activity patterns, water consumption, and food intake.

As the most studied portion of the limbic system, the hypothalamus has diversified functions. The various parts control water balance, appetite, predatory attack, sexual behavior, and the sleep-wake cycle. Some emotions also are associated with this area, among them being fear, anger, aggression, and rage with its defensive threat postures. The septal nuclei of the limbic system moderate sensory stimuli to prevent hyper-reactivity, moderate water consumption, and control emotional responses. In the latter situation septal nuclei suppress aggressive behavior of either amygdaloid or hypothalamic origin. Sensory input into the thalamus is directed to specific cortical areas; thus this area serves as the chief sensory integrating mechanism.[94] The thalamus also regulates states of consciousness and the hypothalamus.[94, 119]

The brain directly affects the behaviors of illness, particularly those associated with fever.[79–81] Depression is one method to conserve energy that would otherwise be lost from movement or when the cat is not curled up to rest. Anorexia also reduces the amount of movement for energy and body heat conservation and has the added benefit of reducing the intake of iron, depriving iron-using bacteria of their nutrition.

Numerous other neural-behavioral interrelations have been investigated with less specific conclusions drawn. Each is dealt with in the appropriate chapter.

SENSORY AND NEURAL BEHAVIOR PROBLEMS

Behavior Problems and the Senses

Problem behaviors that involve the cat's senses occur in a few types of circumstances. Cats that are fondled a great deal have shown persistent mobilization of the third eyelid, indicative of vagal nerve over-stimulation.[33, 142] Recovery requires separation of owner and cat for a prolonged period.

White, blue-eyed cats, except those with Burmese or Siamese dilutions, usually are deaf. In affected individuals degeneration of the organ of Corti starts at about 5 days of age, so that the kitten never hears. As with most deaf cats, bilaterally affected individuals exhibit characteristic hyperalertness. The gene producing this blue-eyed, deaf cat also is responsible for the absence of the reflective tapetal area of the eye, so that nocturnal vision is reduced.

Behavior Problems and Development

Malnutrition can have an especially strong influence on neonatal learning abilities. There is evidence that deprivation may result in changes in food-related emotional behavior.[68] The mildly deprived male kitten's brain undergoes compensatory growth if he is returned to an adequate plane of nutrition.[148] In severer deprivation during the early postnatal period, such as occurs at a 20 per cent nutritional plane for the nursing mother, neuron development and learning ability are permanently affected.[68] Runts in a normal litter may suffer neurologically because of nutritional problems in addition to possible psychological difficulties induced by intimidation from normal littermates.[68]

Early separation from the mother, at 2 weeks of age, for example, can affect a kitten in other ways as well. Commonly the amount of random, non–goal-oriented activity increases.[144] These kittens are more emotional in various situations and slower to calm down later.[144]

Changing Behavior Through Learning

Aversion. Use of an obnoxious stimulus to teach avoidance works well on oral behavior problems. Success in taste or smell aversion requires that the stimulus be coupled with a previously bad experience. A foul-tasting product placed on an item being chewed often is ignored because its potency has been diluted. If the cat has had an oral dose previously, the odor and mild taste bring back negative memories. Aversion is discussed in Chapter 7.

Desensitization. Management of fear or anxiety can be done through desensitization.[165] The process is one in which the cat is gradually exposed to weak or nonfearful stimuli that are increased in intensity over time at such a rate that a fearful response is avoided. For some individuals that are extremely stressed, antianxiety drugs are helpful in the initial desensitization process.

Flooding. Flooding is a technique whereby the problem stimulus is used continuously until the cat no longer shows the fear or stress reaction.[165] The stimulus should be continued for a while even after the problem behavior is stopped, until the animal has reverted to a relaxed state. To stop before relaxation might actually reinforce the undesired behavior.

Punishment. Punishment is the application of an aversive stimulus that reduces the probability that a particular behavior will recur. Techniques for punishment of cats must differ from those for dogs because of the species differences.[21] Typically, techniques that require the owner's presence, such as yelling or throwing something, teach the cat to avoid the behavior in the owner's presence. If the aversive stimulus can be associated with a location or an event, it is more effective against the specific problem. Squirting the cat with water, scaring it with a rattle thrown nearby, and blasting it with a remote-controlled hair dryer are but a few techniques used.[21, 78]

Shaping. Rewards are used for a natural behavior that resembles the behavior ultimately desired.[164] The criteria for the reward gradually become more strict as the cat successfully masters the general behavior and works on the more specific aspects of the desired outcome.

Stress-Related Behavior Problems

Generalized Stress. Stress is probably the most common initiator of behavior changes in cats. Hospitalization or other variations in environment, forced confinement, physical trauma, crowding, changes in routine, continued exposure to high-frequency sounds like those from television remote controls, prolonged anticipatory waiting, mourning, and restraint are but a few causes of frustration. Signs of abnormalities caused by stress vary even more than the causes because they affect a number of body systems. Included in this gamut of signs are convulsions, hyster-oepilepsy, sudden depigmentation, fear, restlessness, excitability, depression, changes in taste preferences, anorexia, aversion to locations, catatonia, eliminations, fever, vomition, diarrhea, shyness, colic, hair loss, bronchospasm, ulcers, paroxysmal hypotonia, aggression, psychological neutering, excessive grooming, and nongrooming. In general, these signs can be classified as inhibitory or excitatory.[54] The signs in the cat, however, are of a narrower spectrum than those seen in the dog or human because the cat is at a neurophylogenetically lower level.[54] Stress can produce intense sympathetic stimulation, which, in turn, can extend to the neurosecretory hypothalamus and the hormone system, particularly the suprarenal (adrenal) glands. Under prolonged stressful conditions, then, resistance to disease usually decreases.[77] Sympathetic system changes may be particularly severe in older cats, and failure of the cat to adapt can result in a rapid psychological and physiologic decline.[54, 121]

There are several methods for controlling stress-related problems. If the cat's environment cannot be changed, a small, dark enclosure, such as a paper box or sack, can provide security. Tranquilizers are widely used and are most effective when they only alleviate mental anxiety. While tranquilized, the cat may be desensitized if behavioral modification, with its controlled repeated introduction of the problem stimulus, is used. After several weeks the drug dosage may be gradually reduced until it is no longer needed. The phenothiazine derivatives and haloperidol of the butyrophenone derivatives are neuroleptics and can reverse impaired thought processes in psychotic humans.[66, 98] The benzodiazepine family, including diazepam (Valium) and chlordiazepoxide (Librium), as well as meprobamate are effective in cases of human anxiety and nervousness in which psychosis is not a major problem.[66, 98] Cat dosages for these drugs are about three times the human dosage (mg/kg).[66] Antidepressants and mood elevators, especially iminodibenzyl derivatives and amitriptyline, also have been used in management of stress-related problems.[66] These drugs, however, can produce pronounced individual reactions.[65]

Cats that show extreme displeasure with veterinarians during office calls may have learned to associate the sight of a syringe with pain. The remedy may simply be to hide the syringe while approaching the cat.[70] The same principle, eliminating the stimulus cue that causes stress, can work successfully for a wide range of situations.

Psychogenic Shock. Cats, especially nervous individuals, are particularly vulnerable to psychogenic shock. This condition can be initiated by preparation for surgery, war conditions, or severe fights with cats, dogs, or humans.[15, 33, 97] Affected cats tend to hide in dark corners, showing depression, salivation, anorexia, pupil dilation, and hyperesthesia.[15, 97, 183] Hallucinatory behavior, such as jumping into the air to catch imaginary objects, also has been reported in affected adults.[97, 183] The shock syndrome may have developed as a method for survival, since lack of motion inhibits attack by a predator.[15] Treatment is the same as that for any shock condition.

Inappropriate Behaviors

Certain natural behaviors of the adult cat appear at inappropriate times, and artificial environments are causing the incidence of this abnormality to increase. Each normal behavior pattern is allotted a given amount of natural energy.[158] If one of these normal behavior patterns is not expressed over a period of time because an appropriate stimulus is lacking, the energy produced for it builds up within the individual. Cats kept in tidy homes often do not have the opportunity to stalk and kill prey. As these energies build up, the threshold stimulus to initiate the behavioral expression decreases to the point that minor stimuli can result in the behavior in situations that seem inappropriate. The motion of human feet can initiate a prey-killing attack directed at the ankles. In another situation, when hearing the mailman, a cat may wait under the door-type mail slot to attack the incoming mail. Even after being hit on the head by a large magazine or catalogue, the cat may continue the inappropriate prey-killing attack. For other cats, the barren environment could result in masturbation, digging motions around the outside of the food bowl or litter box, and aggressive extremes in play behavior because of the lack of sexual, normal digging, and play activities, respectively. Kittens raised with minimal social play bite more often and harder than those allowed to interact with littermates.[63] Although they could play well by themselves, their social skills were rudimentary. Stereotyped behaviors, rhythmic pacing and head-swinging, and prolonged sniffing of the air in one location also can be seen when the cat's normal energies are not released.[57, 167] These behaviors are displacement activities. Displacement activities and stereotyped behavior are managed most easily by encouraging activity, usually play, with another cat or a toy. Neutering and progestins also are helpful because of their calming effect.

Behavior Problems and the Brain

Abnormalities in the central nervous system are not completely understood, but certain generalizations can be made. Irritative lesions, such as encephalitis and atrophying scar tissue, frequently are unilateral.[41, 67, 72] Suppressive changes of parts of the central nervous system usually are bilateral, and thus often involve a midline lesion.[67, 72] Included in the latter category are septal or ventral hypothalamic lesions, which precipitate aggression, hyperreactivity, and increased or decreased ingestive behavior; amygdala lesions, which prevent male copulatory behavior; and hippocampal abnormalities, which cause staring, excessive grooming, excessive vocalization, and seizures.[30, 41, 45, 67] Localized twitching of the skin, along with tail-lashing, urination, and vocalization, have been controlled with anticonvulsants.[26]

Drugs can alter the mental state of the cat. Ketamine hydrochloride in combination with xylazine has been reported to cause hallucinations during recovery.[123] Ketamine hydrochloride is known to produce hallucinations, irritability, and mental confusion in humans and may cause similar reactions in cats, especially if the anesthetic recovery period includes many external stimuli. This could account for individual cats becoming extremely withdrawn for varying periods after anesthetization.

Behavior Problems and Breed Variations

Breed variations in behavior and reactions to situations are not well known. Cat lines that have undergone a great deal of concentrated inbreeding or line-breeding may experience more behavior problems: many Abyssinian, Russian blue, and Siamese cats exhibit excessive restlessness, nervousness, and an unreliable disposition.[27, 154]

CASE PRESENTATIONS ▬▬▬▬▬▬▬▬▬▬▬▬▬▬▬▬▬▬▬▬▬▬▬

CASE 2–1. Ten-week-old domestic shorthair female. The kitten belonged to a working couple and was their only pet. Since they got the cat 4 weeks earlier, it "took off" at irregular intervals, running full speed around the house, biting and clawing at people or things in its path. Just before one of these "attacks," the owners noticed that its pupils rapidly dilated. Suddenly, after a few minutes of frantic activity, the "attack" stopped and the kitten appeared perfectly normal. Previous antiepileptic therapy was unsuccessful.

Diagnosis. Normal. The kitten was exhibiting normal chase and fight social play behaviors except that there was no other kitten to participate.

Treatment. None. No therapy was necessary for this kitten; however, it should be provided with another kitten or movable toys to play with.

CASE 2–2. Three-year-old Persian male. About 8 months ago the cat began to have nocturnal grand mal seizures. At first, there was one seizure a month, but by this visit there were two each night. These seizures occurred between 3 and 5 A.M., and each lasted for about 2 minutes, with a 4- to 5-minute postseizural disorientation. The cat was a show animal and was fed a good-quality commercial canned diet in the evening. The animal's disposition was calm, and its usual routine had not been changed. Medication did not control the problem.

Diagnosis. Seizures caused by a food allergy. The cat's home diet was changed to the same commercial diet used in the hospital, and the seizures stopped.

Treatment. Maintain the cat on the new diet.

CASE 2–3. Fourteen-month-old Siamese neutered male. About 2 weeks ago the cat fell 3 to 4 feet, and the owners thought that it might have hit its head. There was some immediate discomfort, but the attending veterinarian found no problems. Over the next 4 days the cat became increasingly mean, biting at its tail, especially after waking.

Medical Workup. The physical and radiographic examinations were normal.

Diagnosis. Probable pinched nerve.

Treatment. Use of a pain reliever brought almost immediate return to normal.

CASE 2–4. Four-and-one-half-year-old domestic longhair neutered female. During the past few months the cat had become increasingly aggressive toward people. It was the only pet of a retired couple and had become so aggressive that they could no longer hold it to pet it. The cat also attacked the arms and legs of friends who came to visit.

Medical Workup. The physical examination was unremarkable. Laboratory data included a normal urinalysis, blood analysis, fecal analysis, and electroencephalogram. The T_4-thyroid value was very low.

Diagnosis. Hypothyroidism.

Treatment. Thyroid hormone replacement therapy brought a gradual return to normal behavior within 2 weeks.

CASE 2–5. Three-year-old Siamese-cross neutered male. During the entire time these owners had the cat, it would bite them if it did not get immediate or constant attention. The owners put up with the behavior on a daily basis but were now tired of it and thinking of euthanasia for the cat.

Diagnosis. Learned aggression.

Treatment. Consistent punishment by squirting the cat in the face with a water spray bottle each time it bit decreased the severity of the problem to an occasional one. At first the cat avoided the owners, but then it gradually learned what was acceptable and what was not.

CASE 2–6. Nine-month-old domestic shorthair male. Most of the time the owner reported that the cat was an acceptable pet; however, for the past month there had been times of aggression. The attack started with the hair standing up and a stiff-legged approach; then the cat ran and pounced, usually on the owner's roommate.

Diagnosis. Play aggression.

Treatment. The roommate started carrying a water spray bottle with him to spray the cat as it approached aggressively. This worked well for a few days and then the cat directed the same behavior to the owner. He was successful at stopping the problem by punishing the cat with the water spray.

CASE 2–7. Eleven-year-old domestic longhair neutered male. The cat had lived with the owner's grandmother until 3 weeks ago. After the move the cat was kept inside for 2 weeks and then let outside occasionally on a leash. Five days earlier the cat had been let out unleashed in the morning and was still there at noon. By late afternoon the cat was gone. It was found in the old neighborhood the morning of presentation.

Medical Workup. No abnormalities were found.

Diagnosis. Return to old territory.

Treatment. The owner was concerned for the cat's safety and decided to make the cat an indoor pet. Because this animal is older, the length of confinement to help it establish a new territory was going to be great, and by then it would probably be a well-adjusted indoor cat anyway.

CASE 2–8. Five-month-old domestic shorthair female. While in for the cat's vaccinations the owner had described the cat as "hyper," meaning that it would have occasional periods of suddenly taking off and running around the house. Most of the time it was fine.

Diagnosis. Normal play behavior.

Treatment. It is important for the owner to recognize this as normal behavior for a young kitten, with no treatment indicated.

CASE 2–9. Two-year-old domestic shorthair neutered female. Ever since this cat was a kitten it has been close to the owner, both physically and behaviorally. It went into the shower, let the owner brush its teeth, and played fetch. To get picked up and carried, this cat bit the owner's feet. If it was kept out of the shower, it shredded the curtain or clawed the closed bathroom door.

Diagnosis. Learned aggression and destructive clawing.

Treatment. The unaccepted behaviors were punished either by shaking a rattle made of a soda can containing rocks or by blasting the cat with an air jet from a gun-shaped hair dryer. The behaviors gradually decreased in frequency and finally disappeared by 6 months.

CASE 2–10. Two-year-old domestic shorthair male. The cat was bottle-raised and gradually became mean to the owners. It had recently started to attack itself, growling and biting at its side and tail. The episodes of human attacks had not changed, but the self-directed attacks were increasing in severity and frequency. When they first started 6 months ago, they were occasional, lasting for only a few seconds. By this visit they occurred four times a day and lasted for 15 to 20 minutes.

Medical Workup. The physical examination was unremarkable. There was no evidence of skin lacerations or abrasions. Laboratory data included a normal urinalysis, blood analysis, and fecal analysis. The owner declined an electroencephalogram.

Diagnosis. Play aggression toward the owner and probable epileptic self-directed aggression.

Treatment. The owner was concerned about the safety of a 7-month-old child, especially since the boy was now crawling, and opted for euthanasia of the cat.

Also see cases 3–2, 5–2, 5–3, 8–1, 10–1, and 10–2.

REFERENCES

1. Adamec, R. E., Stark-Adamec, C., and Livingston, K. E.: The expression of an early developmentally emergent defensive bias in the adult domestic cat (*Felis catus*) in non-predatory situations. Appl. Anim. Ethol. 10:89, 1983.
2. Adey, W. R.: Hippocampal states and functional relations with corticosubcortical systems in attention and learning. Prog. Brain Res. 27:228, 1967.

3. Adler, H. E.: Some factors of observational learning in cats. J. Genet. Psychol. 86:159, 1955.
4. Albone, E. S., and Shirley, S. G.: Mammalian Semiochemistry: The Investigation of Chemical Signals Between Mammals. Somerset, NJ: John Wiley & Sons, 1984.
5. Allison, A. C.: The morphology of the olfactory system in vertebrates. Biol. Rev. 28:195, 1953.
6. Altman, J., Brunner, R. L., and Bayer, S. A.: The hippocampus and behavioral maturation. Behav. Biol. 8:557, 1973.
7. Animal behavior may predict earthquakes. Vet. Med. Small Anim. Clin. 73:834, 1978.
8. Bacon, W. D.: Aversive conditioning in neonatal kittens. J. Comp. Physiol. Psychol. 83:306, 1973.
9. Barlow, H. B., Blakemore, C., and Pettigrew, J. D.: The neural mechanism of binocular depth discrimination. J. Physiol. 193:327, 1967.
10. Barrett, R. P.: The "calming response." Fel. Pract. 7:46, Jan. 1977.
11. Bateson, P., and Young, M.: Separation from the mother and the development of play in cats. Anim. Behav. 29:173, 1981.
12. Bateson, P., Mendl, M., and Feaver, J.: Play in the domestic cat is enhanced by rationing of the mother during lactation. Anim. Behav. 40:514, 1990.
13. Beadle, M.: The Cat: History, Biology, and Behavior. New York: Simon & Schuster, 1977.
14. Beaver, B. V.: Reflex development in the kitten. Appl. Anim. Ethol. 4:93, 1978.
15. Beaver, B. V. G.: Feline behavioral problems. Vet. Clin. North Am. 6:333, 1976.
16. Beaver, B. V. G., and Knauer, K. W.: The ear. In Catcott, E. J., ed.: Feline Medicine and Surgery. 2nd ed. Santa Barbara, CA: American Veterinary Publications, 1975.
17. Beddard, F. E.: Observations upon the carpal vibrissae in mammals. Proc. Zool. Soc. (Lond.) 1:127, 1902.
18. Berry, C. S.: An experimental study of imitation in cats. J. Comp. Neurol. Psychol. 18:1, 1908.
19. Bishop, P. O., Kozak, W., and Vakkur, G. J.: Some quantitative aspects of the cat's eye: Axis and plane of reference, visual field co-ordinates, and optics. J. Physiol. (Lond.) 163:466, 1962.
20. Blake, R., Cool, S. J., and Crawford, M. L. J.: Visual resolution in the cat. Vision Res. 14:1211, 1974.
21. Borchelt, P. L., and Voith, V.: Punishment. Compendium on Continuing Education 7:780, 1985.
22. Boudreau, J. C., and Tsuchitani, C.: Binaural interaction in the cat superior olive S segment. J. Neurophysiol. 31:442, 1968.
23. Boudreau, J. C., and Tsuchitani, C.: Sensory Neurophysiology. New York: Van Nostrand Reinhold, 1973.
24. Boyd, B. O., and Warren, J. M.: Solution of oddity problems by cats. J. Comp. Physiol. Psychol. 50:258, 1957.
25. Brearley, E. A., and Kenshalo, D. R.: Behavioral measurements of the sensitivity of cat's upper lip to warm and cool stimuli. J. Comp. Physiol. Psychol. 70:1, 1970.
26. Brunner, F.: The application of behavior studies in small animal practice. In Fox, M. W., ed.: Abnormal Behavior in Animals. Philadelphia: W. B. Saunders Co., 1968.
27. Bryant, D.: The Care and Handling of Cats. New York: Ives Washburn, 1944.
28. Burkhardt, D., Schleidt, W., and Altner, H.: Signals in the Animal World. New York: McGraw-Hill Book Co., 1967.
29. Burton, M.: The Sixth Sense of Animals. New York: Taplinger Publishing Co., 1973.
30. Caplan, M.: An analysis of the efforts of septal lesions on negatively reinforced behavior. Behav. Biol. 9:129, 1973.
31. Caro, T. M.: The effects of experience on the predatory patterns of cats. Behav. Neural Biol. 29:1, 1980.
32. Caro, T. M.: Sex differences in the termination of social play in cats. Anim. Behav. 29:271, 1981.
33. Chertok, L., and Fontaine, M.: Psychosomatics in veterinary medicine. J. Psychosom. Res. 7:229, 1963.
34. Chesler, P.: Maternal influence in learning by observation in kittens. Science 166:901, 1969.

35. Cohen, M. J., Hagiwara, S., and Zotterman, Y.: The response spectrum of taste fibers in the cat: A single fiber analysis. Acta Physiol. Scand. 33:316, 1955.
36. Craig, D.: Personal communication, 1977.
37. Crescitelli, F.: The Visual System in Vertebrates. New York: Springer-Verlag, 1977.
38. Cruickshank, R. M.: Animal infancy. In Carmichael, L., ed.: Manual of Child Psychology. New York: John Wiley & Sons, 1946.
39. DeLahunta, A.: Veterinary Neuroanatomy and Clinical Neurology. Philadelphia: W. B. Saunders Co., 1977.
40. De Reuck, A. V. S., and Knight, J.: Hearing mechanisms in vertebrates. Boston: Little, Brown & Co., 1968.
41. Dhume, R. A., Gogate, M. G., deMascarenhas, J. F., and Sharma, K. N.: Functional dissociation within hippocampus: Correlates of visceral and behavioral patterns induced on stimulation of ventral hippocampus in cats. Indian J. Med. Res. 64:33, 1976.
42. Dodson, J. D.: The relation of strength of stimulus to rapidity of habit-formation in the kitten. J. Anim. Behav. 5:330, 1915.
43. Dodwell, P. C., Timney, B. N., and Emerson, V. F.: Development of visual stimulus-seeking in dark-reared kittens. Nature 260:777, 1976.
44. Doty, R. L.: Mammalian Olfaction, Reproductive Processes, and Behavior. New York: Academic Press, 1976.
45. Egger, M. D., and Flynn, J. P.: Effects of electrical stimulation of the amygdala on hypothalamically elicited attack behavior in cats. J. Neurophysiol. 26:705, 1963.
46. Eisenberg, J. F., and Kleiman, D. G.: Olfactory communication in mammals. Annu. Rev. Ecol. System 3:1, 1972.
47. Elberger, A. J.: The effect of neonatal section of the corpus callosum on the development of depth perception in young cats. Vision Res. 20:177, 1980.
48. Elul, R., and Marchiafava, P. L.: Accommodation of the eye as related to behaviour in the cat. Arch. Ital. Biol. 102:616, 1964.
49. Ewer, R. F.: Further observations on suckling behaviour in kittens, together with some general considerations of interrelations of innate and acquired responses. Behaviour 17:247, 1961.
50. Ewer, R. F.: The Carnivores. Ithaca, NY: Cornell University Press, 1973.
51. Ewert, J. P.: Neuroethology. New York: Springer-Verlag, 1980.
52. Fitzgerald, O.: Discharges from the sensory organs of the cat's vibrissae and the modification of their activity by ions. J. Physiol. (Lond.) 98:163, 1940.
53. Flynn, W. E., and Elliott, D. N.: Role of the pinna in hearing. J. Acoust. Soc. Am. 38:104, 1965.
54. Fox, M. W.: New information on feline behavior. Mod. Vet. Pract. 56:50, Apr. 1965.
55. Fox, M. W.: Neurobehavioral development and the genotype-environment interaction. Q. Rev. Biol. 45:131, 1970.
56. Fox, M. W.: The behaviour of cats. In Hafez, E. S. E., ed.: The behaviour of Domestic Animals. 3rd ed. Baltimore: Williams & Wilkins Co., 1975.
57. Fox, M. W.: Personal communication, 1977.
58. Galambos, R.: Processing of auditory information. In Brazier, M. A. B., ed.: Brain and Behavior. Vol. 1. Washington, DC: American Institute of Biological Sciences, 1961.
59. Ganz, L., and Fitch, M.: The effects of visual deprivation on perceptual behavior. Exp. Neurol. 22:638, 1968.
60. Giammanco, S., Paderni, M. A., and Carollo, A.: The effect of thermic stress on the somatic reaction of rage and on rapid circling turns, in the cat. Arch. Int. Physiol. Biochem. 84:787, 1976.
61. Gottlieb, G.: Ontogenesis of sensory function in birds and mammals. In Tobach, E., Aronson, L. R., and Shaw, E., eds.: The Biopsychology of Development. New York: Academic Press, 1971.
62. Guillery, R. W.: Visual pathways in albinos. Sci. Am. 230:44, 1974.
63. Guyot, G. W., Cross, H. A., and Bennett, T. L.: The domestic cat. In Roy, M. A., ed.: Species Identity and Attachment: A phylogenetic Evaluation. New York: Garland STPM Press, 1980.
64. Hamilton, G. V.: A study of trial and error reactions in mammals. J. Anim. Behav. 1:33, 1911.

65. Hart, B. L.: Psychopharmacology in feline practice. Fel. Pract. 3:6, May-June 1973.
66. Hart, B. L.: Drug choice in feline psychopharmacology. Fel. Pract. 3:8, July-Aug. 1973.
67. Hart, B. L.: The brain and behavior. Fel. Pract. 3:4, Sept.-Oct. 1973.
68. Hart, B. L.: Behavior of the litter runt. Fel. Pract. 4:14, Sept.-Oct. 1974.
69. Hart, B. L.: The catnip response. Fel. Pract. 4:8, Nov.-Dec. 1974.
70. Hart, B. L.: Handling and restraint of the cat. Fel. Pract. 5:10, Mar.-Apr. 1975.
71. Hart, B. L.: Learning ability in cats. Fel. Pract. 5:10, Sept.-Oct. 1975.
72. Hart, B. L.: The medical interview and clinical evaluation of behavioral problems. Fel. Pract. 5:6, Dec. 1975.
73. Hart, B. L.: Quiz on feline behavior. Fel. Pract. 6:10, May 1976.
74. Hart, B. L.: Behavioral aspects of selecting a new cat. Fel. Pract. 6:8, Sept. 1976.
75. Hart, B. L.: Olfaction and feline behavior. Fel. Pract. 7:8, Sept. 1977.
76. Hart, B. L.: Sensory capacities and behavioral feats. Fel. Pract. 7:8, Nov. 1977.
77. Hart, B. L.: Psychosomatic aspects of feline medicine. Fel. Pract. 8:8, July-Aug. 1978.
78. Hart, B. L.: Water sprayer therapy. Fel. Pract. 8:13, Nov. 1978.
79. Hart, B. L.: Animal behavior and the fever response: Theoretical considerations. J. Am. Vet. Med. Assoc. 187:998, 1985.
80. Hart, B. L.: Behavior of sick animals. Vet. Clin. North Am. [Food Anim. Pract.] 3:383, 1987.
81. Hart, B. L.: Biological basis of the behavior of sick animals. Neurosc. Biobehav. Rev. 12:123, 1988.
82. Hatch, R. C.: Effect of drugs on catnip (Nepeta cataria)–induced pleasure behavior in cats. Am. J. Vet. Res. 33:143, 1972.
83. Heffner, R. S., and Heffner, H. E.: Hearing range of the domestic cat. Hearing Res. 19:85, 1985.
84. Hein, A., Vital-Durand, F., Salinger, W., and Diamond, R.: Eye movements initiate visual-motor development in the cat. Science 204:1321, 1979.
85. Herbert, J. M., and Harsh, C. M.: Observational learning by cats. J. Comp. Psychol. 37:81, 1944.
86. Houpt, K. A.: Companion animal behavior: A review of dog and cat behavior in the field, the laboratory and the clinic. Cornell Vet. 75:248, 1985.
87. Houpt, K. A., and Wolski, T. R.: Domestic Animal Behavior for Veterinarians and Animal Scientists. Ames: Iowa State University Press, 1982.
88. Hubel, D. H., and Wiesel, T. N.: Receptive fields, binocular interaction, and functional architecture in the cat's visual cortex. J. Physiol. (Lond.) 160:106, 1962.
89. Hughes, A.: Vergence in the cat. Vision Res. 12:1961, 1972.
90. Hughes, A.: Observing accommodation in the cat. Vision Res. 13:481, 1973.
91. Hughes, C. P., and Chi, D. Y.: Visual function in the ventral lateral geniculate nucleus of the cat. Exp. Neuro. 79:611, 1983.
92. Jacobs, G. H.: Comparative Color Vision. New York: Academic Press, 1981.
93. Jacobson, S. G., Franklin, K. B. J., and McDonald, W. I.: Visual acuity of the cat. Vision Res. 16:1141, 1976.
94. Jenkins, T. W.: Functional Mammalian Neuroanatomy. Philadelphia: Lea & Febiger, 1972.
95. Jewett, D. L.: Volume-conducted potentials in response to auditory stimuli as detected by averaging in the cat. Electroencephalogr. Clin. Neurophysiol. 28:609, 1970.
96. Jewett, D. L., and Romano, M. N.: Neonatal development of auditory system potentials averaged from the scalp of rat and cat. Brain Res. 36:101, 1972.
97. Joshua, J. O.: Abnormal behavior in cats. In Fox, M. W., ed.: Abnormal Behavior in Animals. Philadelphia: W. B. Saunders Co., 1968.
98. Kakolewski, J. W.: Psychopharmacology: Clinical and experimental aspects. In Fox, M. W., ed.: Abnormal Behavior in Animals. Philadelphia: W. B. Saunders Co., 1968.
99. Kasprzak, H., Tapper, D. N., and Craig, P. H.: Functional development of the tactile pad receptor system. Exp. Neurol. 26:439, 1970.
100. Kemp, I. R., and Kaada, B. R.: The relation of hippocampal theta activity to arousal, attentive behaviour and somato-motor movements in unrestrained cats. Brain Res. 95:323, 1975.
101. Kennedy, J. L., and Smith, K. U.: Visual thresholds of real movement in the cat. J. Gen. Psychol. 46:470, 1935.

102. Kenshalo, D. R.: The temperature sensitivity of furred skin of cats. J. Physiol. (Lond.) 172:439, 1964.

103. Kenshalo, D. R.: Cutaneous temperature sensitivity. In Dawson, W. W., and Enoch, J. M., eds.: Foundations of Sensory Science. New York: Springer-Verlag, 1984.

104. Kenshalo, D. R., Duncan, D. G., and Weymark, C.: Thresholds for thermal stimulation of the inner thigh, footpad, and face of cats. J. Comp. Physiol. Psychol. 63:133, 1967.

105. Kenshalo, D. R., Hensel, H., Graziadei, P., and Fruhstorfer, H.: On the anatomy, physiology, and psychophysics of the cat's temperature-sensing system. In Dubner, R., and Kawamura, Y., eds.: Oral-Facial Sensory and Motor Mechanisms. New York: Appleton-Century-Crofts, 1971.

106. Kolb, B., and Nonneman, A. J.: The development of social responsiveness in kittens. Anim. Behav. 23:368, 1975.

107. Konrad, K. W., and Bagshaw, M.: Effect of noval stimuli on cats reared in a restricted environment. J. Comp. Physiol. Psychol. 70:157, 1970.

108. Kruger, S., and Boudreau, J. C.: Responses of cat geniculate ganglion tongue units to some salts and physiological buffer solutions. Brain Res. 47:127, 1972.

109. Leventhal, A. G., Vitek, D. J., and Creel, D. J.: Abnormal visual pathways in normally pigmented cats that are heterozygous for albinism. Science 229:1395, 1985.

110. Lubar, J. F., and Numan, R.: Behavioral and physiological studies of septal function and related medial cortical structures. Behav. Biol. 8:1, 1973.

111. Martin, P., and Bateson, P.: The ontogeny of locomotory play behaviour in the domestic cat. Anim. Behav. 33:502, 1985.

112. Martin, P., and Bateson, P.: The influence of experimentally manipulating a component of weaning on the development of play in domestic cats. Anim. Behav. 33:511, 1985.

113. Marzi, C. A., and Stefano, M.: Role of Siamese cat's crossed and uncrossed retinal fibres in pattern discrimination and interocular transfer. Arch. Ital. Biol. 116:330, 1978.

114. Masterton, B., Thompson, G. C., Bechtold, J. K., and RoBards, M. J.: Neuroanatomical basis of binaural phase-difference analysis for sound localization: A comparative study. J. Comp. Physiol. Psychol. 89:379, 1975.

115. Mead, L. C.: Visual brightness discrimination in the cat as a function of illumination. J. Genet. Psychol. 60:223, 1942.

116. Mendl, M.: The effects of litter-size variation on the development of play behaviour in the domestic cat litters of one and two. Anim. Behav. 36:20, 1988.

117. Miles, R. C.: Learning in kittens with manipulatory, exploratory, and food incentives. J. Comp. Physiol. Psychol. 51:39, 1958.

118. Mitchell, D. E., Giffin, F., Wilkinson, F., et al.: Visual resolution in young kittens. Vision Res. 16:363, 1976.

119. Moore, C. N., Casseday, J. H., and Neff, W. D.: Sound localization: The role of the commissural pathways of the auditory system of the cat. Brain Res. 82:13, 1974.

120. Morgenson, G. J., and Huang, Y. H.: The neurobiology of motivated behavior. Prog. Neurobiol. 1:55, 1973.

121. Mosier, J. E.: Common medical and behavioral problems in cats. Mod. Vet. Pract. 56:699, 1975.

122. Movshon, J. A.: Reversal of the physiological effects of monocular deprivation in the kitten's visual cortex. J. Physiol. (Lond.) 261:125, 1976.

123. Muir, W. W.: Hallucinations caused by xylazine-ketamine. Mod. Vet. Pract. 58:654, 1977.

124. Nagaki, J., Yamashita, S., and Sato, M.: Neural response of cat to taste stimuli of varying temperatures. Jpn. J. Physiol. 14:67, 1964.

125. Neff, W. D.: Discriminatory capacity of different divisions of the auditory system. In Brazier, M. A. B., ed.: Brain and Behavior. Vol. 1. Washington, DC: American Institute of Biological Science, 1961.

126. Neff, W. D., and Diamond, I. T.: The neural basis of auditory discrimination. In Harlow, H. F., and Woolsey, C. N., eds.: Biological and Biochemical Bases of Behavior. Madison: University of Wisconsin Press, 1958.

127. Nelson, P. G., and Erulkar, S. D.: Synaptic mechanisms of excitation and inhibition in the central auditory pathway. J. Neurophysiol. 26:908, 1963.

128. Nilsson, B. Y.: Structure and function of the tactile hair receptors on the cat's foreleg. Acta Physiol. Scand. 77:396, 1969.
129. Nilsson, B. Y., and Skoglund, C. R.: The tactile hairs on the cat's foreleg. Acta Physiol. Scand. 65:364, 1965.
130. Nonneman, A. J., and Kolb, B. E.: Lesions of hippocampus or prefrontal cortex alter species-typical behaviors of the cat. Behav. Biol. 12:41, Sept. 1974.
131. Peters, G., and Wozencraft, W. C.: Acoustic communication in fissiped carnivores. In Gittleman, J. L., ed.: Carnivore Behavior, Ecology, and Evolution. Ithaca, NY: Cornell University Press, 1989.
132. Pfaffmann, C.: Differential responses of the new-born cat to gustatory stimuli. J. Genet. Psychol. 49:61, 1936.
133. Rhine, J. B., and Feather, S. R.: The study of cases of "psi-trailing" in animals. J. Parapsychol. 26:1, Mar. 1962.
134. Romanes, G. J.: Mental Evolution in Animals. New York: AMS Press, 1969.
135. Rose, G. H., and Lindsley, D. B.: Development of visually evoked potentials in kittens: Specific and nonspecific responses, J. Neurophysiol. 31:607, 1968.
136. Rose, J. E., Gross, N. B., Geisler, C. D., and Hind, J. E.: Some neural mechanisms in the inferior colliculus of the cat which may be relevant to localization of a sound source. J. Neurophysiol. 29:288, 1966.
137. Rosenblatt, J. S.: Suckling and home orientation in the kitten: A comparative development study. In Tobach, E., Aronson, L. R., and Shaw, E., eds.: The Biopsychology of Development. New York: Academic Press, 1971.
138. Rosenblatt, J. S.: Learning in newborn kittens. Sci. Am. 227:18, 1972.
139. Rosenblatt, J. S., Turkewitz, G., and Schneirla, T. C.: Development of home orientation in newly born kittens. Trans. N.Y. Acad. Sci. 31:231, 1969.
140. Rosenzweig, M. R., and Bennett, E. L.: Neural mechanisms of learning and memory. Cambridge, MA: M.I.T. Press, 1976.
141. Schiffman, H. R.: Evidence for sensory dominance: Reactions to apparent depth in rabbits, cats, and rodents. J. Comp. Physiol. Psychol. 71:38, Apr. 1970.
142. Schmidt, J. P.: Psychosomatics in veterinary medicine. In Fox, M. W., ed.: Abnormal Behavior in Animals. Philadelphia: W. B. Saunders Co., 1968.
143. Schweikert, G. E., III, and Treichler, F. R.: Visual probability learning and reversal in the cat. J. Comp. Physiol. Psychol. 67:269, 1969.
144. Seitz, P. F. D.: Infantile experience and adult behavior in animal subjects. Psychosom. Med. 21:353, 1959.
145. Shapley, R., and Victor, J.: Hyperacuity in cat retinal ganglion cells. Science 231:999, 1986.
146. Sherman, S. M.: Visual field defects in monocularly and binocularly deprived cats. Brain Res. 49:25, 1973.
147. Simoni, A., and Sprague, J. M.: Perimetric analysis of binocular and monocular visual fields in Siamese cats. Brain Res. 111:189, 1976.
148. Smith, B. A., and Jansen, G. R.: Behavior and brain composition of offspring of underfed cats. Fed. Proc. 36:1108, 1977.
149. Smith, K. U.: Visual discrimination in the cat. III. The relative effect of paired and unpaired stimuli in the discriminative behavior of the cat. J. Genet. Psychol. 48:29, 1936.
150. Smith, K. U.: Visual discrimination in the cat. IV. The visual acuity of the cat in relation to stimulus distance. J. Genet. Psychol. 49:297, 1936.
151. Smith, K. U.: The relation between visual acuity and the optic projection centers in the brain. Science 86:564, 1937.
152. Smith, R. C.: The Complete Cat Book. New York: Walker & Co., 1963.
153. Starr, A.: Suppression of single unit activity in cochlear nucleus of the cat following sound stimulation. J. Neurophysiol. 28:850, 1965.
154. Suehsdorf, A.: The cats in our lives. National Geographic 125:508, 1964.
155. Sutherland, N. S., and Mackintosh, N. J.: Mechanisms of Animal Discrimination Learning. New York: Academic Press, 1971.
156. Thompson, R. F., Johnson, R. H., and Hoopes, J. J.: Organization of auditory, somatic sensory, and visual projection to association fields of cerebral cortex in the cat. J. Neurophysiol. 26:343, 1963.

157. Thorn, F., Gollender, M., and Erikson, P.: The development of the kitten's visual optics. Vision Res. 16:1145, 1976.
158. Thorpe, W. H.: Learning and Instinct in Animals. Cambridge, MA: Harvard University Press, 1963.
159. Tilney, F., and Casamajor, L.: Myelinogeny as applied to the study of behavior. Arch. Neurol. Psychiatry 12:1, July 1924.
160. Tucker, A. O., and Tucker, S. S.: Catnip and the catnip response. Econ. Botany 42:214, 1988.
161. Vakkur, G. J., and Bishop, P. O.: The schematic eye in the cat. Vision Res. 3:357, 1963.
162. Villablanca, J. R., and Olmstead, C. E.: Neurological development of kittens. Dev. Psychobiol. 12:101, 1979.
163. Voith, V. L.: Personal communication, 1978.
164. Voith, V. L.: You, too, can teach a cat tricks (examples of shaping, second-order reinforcement, and constraints on learning). Mod. Vet. Pract. 62:639, 1981.
165. Voith, V., and Borchelt, P.: Fears and phobias in companion animals. Compendium on Continuing Education 7:209, 1985.
166. Volokhov, A. A.: The ontogenetic development of higher nervous activity in animals. In Himwich, W. A., ed.: Developmental Neurobiology. Springfield, IL: Charles C Thomas, 1970.
167. Wallach, M. B., and Gershon, S.: The induction and antagonism of central nervous system stimulant-induced stereotyped behavior in the cat. Eur. J. Pharmacol. 18:22, 1972.
168. Warkentin, J., and Smith, K. U.: The development of visual acuity in the cat. J. Genet. Psychol. 50:371, 1937.
169. Warren, J. M.: Oddity learning set in a cat. J. Comp. Physiol. Psychol. 53:433, 1960.
170. Warren, J. M.: Overtraining, extinction, and reversal learning by kittens. Anim. Learn. Behav. 3:340, 1975.
171. Warren, J. M.: Irrelevant cues and shape discrimination learning by cats. Anim. Learn. Behav. 4:22, 1976.
172. Warren, J. M., and Baron, A.: The formation of learning sets by cats. J. Comp. Physiol. Psychol. 49:227, 1956.
173. Washburn, M. F.: The Animal Mind. 3rd ed. New York: Macmillan, 1976.
174. Wassle, H.: Optical quality of the cat eye. Vision Res. 11:995, 1971.
175. Weigel, I.: Small cats and clouded leopards. In Grzimek, H. C. B., ed.: Grzimek's Animal Life Encyclopedia. Vol. 12. New York: Van Nostrand Reinhold Co., 1975.
176. West, M.: Social play in the domestic cat. Am. Zool. 14:427, 1974.
177. Wever, E. G., Vernon, J. A., Rahm, W. E., and Strother, W. F.: Cochlear potentials in the cat in response to high-frequency sounds. Proc. Natl. Acad. Sci. USA 44:1087, 1958.
178. Widdowson, E. M.: Food, growth, and development in the suckling period. In Graham-Jones, O., ed.: Canine and Feline Nutritional Requirements. New York: Pergamon Press, 1965.
179. Wienrich, M., and Zrenner, E.: Colour-opponent mechanisms in cat retinal ganglion cells. In Mollon, J., and Sharpe, L. T., eds.: Colour Vision: Physiology and Psychophysics. New York: Academic Press, 1983.
180. Wiesel, T. N., and Hubel, D. H.: Effects of visual deprivation on morphology and physiology of cells in the cat's lateral geniculate body. J. Neurophysiol. 26:978, 1963.
181. Wilson, M., Warren, J. M., and Abbott, L.: Infantile stimulation, activity and learning by cats. Child Dev. 36:843, 1965.
182. Windle, W. F., and Griffin, A. M.: Observations on embryonic and fetal movements of the cat. J. Comp. Neurol. 52:149, 1931.
183. Worden, A. N.: Abnormal behaviour in the dog and cat. Vet. Rec. 71:966, 1959.

ADDITIONAL READINGS

Adamec, R. Behavioral and epileptic determinants of predatory attack behavior in the cat. Can. J. Neurol. Sci. 2:457, 1975.

Adamec, R. E. Hypothalamic and extrahypothalamic substrates of predatory attack: Suppression and the influence of hunger. Brain Res. 106:57, 1976.

Albus, K. The detection of movement direction and effects of contrast reversal in the cat's striate cortex. Vision Res. 20:289, 1980.

Algers, B. T.V. apparatus upsets cats. Friskies Res. Dig. 13:14, Fall 1977.

Allikmets, L. H. Cholinergic mechanisms in aggressive behaviour. Med. Biol. 52:19, 1974.

Anderson, H. T. Problems of taste specificity. In Wolstenholme, G. E. W., and Knight, J., eds.: Taste and Smell in Vertebrates. London: Churchill, Ltd., 1970.

Appelle, S. Perception and discrimination as a function of stimulus orientation: The "oblique effect" in man and animals. Psychol. Bull. 78:266, 1972.

Baccelli, G., Albertini, R., Mancia, G., and Zanchetti, A. Interactions between sino-aortic reflexes and cardiovascular effects of sleep and emotional behavior in the cat. Circ. Res. 38 (Suppl. 1):30, 1976.

Bateson, P. The development of play in cats. Appl. Anim. Ethol. 4:290, 1978.

Baumgartner, G., Brown, J. L., and Schulz, A. Responses of single units of the cat visual system to rectangular stimulus patterns. J. Neurophysiol. 28:1, 1965.

Beach, F. A. Current concepts of play in animals. American Naturalist 79:523, 1945.

Bergsma, D. R., and Brown, K. S. White fur, blue eyes, and deafness in the domestic cat. J. Hered. 62:171, 1971.

Berkley, K. J., and Parmer, R. Somatosensory cortical involvement in responses to noxious stimulation in the cat. Exp. Brain Res. 20:363, 1974.

Berkley, M. A. A system for behavioral evaluation of the visual capacities of cats. Behav. Res. Methods Instrumentation 11:545, 1979.

Berkson, G. Maturation defects in kittens. Am. J. Ment. Defic. 72:757, 1959.

Berman, A. L. Interaction of cortical responses to somatic and auditory stimuli in anterior ectosylvian gyrus of cat. J. Neurophysiol. 24:608, 1961.

Berman, A. L. Overlap of somatic and auditory cortical response fields in anterior ectosylvian gyrus of cat. J. Neurophysiol. 24:595, 1961.

Berntson, G. G., Hughes, H. C., and Beattie, M. S. A comparison of hypothalamically induced biting attack with natural predatory behavior in the cat. J. Comp. Physiol. Psychol. 90:167, 1976.

Berntson, G. G., and Leibowitz, S. F. Biting attack in cats: Evidence for central muscarinic mediation. Brain Res. 51:366, 1973.

Bjursten, L. M., Norrsell, K., and Norrsell, U. Behavioral repertory of cats without cerebral cortex from infancy. Exp. Brain Res. 25:115, 1976.

Blake, R., and DiGianfilippo, A. Spatial vision in cats with selective neural deficits. J. Neurophys. 43:1197, 1980.

Bland, K. P. Tom-cat odour and other pheromones in feline reproduction. Vet. Sci. Comm. 3:125, 1979.

Bogen, J. E., Suzuki, M., and Campbell, B. Paw contact placing in the hypothalamic cat given caffeine. J. Neurobiol. 6:125, 1975.

Bosher, S. K., and Hallpike, C. S. Observations on histological features, development and pathogenesis of the inner ear degeneration of the deaf white cat. Proc. R. Soc. Lond. [Biol.] 162:147, 1965.

Brogden, W. J., Girden, E., Mettler, F. A., and Culler, E. Acoustic value of the several components of the auditory system in cats. Am. J. Physiol. 116:252, 1936.

Brooks, C. Teaching tricks to your cat. Pet News 3:40, Sept.-Oct. 1977.

Brooks, V. B., Rudomin, P., and Slayman, C. L. Sensory activation of neurons in the cat's cerebral cortex. J. Neurophysiol. 24:286, 1961.

Buser, P., and Bignall, K. E. Nonprimary sensory projections on the cat neocortex. Int. Rev. Neurobiol. 10:111, 1967.

Cain, D. P. The role of the olfactory bulb in limbic mechanisms. Psychol. Bull. 81:654, 1974.

Caro, T. M. Effects of the mother, object play, and adult experience on predation in cats. Behav. Neural Biol. 29:29, 1980.

Carpenter, J. A. Species differences in taste preferences. J. Comp. Physiol. Psychol. 49:139, 1959.

Carreras, M., and Andersson, S. A. Functional properties of neurons of the anterior ectosylvian gyrus of the cat. J. Neurophysiol. 26:100, 1963.

Celesia, G. G. Segmental organization of cortical afferent areas in the cat. J. Neurophysiol. 26:193, 1963.

Chi, C. C., Bandler, R. J., and Flynn, J. P. Neuroanatomic projections related to biting attack elicited from ventral midbrain in cats. Brain Behav. Evol. 13:91, 1976.

Chow, K. L., and Stewart, D. L. Reversal of structural and functional effects of long-term visual deprivation in cats. Exp. Neurol. 34:409, 1972.

Clemente, C. D., and Chase, M. H. Neurological substrates of aggressive behavior. Annu. Rev. Physiol. 35:329, 1973.

Cohen, D. H., and Obrist, P. A. Interactions between behavior and the cardiovascular system. Circ. Res. 37:693, 1975.

Colpaert, F. C. The ventromedial hypothalamus and the control of avoidance behavior and aggression: Fear hypothesis versus response-suppression theory of limbic system function. Behav. Biol. 15:27, Sept. 1975.

Cornwell, A. C. Electroretinographic responses following monocular visual deprivation in kittens. Vision Res. 14:1223, 1974.

Cornwell, P., Overman, W., Levitsky, C., et al. Performance on the visual cliff by cats with marginal gyrus lesions. J. Comp. Physiol. Psychol. 90:996, 1976.

Cragg, B. G. The development of synapses in kitten visual cortex during visual deprivation. Exp. Neurol. 46:445, 1975.

Daves, W. F., and Boostrom, E. Object properties mediating visual object discrimination in the cat. Percept. Mot. Skills 19:343, 1964.

DeMolina, A. F., and Hunsperger, R. W. Organization of subcortical systems governing defence and flight reactions in the cat. J. Physiol. (Lond.) 160:200, 1962.

Derdzinski, D., and Warren, J. M. Perimeter, complexity, and form discrimination learning by cats. J. Comp. Physiol. Psychol. 68:407, 1969.

Dews, P. B., and Wiesel, T. N. Consequences of monocular deprivation on visual behaviour in kittens. J. Physiol. (Lond.) 206:437, 1970.

Diamond, I. T., and Neff, W. D. Ablation of temporal cortex and discrimination of auditory patterns. J. Neurophysiol. 20:300, 1957.

Dürsteler, M. R., Garey, L. J., and Movshon, J. A. Reversal of the morphological effects of monocular deprivation in the kitten's lateral geniculate nucleus. J. Physiol. (Lond.) 261:189, 1976.

Dworkin, S. Conditioned motor reflexes in cats. Am. J. Physiol. 109:31, 1934.

Eleftheriou, B. E., and Scott, J. P. The Physiology of Aggression and Defeat. New York: Plenum Publishing Corp., 1971.

Ewer, R. F. Ethology of Mammals. London: Paul Elek, Ltd., 1968.

Fox, M. W. Natural environment: Theoretical and practical aspects for breeding and rearing laboratory animals. Lab. Anim. Care 16:316, 1966.

Fox, M. W. Psychomotor disturbances. In Fox, M. W., ed. Abnormal Behavior in Animals. Philadelphia: W. B. Saunders Co., 1968.

Fox, M. W. Psychopathology in man and lower animals. J. Am. Vet. Med. Assoc. 159:66, 1971.

Fox, M. W. Understanding Your Cat. New York: Coward, McCann & Geoghegan, 1974.

Fraser, A. F. Behavior disorders in domestic animals. In Fox, M. W., ed. Abnormal Behavior in Animals. Philadelphia: W. B. Saunders Co., 1968.

Fried, P. A. Septum and behavior: A review. Psychol. Bull. 78:292, 1972.

Fukada, Y. Receptive field organization of cat optic nerve fibers with special reference to conduction velocity. Vision Res. 11:209, 1971.

Ganz, L., Hirsch, H. V. B., and Tieman, S. B. The nature of perceptual deficits in visually deprived cats. Brain Res. 11:547, 1972.

Gibbs, E. L., and Gibbs, F. A. A purring center in the brain of the cat. J. Comp. Neurol. 64:209, 1936.

Gibson, E. J., and Walk, R. D. The visual cliff. Sci. Am. 202:64, 1960.

Glassman, R. B. Cutaneous discrimination and motor control following somatosensory cortical ablation. Physiol. Behav. 5:1009, 1970.

Glusman, M. The hypothalamic "savage" syndrome. Res. Publ. Assoc. Res. Nerv. Ment. Dis. 52:52, 1974.

Goldberg, J. M., and Neff, W. D. Frequency discrimination after bilateral ablation of cortical auditory areas. J. Neurophysiol. 24:119, 1961.

Gorham, M. E., and Mitchell, R. Classifying the catnip response: The low-down on feline highs. D.V.M. 10:32, Jan. 1979.

Gruber, S. H. Mechanisms of color vision; an ethologist's primer. In Burtt, E. H., Jr., ed. The Behavioral Significance of Color. New York: Garland Publishing, Inc., 1979.

Gunter, R. The absolute threshold for vision in the cat. J. Physiol. (Lond.) 114:8, 1951.

Hamilton, L. W. Active avoidance impairment following septal lesions in cats. J. Comp. Physiol. Psychol. 69:420, 1979.

Hara, K., Cornwell, P. R., Warren, J. M., and Webster, I. H. Posterior extramarginal cortex and visual learning by cats. J. Comp. Physiol. Psychol. 87:884, 1974.

Hart, B. L. Disease processes and behavior. Fel. Pract. 3:6, Nov.-Dec. 1973.

Hart, B. L. A quiz on feline behavior. Fel. Pract. 5:12, May-June 1975.

Hart, B. L. Quiz on feline behavior. Fel. Pract. 7:20, May 1977.

Hekmatpanah, J. Organization of tactile dermatomes C1 through L4, in cat. J. Neurophysiol. 24:129, 1961.

Hemmer, H. Gestation period and postnatal development in felids. In Eaton, R. L., ed. The World's Cats. Vol. 3. Seattle: Carnivore Research Institute, 1976.

Hendersen, R. W. Learning in Animals. Stroudsburg, PA: Hutchinson Ross Publishing Co., 1982.

Henry, J. P. Mechanisms of psychosomatic disease in animals. Adv. Vet. Sci. Comp. Med. 20:115, 1976.

Hirsch, H. V. B., and Spinelli, D. N. Visual experience modifies distribution of horizontally and vertically oriented receptive fields in cats. Science 168:869, 1970.

Horn, G., and Wiesenfeld, Z. Attention in the cat: Electrophysiological and behavioural studies. Exp. Brain Res. 21:67, 1974.

Houpt, K. A. Animal behavior as a subject for veterinary students. Cornell Vet. 66:73, 1976.

Houpt, K. A. Domestic Animal Behavior for Veterinarians and Animal Scientists. 2nd ed. Ames: Iowa State University Press, 1991.

Hubel, D. H., and Wiesel, T. N. Receptive fields of cells in striate cortex of very young, visually inexperienced kittens. J. Neurophysiol. 26:994, 1963.

Hubel, D. H., and Wiesel, T. N. Receptive fields and functional architecture in two nonstriate visual areas (18 and 19) of the cat. J. Neurophysiol. 28:229, 1965.

Hubel, D. H., and Wiesel, T. N. Binocular interaction in striate cortex of kittens reared with artificial squint. J. Neurophysiol 28:1041, 1965.

Jackson, B., and Reed, A. Catnip and the alteration of consciousness. J.A.M.A. 207:1349, 1969.

Jacobs, B. L., Trulson, M. E., and Stern, W. C. An animal behavior model for studying the actions of LSD and related hallucinogens. Science 194:741, 1976.

Johansson, G. G., Kalimo, R., Niskanen, H., and Ruusunen, S. Effects of stimulation parameters on behavior elicited by stimulation of the hypothalamic defense area. J. Comp. Physiol. Psychol. 87:1100, 1974.

John, E. R., Chesler, P., Bartlett, F., and Victor, I. Observation learning in cats. Science 159:1489, 1968.

Kare, M. R., and Halpern, B. P. Physiological and Behavioral Aspects of Taste. Chicago: University of Chicago Press, 1961.

Karmel, B. Z., Miller, P. N., Dettweiler, L., and Anderson, G. Texture density and normal development of visual depth avoidance. Dev. Psychobiol. 3:73, 1970.

Keidel, W. D. The sensory detection of vibrations. In Dawson, W. W., and Enoch, J. M., eds. Foundations of Sensory Science. New York: Springer-Verlag, 1984.

Kling, A., Kovach, J. K., and Tucker, T. J. The behaviour of cat. In Hafez, E. S. E., ed. The Behaviour of Domestic Animals. 2nd ed. Baltimore: Williams & Wilkins Co., 1969.

Kling, A., Orbach, J., Schwartz, N. B., and Towne, J. C. Injury to the limbic system and associated structures in cats. Arch. Gen. Psychiatry 3:391, 1960.

Koepke, J. E., and Pribram, K. H. Effect of milk on the maintenance of sucking behavior in kittens from birth to six months. J. Comp. Physiol. 75:363, 1971.

Kuffler, S. W., Fitzhugh, R., and Barlow, H. B. Maintained activity in the cat's retina in light and darkness. J. Gen. Physiol. 40:683, 1957.

Kuhn, R. A. Organization of tactile dermatomes in cat and monkey. J. Neurophysiol. 16:169, 1953.

Kurtsin, I. T. Pavlov's concept of experimental neurosis and abnormal behavior in animals.

In Fox, M. W., ed. Abnormal Behavior in Animals. Philadelphia: W. B. Saunders Co., 1968.

Kurtsin, I. T. Physiological mechanisms of behavior disturbances and corticovisceral interrelations in animals. In Fox, M. W., ed. Abnormal Behavior in Animals. Philadelphia: W. B. Saunders Co., 1968.

Langworthy, O. R. Behavioral disturbances related to the decomposition of reflex activity caused by cerebral injury: An experimental study of the cat. J. Neuropathol. Exp. Neurol. 3:87, 1944.

Levinson, B. M. Man and his feline pet. Mod. Vet. Pract. 53:35, Nov. 1972.

Levinson, P. K., and Flynn, J. P. The objects attacked by cats during stimulation of the hypothalamus. Anim. Behav. 13:217, 1965.

Loop, M. S., Bruce, L. L., and Petuchowski, S. Cat color vision: The effect of stimulus size, shape and viewing distance. Vision Res. 19:507, 1979.

Lorenz, K., and Leyhausen, P. Motivation of Human and Animal Behavior. New York: Van Nostrand Reinhold Co., 1973.

MacDonnell, M. F., and Flynn, J. P. Control of sensory fields by stimulation of hypothalamus. Science 152:1406, 1966.

Macleod, A. J. Chemistry of odours. In Stoddart, D. M., ed. Olfaction in Mammals. London: Academic Press, 1980.

Mancia, G., Baccelli, G., and Zanchetti, A. Regulation of renal circulation during behavioral changes in the cat. Am. J. Physiol. 227:536, 1972.

Marler, P., and Vandenbergh, J. G. Handbook of Behavioral Neurobiology. Vol. 3. Social Behavior and Communication. New York: Plenum Press, 1979.

Maruyama, N., and Kanno, Y. Experimental study on functional compensation after bilateral removal of auditory cortex in cats. J. Neurophysiol. 24:193, 1961.

Masterton, R. B. Adaptation for sound localization in the ear and brainstem of mammals. Fed. Proc. 33:1904, 1974.

Masterton, R. B., Jane, J. A., and Diamond, I. T. Role of brain-stem auditory structures in sound localization. II. Inferior colliculus and its brachium. J. Neurophysiol. 31:96, 1968.

Mayers, K. S., Robertson, R. T., Rubel, E. W., and Thompson, R. F. Development of polysensory responses in association cortex of kitten. Science 171:1038, 1971.

McAllister, W. G., and Berman, H. D. Visual form discrimination in the domestic cat. J. Comp. Psychol. 12:207, 1931.

McClung, A. W., and Hart, B. L. Olfactory loss affecting behavior? Fel. Pract. 8:17, May 1978.

McFarland, C. A., and Hart, B. L. Aggressive behavior. Fel. Pract. 8:13, July 1978.

Mello, N. K., and Peterson, N. J. Behavioral evidence for color discrimination in cat. J. Neurophysiol. 27:323, 1964.

Meyer, D. R., and Anderson, R. A. Colour discrimination in cats. In de Reuck, A. V. S., and Knight, J., eds. Colour Vision. London: Churchill, Ltd., 1965.

Mignard, M., and Malpeli, J. G. Paths of information flow through visual cortex. Science 251:1249, 1991.

Miller, J. D., Watson, C. S., and Covell, W. P. Deafening effects of noise on the cat. Acta Otolaryngol. [Stockh.] 176(Suppl.):2, 1963.

Morgane, P. J., and Kosman, A. J. Alterations in feline behavior following bilateral amygadalectomy. Nature 180:598, 1957.

Movshon, J. A. Reversal of the behavioural effects of monocular deprivation in the kitten. J. Physiol. (Lond.) 261:175, 1976.

Muir, D. W., and Mitchell, D. E. Behavioral deficits in cats following early selected visual exposure to contours of a single orientation. Brain Res. 85:459, 1975.

Murata, K., Cramer, H., and Bach-y-Rita, P. Neuronal convergence of noxious, acoustic, and visual stimuli in the visual cortex of the cat. J. Neurophysiol. 28:1223, 1965.

Neff, W. D., Fisher, J. F., Diamond, I. T., and Yela, M. Role of auditory cortex in discrimination requiring localization of sound in space. J. Neurophysiol. 19:500, 1956.

Neff, W. D., and Hind, J. E. Auditory thresholds of the cat. J. Acoust. Soc. Am. 27:480, 1955.

Negus, V. E. The organ of Jacobson. J. Anat. 90:515, 1956.

Oliver, J. Determinants of experimental neurosis in cats. J. Clin. Psychol. 31:594, 1975.

Oswaldo-Cruz, E., and Kidd, C. Functional properties of neurons in the lateral cervical nucleus of the cat. J. Neurophysiol. 27:1, 1964.

Paden, G. F., and Goddard, G. V. Catnip and oestrous behaviour in the cat. Anim. Behav. 14:372, 1966.

Quilliam, T. A. Non-auditory vibration receptors. Int. Audiol. 7:311, 1968.

Reis, D. J. Central neurotransmitters in aggression. Res. Publ. Assoc. Res. Nerv. Ment. Dis. 52:119, 1974.

Rheingold, H. L., and Eckerman, C. O. Familiar social and nonsocial stimuli and the kitten's response to a strange environment. Dev. Psychobiol. 4:71, 1971.

Roberts, W. W., and Bergquist, E. H. Attack elicited by hypothalamic stimulation in cats raised in social isolation. J. Comp. Physiol. Psychol. 66:590, 1968.

Roberts, W. W., and Keiss, H. O. Motivational properties of hypothalamic aggression in cats. J. Comp. Physiol. Psychol. 58:187, 1964.

Robinson, J. S., and Voneida, J. Central cross-integration of visual inputs presented simultaneously to the separate eyes. J. Comp. Physiol. Psychol. 57:22, 1964.

Rodieck, R. W., and Stone, J. Response of cat retinal ganglion cells to moving visual patterns. J. Neurophysiol. 28:819, 1965.

Roldán, E., Alvarez-Pelaez, R., and de Molina, A. F. Electrographic study of the amygdaloid defense response. Physiol. Behav. 13:779, 1974.

Rose, J. E., and Woolsey, C. N. Cortical connections and functional organization of the thalamic auditory system of the cat. In Harlow, H. F., and Woolsey, C. N., eds. Biological and Biochemical Bases of Behavior. Madison: University of Wisconsin Press, 1958.

Rosenkilde, C. E., and Divac, I. Time-discrimination performance in cats with lesions in prefrontal cortex and caudate nucleus. J. Comp. Physiol. Psychol. 90:343, 1976.

Rosenzweig, M. Discrimination of auditory intensities in the cat. Am. J. Psychol. 59:127, 1946.

Rothfield, L., and Harman, P. J. On the relation of the hippocampal-fornix system to the control of rage responses in cats. J. Comp. Neurol. 101:265, 1954.

Rubel, E. W. A comparison of somatotropic organization in sensory neocortex of newborn kittens and adult cats. J. Comp. Neurol. 143:447, 1971.

Scharlock, D. P., Neff, W. D., and Strominger, N. L. Discrimination of tone duration after bilateral ablation of cortical auditory areas. J. Neurophysiol. 28:673, 1965.

Scharlock, D. P., Tucker, T. J., and Strominger, N. L. Auditory discrimination by the cat after neonatal ablation of temporal cortex. Science 141:1197, 1963.

Schilder, P. Loss of a brightness discrimination in the cat following removal of the striate area. J. Neurophysiol. 29:888, 1966.

Schwartz, A. S., and Whalen, R. E. Amygdala activity during sexual behavior in the male cat. Life Sci. 4:1359, 1965.

Scott, J. P. Aggression. 2nd ed. Chicago: University of Chicago Press, 1975.

Sechzer, J. A., and Brown, J. L. Color discrimination in the cat. Science 144:427, 1964.

Seward, J. P., and Humphrey, G. L. Changes in heart rate during avoidance training and extinction in the cat. J. Comp. Physiol. Psychol. 66:764, 1968.

Shapley, R., and Victor, J. D. The contrast gain control of the cat retina. Vision Res. 19:431, 1979.

Sherman, S. M. Visual development in cats. Invest. Ophthalmol. 11:394, 1972.

Shipley, C., Buchwald, J. S., Norman, R., and Guthrie, D. Brain stem auditory evoked response development in the kitten. Brain Res. 182:313, 1980.

Siegel, A., Edinger, H., and Dotto, M. Effects of electrical stimulation of the lateral aspect of the prefrontal cortex upon attack behavior in cats. Brain Res. 93:473, 1975.

Smith, B. A., and Jansen, G. R. Early undernutrition and subsequent behavior patterns in cat. J. Nutr. 103:xxix, 1973.

Smith, K. U. Visual discrimination in the cat. I. The capacity of the cat for visual figure discrimination. J. Genet. Psychol. 44:301, 1934.

Smith, K. U. Visual discrimination in the cat. II. A further study of the capacity of the cat for visual figure discrimination. J. Genet. Psychol. 45:336, 1934.

Squires, R. D., Jacobson, F. H., and Bergey, G. E. Hypothermia in cats during physical restraint. National Technical Information Service AD-735:883, 1971.

Sutin, J., Rose, J., Van Atta, L., and Thalmann, R. Electrophysiological studies in an animal model of aggressive behavior. Res. Publ. Assoc. Res. Nerv. Ment. Dis. 52:93, 1974.

Thomas, G. J., Fry, W. J., Fry, F. J., et al. Behavioral effects of mammillothalamic tractotomy in cats. J. Neurophysiol. 26:857, 1963.

Thompson, R. F., Smith, H. E., and Bliss, D. Auditory, somatic sensory, and visual response interactions and interrelations in association and primary cortical fields of the cat. J. Neurophysiol. 26:365, 1963.

Thorn, F. Detection of luminance differences by the cat. J. Comp. Physiol. Psychol. 70:326, 1970.

Thorndike, E. L. Animal Intelligence. New York: Hafner Publishing Co., 1970.

Tucker, T., and Kling, A. Differential effects of early vs. late brain damage on visual duration discrimination in cat. Fed. Proc. 25:207, 1966.

Van Hof-Van Duin, J. Development of visuomotor behavior in normal and dark-reared cats. Brain Res. 104:233, 1976.

Verberne, G. Beobachtungen und Versuche Über das Flehmen Katzenartiger Raubtiere. Z. Tierpsychol. 27:807, 1970.

Verberne, G. Chemocommunication among domestic cats, mediated by the olfactory and vomeronasal senses. II. The relation between the function of Jacobson's organ (vomeronasal organ) and flehmen behaviour. Z. Tierpsychol. 42:113, 1976.

Verberne, G., and DeBoer, J. Chemocommunication among domestic cats, mediated by the olfactory and vomeronasal senses. I. Chemocommunication. Z. Tierpsychol. 42:86, 1976.

Vital-Durand, F., and Jeannerod, M. Eye movement related activity in the visual cortex of dark-reared kittens. Electroencephalogr. Clin. Neurophysiol. 38:295, 1975.

Wada, J. A., and Sato, M. Directedness of defensive emotional behavior and motivation for aversive learning. Exp. Neurol. 40:445, 1973.

Walk, R. D. The study of visual depth and distance perception in animals. In Lehrman, D. S., Hinde, R. A., and Shaw, E., eds. Advances in the Study of Behavior. Vol. 1. New York: Academic Press, 1965.

Walker, A. D. Taste preferences in the domestic dog and cat. Gaines Dog Res. Prog., Summer 1975.

Waller, G. R., Price, G. H., and Mitchell, E. D. Feline attractant, cis, trans-nepetalactone: Metabolism in the domestic cat. Science 164:1281, 1969.

Warkentin, J., and Carmichael, L. A study of the development of the air-righting reflex in cats and rabbits. J. Genet. Psychol. 55:67, 1939.

Warren, J. M. Discrimination of mirror images by cats. J. Comp. Physiol. Psychol. 69:9, 1969.

Warren, J. M. Transfer of responses to open and closed shapes in discrimination by cats. Percept. Psychophys. 12:449, 1972.

Warren, J. M., Warren, H. B., and Akert, K. Orbitofrontal cortical lesions and learning in cats. J. Comp. Neurol. 118:17, 1962.

Wemmer, C., and Scow, R. Communication in the Felidae with emphasis on scent marking and contact patterns. In Sebeok, T. A., ed. How Animals Communicate. Bloomington: Indiana University Press, 1977.

Wenzel, B. M. Tactile stimulation as reinforcement for cats and its relation to early feeding experience. Psychol. Rep. 5:297, 1959.

West, C. D., and Harrison, C. D. Transneuronal cell atrophy in the congenitally deaf white cat. J. Comp. Neurol. 151:377, 1973.

Wickelgren, W. O. Effects of walking and flash stimulation on click-evoked responses in cats. J. Neurophysiol. 31:769, 1968.

Wiesel, T. N., and Hubel, D. H. Comparison of the effects of unilateral and bilateral eye closure on cortical unit responses in kittens. J. Neurophysiol. 28:1029, 1965.

Wiesel, T. N., and Hubel, D. H. Extent of recovery from the effects of visual deprivation in kittens. J. Neurophysiol. 28:1060, 1965.

Winans, S. S. Visual form discrimination after removal of the visual cortex in cats. Science 158:944, 1967.

Zetterstrom, B. The effect of light on the appearance and development of the electroretinogram in newborn kittens. Acta Physiol. Scand. 35:272, 1956.

Zvartau, E. E., and Patkina, N. A. Motivational properties of hypothalamic stimulation in cats. Bull. Exp. Biol. Med. 75:233, 1973.

3

Feline Communicative Behavior

Intraspecies communication takes three major forms: vocal expression, body postures, and visual and olfactory marks. Interspecies communication is more complicated because animals of different species, such as dogs and cats, are not considered to have the innate ability to understand the communications of each other. Because humans can learn many feline signals, better understanding and communication between people and cats are possible.

VOCAL COMMUNICATION

Vocal communication, in addition to marking behavior, which is discussed later in the chapter, is important to the cat for the spacing of individuals. It prevents direct confrontations between these basically asocial animals. Distance-reducing vocal patterns in response to humans usually do not occur if the distance from the human is greater than 8 feet.[34] The variations of tonal elements during specific-goal emotional states result from changes in the laryngopharynx because of touch reception and tension variation rather than from oral position variations.[34, 42] Phonetically distinct sounds have been carefully differentiated and placed into one of three groups, according to how the sound is produced. (See Appendix A.) Although kittens can recognize familiar voices by 4 weeks of age, they usually do not take specific notice of one another's vocal communication patterns until their 9th week.[34]

Murmur Patterns

Murmur vocalizations involve sounds a cat produces while its mouth is closed.[34]

Grunt. The "grunt" sound, present at birth, normally disappears at maturity, but an occasional adult will voice a grunt when particularly baffled by a difficult obstacle.[34]

Purr. By 2 days of age, the "purr" is present and is produced by both nursing kittens and queen. It initially serves as a form of communication between them, vocal for her and tactile for the kittens, which stop the purr only for swallowing.[34]

A "greeting" or request vocalization is an expanded form of a single inhalation segment of the purr. In the kitten, this purring vocalization increases in intensity until it reaches the greeting level by about the 3rd week of life, when it may alert other kittens as the first reaches the queen to nurse.[11, 34] This sound, though usually short, can be prolonged, as when the cat approaches from a distance. As the kitten matures, the purr can develop several other inflections and meanings. The request purr for food or attention develops after the 12th week.[34]

A cat may purr in almost any situation, including just before death, which probably reflects a state of euphoria similar to that experienced by terminally ill humans. Experiences that are interpreted to be either pleasurable or anxious also may be accompanied by purring vocalizations. Studies show that it is common for the cat to produce an inaudible purr in the presence of humans.[36]

There are many descriptions of how the purr is generated. Theories include fremitus of blood passing through kinetic angulation in major vessels and soft palate vibrations. Electromyographic studies show, however, that the purr results from activation of the intrinsic laryngeal muscles by partial glottal closure and increased transglottal pressure for 20- to 30-millisecond bursts.[36, 44] That, in turn, is controlled by the neural infundibulum.[15] The diaphragm is alternately activated to produce the more or less continuous sound.[36, 44] The inhalation component of the purr frequently is the louder, longer, and lower-pitched component, although there is considerable individual variation. In some cats, the exhalation portion of the purr may be the major component. The purring interval is variable and depends on the cat's intensity of interest.

Call. The feline "call" sound, which is primarily to draw someone or something toward the cat, is used as a female's signal of readiness to mate.[12, 13, 34] Variations include the coaxing sounds used by a tomcat to notify females that he is ready to mate, to invite young males out to fight, and to announce his presence to other males. This advertising sound is not used by all South American domestic cats, indicating that a learning component may be present in vocalization.[38]

Acknowledgment. The cat that is close to its owner may use a single short murmur of "acknowledgment" when it visualizes something it is about to receive.[34] This vocalization does not occur until sometime after the 12th week of age.

Vowel Patterns

The five types of sounds produced when the mouth is first opened and then gradually closed are called vowel patterns.[34]

Demand. "Demand," like several other patterns, often is the intermediate form of a series of vocalizations that increase in intensity with time. Kittens do not acquire this pattern until after 79 days of age.[34] Variations by means of voice inflections allow the cat to indicate different moods. In tense situations, more stress is given to the initial sound, whereas the opposite occurs in situations of hopelessness.[34] A coaxing variation is soft and begins with a closed mouth. The "whisper" occurs when the cat is aware that it is not advisable to make noise but is unable to suppress the demand.[34] That results in a mouthing movement with little or no noise, a "silent meow." A chirping variation of demand is commonly expressed, accompanied by intense tail-flicking, when the cat is highly aroused by the sight of prey. Queens use another form of demand to call their kittens to see prey.[2] A slower, more drawn-out vocalization is expressed when the cat is absorbed in a goal pursuit. The demand then becomes a "begging demand."[34]

Bewilderment. "Bewilderment" is a minor vowel pattern that first occurs after 79 days of age and has a prolonged or more intense terminal sound. The initial portion of this sound also can indicate a high expectancy or confidence if it is stressed.[34]

Complaint. Vocalizations of "complaint" also begin sometime after 79 days of age.[8, 34] Some cats that express a vocal complaint are satisfied with a human's verbal sympathy.[34]

Mating Cry. Mild forms of the "mating cry" can be expressed by gradually closing an open mouth.[34] It is a characteristic two-syllable call used by an estrous female.[24]

Anger Wail. A common form of vocalization for the young kitten has been termed the "anger wail."[34] These distress vocalizations can be heard as early as the 1st day of life and seem to be related to the absence of the smell of the mother or littermates, or both. During the first few days, the mean number of distress cries is one or two during a 3-minute period, but the number rapidly increases during the first 5 days of life. It reaches a peak soon after the 2-week-old period, which is the most vocal period of the kitten's life.[37, 40] Although this sound is first associated with competition during nursing, it later becomes individualized and associated with rough forms of play, fights, and protests.[12, 34, 37]

Siamese Vocalizations. Most of the unusual, excessive, and loud vocalizations associated with the Siamese cat are classified as vowel patterns. The distinctive qualities of these sounds are apparently associated with the same recessive gene that carries their typical pigmentation.[47]

Strained Intensity Patterns

Sounds that express an intense emotional state are produced with the mouth held open.[34]

Growl. The warning "growl" occurs during a slow, steady exhalation. The queen uses this vocalization to scatter her kittens and warn them to seek immediate shelter. If necessary, she reinforces the warning with a bat from her paw. When the queen is especially alarmed, this vocalization takes on a dog-bark quality.[12, 13] Young kittens can produce this sound, and usually first express it when they have matured enough to escape with pieces of food.[34] During a fight, the growl is 400 to 800 Hz.[24]

Snarl. Active fighting, especially between males, is accompanied by a "snarl." After a noisy inhalation, the vocalization is expressed and abruptly stopped.[34] The amount of noise is intense but usually out of proportion to the amount of actual physical damage.

Hiss. The "hiss" and its more intense variation, the "spit," are involuntary reactions to surprise by an enemy. The sound is produced as air is forced through a small oral opening while the cat is changing positions to view the approacher.[34] These vocalizations can occur even before the eyes open in the kitten and are controlled, along with other forms of defensive behavior, by the amygdala and the hypothalamus.

Mating Cry. The "mating cry" of the tomcat is an intense form of vocalization, which is probably a highly modified form of demand. Often accompanying this caterwauling cry is the parasympathetic reaction of drooling, with increased swallowing and licking.[34]

Scream. As copulation ends, the female cat vocalizes a form of "scream." This sudden loud pattern, also termed "pain shriek," probably represents an intense variation of the complaint vocal pattern.[34, 36] Vaginal stimulation by the penile spines normally is the initiating factor.

Refusal. "Refusal," a minor sound, low and rasping, usually is associated with occasions when a cat draws back from something forced on it.[34]

POSTURAL COMMUNICATION

The cat uses various body postures as primary methods of communication, but these postures are probably less significant for the cat than for more social animals because the cat's existence does not rely on maintaining harmony within a social group. Nevertheless, the cat uses certain patterns to indicate whether or not another individual may approach.

Distance-Reducing Postures

Submissive Postures. Because the cat is asocial, submissive postures are of minimal significance and, if present, are less highly developed than those of a social species. Submission involves postures that mainly serve to inhibit an attack if flight is not possible. The ears may be flattened back against its head. This posture frequently is shown by a nonterritorial male or female when approached by the territorial male, which may then use the mounting postures associated with mating on the lower-ranking individual. The mounted individual tolerates mounting only until it can escape. Crouching also may be an invitation to approach, as with a female in heat.[13]

Active Approaches. In an active approach to one cat by another, the tail is held vertically.[27] When a cat approaches a friendly being or when a kitten approaches the queen, the vertical tail position is particularly obvious (Fig. 3–1).

This tail position may have been derived from the queen's licking of the anogenital area of the kittens.[12, 13] In addition, when petted, a friendly cat responds by pushing the petted part of its body closer to the person for contact (Fig. 3–2). Thus the cat will extend its pelvic limbs when the

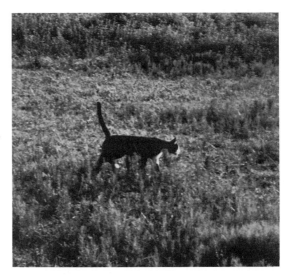

FIGURE 3–1. The vertical tail posture of a friendly approach.

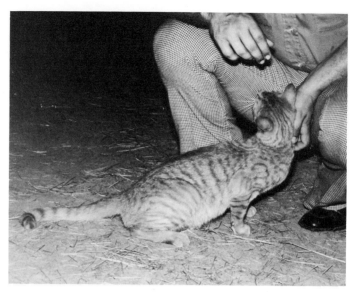

FIGURE 3–2. A cat responds to petting by pushing the petted area closer.

base of the tail is rubbed or flex its forelimbs and turn its head for a neck massage.

Play Postures. Play postures, described in Chapter 2, are distance-reducing, as are play-soliciting postures, such as rolling over to expose the abdominal area. In the dog, that is a submissive posture, but it is seen in the cat only in play-solicitation, courtship, and extreme defense.[12, 13]

Other Postures. Facial expressions and tail postures without piloerection have a come-closer meaning. Arching of the tail over the cat's back indicates a high arousal, as in play (Fig. 3–3). An inverted U shape to the tail is most significant in the play chase (Fig. 3–4). Extreme excitement, as when watching a bird, can result in a twitching tail movement often accompanied by a chirping vocalization. Facial expressions that involve half-closed eyes, protrusion of the third eyelid, or both most frequently are associated with the performance of a natural body function, such as eating, defecating, social grooming, and copulating.[13, 41] The play face usually includes dilated pupils and forward-pointing ears (Fig. 3–5).

Distance-Increasing Postures

Interactions between cats frequently involve certain patterns of silent communication that indicate when the cat prefers minimal social contact. Thus many body signs are used to convey a distance-increasing message.

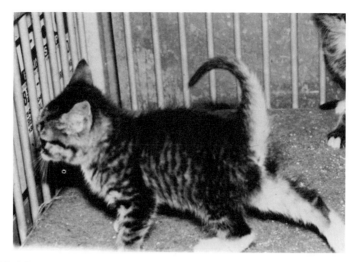

FIGURE 3–3. Arching of the tail over the back is a distance-reducing posture.

The cat always gives adequate warning before an attack. Humans and other species unfortunately do not always interpret the threat postures accurately.

Offensive Threat. In the offensive threat, direct eye contact with constricted pupils, forward-directed whiskers, and a straightforward body position indicate an intention to attack (Fig. 3–6).[12, 28] This stare technique is used to regulate social distances. A subtler, more deliberate back-and-forth flagging of the tail, especially the tail tip, expresses the cat's disturbance with the situation and its agitation.[27] Threat postures as part

FIGURE 3–4. The inverted U tail posture associated with distance-reducing behavior.

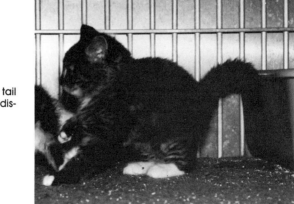

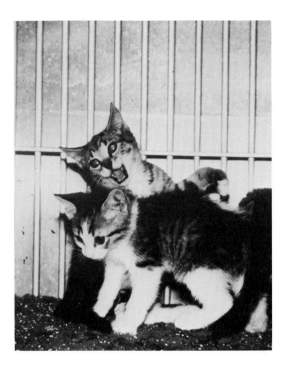

FIGURE 3–5. An intense play facial expression.

of the conditioned defensive reflex can appear before the kitten's eyes have opened, and stabilize by 35 days. Even at this young age, the threat usually involves the optical effect of a rapid approach created by a sudden apparent increase in size owing to piloerection. Tomcats use another variation of this threat.[30] The cat stiffens his rear limbs and straightens his back to slope downhill. Piloerection starts in the thoracolumbar region and increases caudally. The tail comes straight caudal for a short distance and then makes an abrupt bend downward.

Defensive Threat. The typical "Halloween cat" posture is associated with defensive threat (Fig. 3–7). The cat presents to the aggressor an arched lateral display with piloerection rather than a straightforward view, to appear larger in overall size and thus more of a threat. The ears are flattened against the back of the head, the mouth corners are pulled back to bare the teeth, the whiskers are drawn against the side of the head, and the nose is wrinkled. In wild species, males use this posture only in play.[46]

Pariah Threat. The lowest-ranking cat of a group of cats, the pariah, may show a crouched posture whenever approached by the territorial male (Fig. 3–8). This behavior is accompanied by flattened ears, and the cat often bares its teeth, too.

Other Postures. Piloerection is associated with a threat posture for the

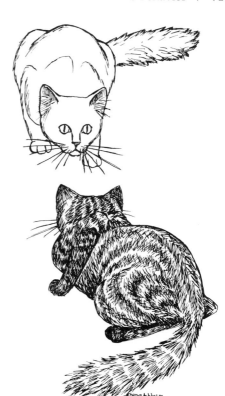

FIGURE 3–6. Offensive threat posture.

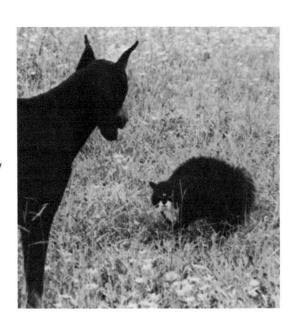

FIGURE 3–7. The lateral display of defensive threat.

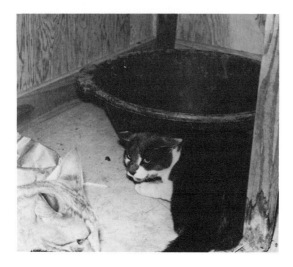

FIGURE 3–8. The crouched display of the pariah threat.

tail. When the tail is vertical with piloerection, a moderately intense offensive threat is indicated (Fig. 3–9). This signal commonly is used when the resident cat chases away an intruder. In defensive threats, the tail is arched over the back with hair erect (Fig. 3–10), while a tail curved into an inverted U with the hair standing is associated with postures that are intermediate between offensive and defensive threats (Fig. 3–11).[12, 13] This posture also is used during defensive withdrawals and during an immobile confrontation, when the ears are back, the pupils dilated, and,

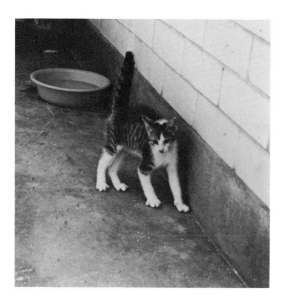

FIGURE 3–9. A vertical tail posture of threat includes piloerection.

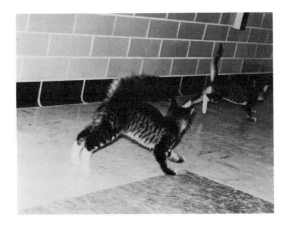

FIGURE 3–10. The tail is arched over the back with the hair standing in play and defensive threats.

except for head movement to closely watch the problem, the cat is motionless.[48] These tail positions are far more common during play behaviors.

Fighting between male cats is ritualized and usually far noisier than injurious. With pupils dilated and claws protruding, the tomcat directs his biting and clawing at the cheeks, neck, and shoulders (Fig. 3–12). This is probably the evolutionary reason for the regional thickening of the skin as a secondary sex characteristic. Initially, the ears, head, and

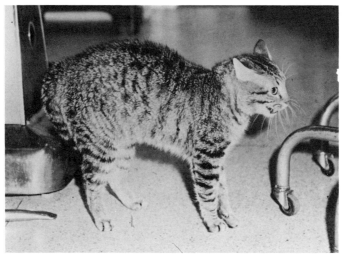

FIGURE 3–11. Piloerection and an inverted U-shaped tail as part of an immobile confrontation.

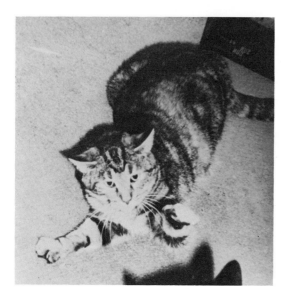

FIGURE 3–12. Clawing is directed toward the head of another.

piloerect tail are raised, but they are lowered as the attack becomes serious. Weight is shifted backward and one forelimb is raised with claws unsheathed. As one cat bites for the other's nape, the response is made by suddenly throwing itself on its back, biting, holding with foreclaws, and lashing with rear claws.[30] Soon both cats are rolling on the ground. They will suddenly leap apart and start the encounter again. Cats usually avoid direct confrontations or fights if at all possible. In attacking a dog that has come within its critical distance, the cat will direct its blows to the eyes and nose and will flee if given the opportunity. If a severe challenge continues, the cat may roll over onto its back so that all four feet can be used as weapons (Fig. 3–13). There is little biting, however, because the cat needs to protect its face.[10, 46]

Fear can be associated with forms of distance-increasing silent communication. In addition to the arched back and piloerection of the other threat postures, the fearful threat includes signs of apprehension, such as salivation, extreme mydriasis, sweating of the footpads, flattened ears, and even panting.[12, 26] The body may be lowered into a crouching position similar to that of the pariah threat, and these cats are best approached from overhead.[26] If the fear stimulus is great enough, the cat may go from the fearful threat reaction into a cataleptic shock syndrome.

Neural Regulation. Distance-increasing behavior is controlled from within the central nervous system. Electrical stimulation of the ventromedial hypothalamus produces behavior typically observed in threat situations as early as 12 days of age.[13] Behavioral alerting, mydriasis, ear retraction, piloerection, hissing, and claw protrusion are some of the

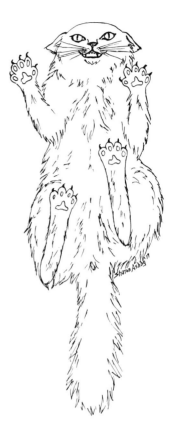

FIGURE 3–13. The extreme defensive posture.

general displays. Extreme ragelike displays include opening the mouth and baring the teeth, curving the tongue, and blowing air.[14] The prefrontal cortex and thalamus apparently play a role in moderating these reactions.[43, 48] In addition, the lateral septal nuclei with their connections into this area are evidently important in overriding the formation of conditioned emotional responses such as fear.[31] A defensive cat personality appears between 30 and 50 days of age, and correlates positively with readiness to adapt defensive immobility and negatively with olfactory exploration and purring during human contact.[1]

Ambivalent Postures

Although most body communication is ambivalent to some degree because of conflicting situations, each attitude usually has one overriding posture, on the basis of which it is classified. Occasionally the cat truly alternates between distance-increasing and distance-reducing behaviors. For example, when approaching an older kitten, the queen may react with maternal grooming when presented a caudal view and with a clawing attack when presented a cranial view.[10] The "Halloween cat" posture of the defensive threat has been classified as ambivalent but probably represents a defensive threat posture rather than a true mental conflict.[13]

MARKING COMMUNICATION

Marking allows more permanent communication. In this way, a cat leaves olfactory and visual messages that remain long after the communicator has gone. Thus individuals can space themselves to prevent meetings and control reproduction. Marking provides information regarding the individual and sexual identity, time spent at the location, and reproduction cycle stage of the marker—all without threat.[5]

Rubbing Behavior

The cat has greatly enlarged sebaceous glands around the mouth, on the chin, in the ear canals, in the perianal area, and at the cranial portion of the base of the tail. These proliferative glands are located in areas that the cat specifically likes to rub or to have rubbed, and this rubbing (or bunting)[24] behavior is directed toward certain individuals and familiar or novel objects. A protruding object or hand often is rubbed first by the very rostral portion of the cat's nose and then by its cheek, such that the cat rubs from the commissure of the mouth toward the lateral commissure of the eye. If the emotion is intense, the cat may open its mouth and draw its lips back to show its teeth. The cat may rub a higher object with the dorsal aspect of its head while standing on its hind feet. It may rub its dorsum and tail along an object such as a chair. Low-lying objects usually are rubbed by a stroke from the chin to the laryngeal area. The sebaceous scent is probably thus transferred to the rubbed object. When rubbing humans, the cat may be using a greeting form of distance-reducing behavior rather than a true marking behavior.[10] Although intact adult males do not rub any more frequently than females, their glands are particularly active.[39, 45] Cats often show facial rubbing on objects when odor deposits have stimulated flehmen. Urine elicits such a response for up to 3 days.[24]

Secretions from the glands of the anal sac also may play an olfactory marking function. This is questioned because the anal sacs are expressed primarily during traumatic experiences and because the anogenital approach is not of major social significance.[45, 47] When petted, the cat may profusely salivate and then rub the corner of its mouth against the individual doing the petting. The saliva transferred may provide another form of olfactory mark.[47]

Wood Scratching

Wood scratching is a second major type of marking behavior, one that uses visual cues. The cat may use either a horizontally or a vertically oriented piece of soft wood or bark, gripping the object with both extended forelimbs (Figs. 3–14 and 3–15). The body may be positioned so that the thorax is lower than the hindquarters if the object is near the ground. On alternating paws, the cat extends and withdraws its claws. These jerky motions vary in length and speed and serve two purposes: to create a visual marker and to condition the claw by removing any thin loose pieces of sheaths.[23] Outer parts of the rear claws are removed by the teeth. Sweat glands in the skin of the foot have been said to leave a secondary olfactory cue,[22] but because these areas are not investigated by other cats, the olfactory function is probably insignificant in territorial marking. Instead, they may provide a reassurance to the resident cat.[5, 23] New objects as well as old favorites frequently are scratched, and the longer the object serves as a scratching medium, the more significance it is likely to have to the individual. Cats are most likely to scratch shortly after awakening and may use the behavior as a form of stretching.[7, 16, 19]

Newborn kittens are unable to completely withdraw their claws until they are about 4 weeks of age. (See Appendix D.) Scratching is an inborn behavior that can be performed by 5 weeks of age. These motions can be observed even if the animal was declawed shortly after birth.[16]

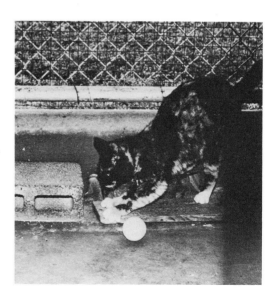

FIGURE 3–14. Scratching a horizontal piece of wood.

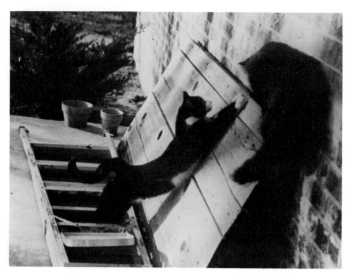

FIGURE 3–15. Scratching a vertically directed object.

Scratching loose soil leaves a disruption that serves as a visual and, possibly, olfactory mark.[9, 47]

Excrement Marking

Urine commonly is used for scent marking, particularly by intact male cats. By spraying the urine, a cat covers a larger area than usual by urinating and at a height convenient for sniffing. Males spend a great deal of time marking their home range, particularly near pathways, crossings, and boundaries.[9, 18] During the marking process, the cat is basically standing and exhibits an erratic twitching motion of the vertical tail (Fig. 3–16). This motion has been described as either neurologically initiated automatic behavior or as voluntary behavior cued for a visual signal.[46, 47]

Besides indicating movement and identity, sprayed urine serves to bring the male and female together during mating season by attracting the female and to acclimate an individual with an area. The latter function usually is served when a tomcat is placed in a new area. Not only does the odor of his own distinct scent provide relief from anxiety and aggression, but it also allows him to establish his own small breeding territory.[17, 18, 20] Urine is sprayed at certain times of the day unless stimulated by an emotional disturbance.[20]

Cats use urine-spraying to leave their own scent, not to cover odors from other cats. Although a cat will smell the urine mark of another, no

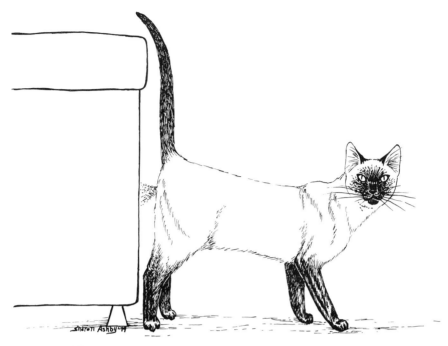

FIGURE 3–16. The marking posture usually used for urine-spraying.

fearful or intimidative responses are evoked, and the animal makes no obvious attempt to cover the odor with his own.[17, 45]

Feces seldom are used by the cat as a scent marker, although situations have been described in which defecation on raised areas served such a purpose.[46, 47] Territorially dominant cats in an untamed population leave feces uncovered in conspicuous places, especially along trails of good hunting areas.[32]

COMMUNICATIVE BEHAVIOR PROBLEMS

Although inability to understand feline communication can be hazardous for humans, the real problem behaviors are associated with marking.

Furniture Clawing

Furniture clawing represents expression of a normal behavior in an atypical environment. Cats confined indoors will mark furniture by clawing if there is nothing else to scratch. Prominent objects and areas are favored, and once scratching on an object is started, the behavior usually continues.[22] Discouragement of scratching without providing an acceptable substitute can lower the scratching threshold, so that the behavior is attempted more frequently and the animal's frustration is increased. It also teaches the cat to run from the owner.

In raising a kitten, the owner can best prevent this behavior problem by providing a scratching post in a prominent location, preferably near the kitten's sleeping area.[7, 16, 33] The physical characteristics of a scratching post or board can affect its suitability. In addition to being stable, the object should be tall enough (at least 12 inches and preferably 2.5 to 3 feet) for the cat to rest on its hind limbs and reach out to claw. The texture of the scratching post is of some significance, with the preferred primary orientation of the fabric weave being longitudinal, thus providing the cat with the most efficient conditioning of each claw.[16, 22, 23] Post usage can be encouraged by placing a favorite toy on top, by leaving the kitten in a room where the post is the only furniture, or by having an older, post-trained cat to provide a source for observational learning.[7, 22] Once the kitten has started using the post, it is best to keep the same one, for just as a cat continues to scratch a favorite tree, so will it continue on another favorite object.

If the owner is not so fortunate as to be able to prevent the problem, behavior modification can be used to retrain the cat. The object scratched should be removed or moved and covered, preferably with plastic, and replaced with an acceptable scratching object.[7, 22] If the cat is scratching the carpet, the owner should place the scratching post over the commonly clawed area. When the cat is seen scratching areas other than the post, "no" should be followed by placing the cat on the post and manipulating its legs as if it were scratching the post.[3, 26] A remotely controlled, water-filled plant sprayer can be effective in behavior modification and has the advantage of obviating the necessity for the owner to physically contact the animal.[21, 25] The cat is then less likely to develop an aversion to the owner. Olfactory cues rather than physical ones also can be used for negative reinforcement. While restraining the cat, the owner holds an aerosol can so that the mist leaves at a 90-degree angle from the cat's face. The spray is released and, at the same moment, a threatening gesture is made toward the cat's face with the can. This introduction, called smell aversion, makes the cat fearful of the particular odor associated with that event. With the cat out of the room, the scratched object should be sprayed well and the mist allowed to settle before the cat returns to the area. A suitable object to be scratched must still be provided. When the cat must be left alone, it should be in a room where scratching has not been a problem.

Many people minimize the scratching problem by clipping the cat's claws. Although there is no correlation between the clipping of claws and frequency of scratching, less damage is done.[7]

Other owners prefer to prevent furniture scratching by having the cat declawed. This can be particularly satisfactory for indoor cats, and even outdoor individuals can relearn defense and climbing if the rear claws remain. Care should be taken, however, because cats that depend on their claws as weapons or for climbing can become psychologically and physically traumatized if they suddenly discover their lack of claws. Even though there is no evidence of long-term problems as a result of this procedure, there remains a moral controversy about the surgery, and a perception exists that other problems, such as biting and jumping on counters or tables, will develop.[6, 29, 33, 35]

Excessive Vocalization

In one study, 2 cats of 23 presented for problem behaviors other than housesoiling or aggression were diagnosed as being excessively vocal.[4] Although this problem often is associated with Siamese or estrous females, it is not restricted to such cats. Excessive vocalization is common after a move or dramatic change in the cat's schedule. For those cats, time and a strict new schedule are helpful.

Urine Spraying

Urine spraying can certainly present problems, and is discussed with all of its ramifications in Chapter 5.

CASE PRESENTATIONS

CASE 3–1. Four-and-one-half-month-old Persian male. The cat was purchased from a Persian breeder at a cat show 4 days before consultation. The cat defecated in the litter box but urinated by spraying two or three times a day. In 4 days, it had not urinated in the litter box, although the breeder said that the cat had always done so in the past. If the current owner keeps the cat, it eventually will be neutered.

Diagnosis. Territorial marking (housesoiling—urine marking).

Treatment. Medroxyprogesterone acetate (75 mg I.M.) stopped the marking behavior until castration.

CASE 3–2. Five-year-old Russian blue neutered male. The cat was fine during the day when the wife of the family was at home. During the past month, the cat meowed constantly during the evenings until the man picked it up and held it. The cat was so persistent that the man was unable to do anything else.

Medical Workup. There were no abnormal findings on the physical examination. The cat tested negative for feline leukemia.

Diagnosis. Excessive vocalization (meowing).

Treatment. Because the behavior was probably learned and rewarded by the owner's attention, it must be discouraged. By squirting the cat with a water sprayer during vocalization and giving attention to it only when it was quiet, the owner was able to break this pattern of noise.

CASE 3–3. Ten-year-old domestic longhair neutered female. The cat had used a scratching post routinely until 3 weeks before presentation, when it had started clawing the furniture. The behavior started on a sofa and two living room chairs shortly after these pieces had been reupholstered.

Diagnosis. Furniture scratching.

Treatment. The old scratching post was placed next to the sofa and all the affected furniture was covered with a plastic sheet. This technique worked while the furniture remained covered, but the problem would recur whenever the plastic was removed. The problem was finally controlled by closing the cat out of the room except when family members were present.

CASE 3–4. Two-year-old domestic shorthair neutered male. The cat woke the owner every morning at 4:30 with a loud meowing noise. It continued the vocalization until the owner got up and fed it. Although the owner tried to ignore the cat, she was afraid that the neighbors in the next apartment would complain.

Diagnosis. Excessive vocalization (demand meowing).

Treatment. Because it was impossible for the owner to ignore the cat and the cat had a weight problem, making free-choice feeding undesirable, it was decided that a remote form of punishment would be used. A gun-type hair dryer was aimed at the area the cat would vocalize from, and it was set up to be turned on remotely. After 1 week of getting blasted by the air, the cat stopped the vocalizing.

Also see cases 2–9 and 4–19.

REFERENCES

1. Adamec, R. E., Stark-Adamec, C., and Livingston, K. C.: The expression of an early developmentally emergent defensive bias in the adult cat (*Felis catus*) in non-predatory situations. Appl. Anim. Ethol. 10:89, 1983.
2. Beadle, M.: The Cat: History, Biology, and Behavior. New York: Simon & Schuster, 1977.
3. Beaver, B. V. G.: Feline behavioral problems. Vet. Clin. North Am. 6:333, 1976.
4. Beaver, B. V.: Feline behavioral problems other than housesoiling. J. Am. Anim. Hosp. Assoc. 25:465, 1989.

5. Beaver, B. V.: Disorders of behavior. In Sherding, R. G., ed.: The Cat: Diseases and Clinical Management. New York: Churchill Livingstone, 1989.
6. Bennett, M., Houpt, K. A., and Erb, H. N.: Effects of declawing on feline behavior. Companion Anim. Pract. 2:7, 1988.
7. Bryant, D.: The Care and Handling of Cats. New York: Ives Washburn, 1944.
8. Dhume, R. A., Gogate, M. G., deMascarenhas, J. F., and Sharma, K. N.: Functional dissociation within hippocampus: Correlates of visceral and behavioral patterns induced on stimulation of ventral hippocampus in cats. Indian J. Med. Res. 64:33, 1976.
9. Eaton, R. L.: The evolution of sociality in the Felidae. In Eaton, R. L., ed.: The World's Cats. Vol. 3. Seattle: Carnivore Research Institute, 1936.
10. Ewer, R. F.: Ethology of Mammals. London: Paul Elek, Ltd., 1968.
11. Ewer, R. F.: The Carnivores. Ithaca, NY: Cornell University Press, 1973.
12. Fox, M. W.: Understanding Your Cat. New York: Coward, McCann & Geoghegan, Inc., 1974.
13. Fox, M. W.: The behaviour of cats. In Hafez, E. S. E., ed.: The Behaviour of Domestic Animals. 3rd ed. Baltimore: Williams & Wilkins Co., 1975.
14. Giammanco, S., Paderni, M. A., and Carollo, A.: The effect of thermic stress on the somatic reaction of rage and on rapid circling turns, in the cat. Arch. Int. Physiol. Biochem. 84:787, 1976.
15. Gibbs, E. L., and Gibbs, F. A.: A purring center in the brain of the cat. J. Comp. Neurol. 64:6, 1936.
16. Hart, B. L.: Behavioral aspects of scratching in cats. Fel. Pract. 2:6, Mar.-Apr. 1972.
17. Hart, B. L.: Normal behavior and behavioral problems associated with sexual function, urination, and defecation. Vet. Clin. North Am. 4:589, 1974.
18. Hart, B. L.: Behavioral patterns related to territoriality and social communication. Fel. Pract. 5:12, Jan.-Feb. 1975.
19. Hart, B. L.: Behavioral aspects of raising kittens. Fel. Pract. 6:8, Nov. 1976.
20. Hart, B. L.: Olfaction and feline behavior. Fel. Pract. 7:8, Sept. 1977.
21. Hart, B. L.: Water sprayer therapy. Fel. Pract. 8:13, Nov. 1978.
22. Hart, B. L.: Starting from scratch: A new perspective on cat scratching. Fel. Pract. 10:8, July-Aug. 1980.
23. Hart, B. L., and Hart, L. A.: Canine and Feline Behavioral Therapy. Philadelphia: Lea & Febiger, 1985.
24. Houpt, K. A., and Wolski, T. R.: Domestic Animal Behavior for Veterinarians and Animal Scientists. Ames: Iowa State University Press, 1982.
25. Jacobs, D. L.: Behavior modification technique. Fel. Pract. 8:6, Mar. 1978.
26. Joshua, J. O.: Abnormal behavior in cats. In Fox, M. W., ed.: Abnormal Behavior in Animals. Philadelphia: W. B. Saunders Co., 1968.
27. Kiley-Worthington, M.: The tail movements of ungulates, canids and felids with particular reference to their causation and function as displays. Behaviour 55:69, 1975.
28. Kleiman, D. G., and Eisenberg, J. F.: Comparisons of canid and felid social systems from an evolutionary perspective. Anim. Behav. 21:637, 1973.
29. Landsberg, G.: Personal communication, 1989.
30. Leyhausen, P.: Cat Behavior: The Predatory and Social Behavior of Domestic and Wild Cats. New York: Garland STPM Press, 1978.
31. Lubar, J. F., and Numan, R.: Behavioral and physiological studies of septal function and related medial cortical structures. Behav. Biol. 8:1, 1973.
32. MacDonald, D. W.: Patterns of scent marking with urine and faeces amongst carnivore communities. Symp. Zool. Soc. Lond. 45:107, 1980.
33. McKeown, D., Luescher, A., and Machum, M.: The problem of destructive scratching by cats. Canad. Vet. J. 29:1017, 1988.
34. Moelk, M.: Vocalizing in the house cat: A phonetic and functional study. Am. J. Psychol. 57:184, 1944.
35. Morgan, M., and Houpt, K. A.: Personal communication, 1989.
36. Remmers, J. E., and Gautier, H.: Neural and mechanical mechanisms of feline purring. Respir. Physio. 16:351, 1972.
37. Rheingold, H. L., and Eckerman, C. O.: Familiar social and nonsocial stimuli and the kitten's response to a strange environment. Dev. Psychobiol. 4:71, 1971.
38. Romanes, G. J.: Mental Evolution in Animals. New York: AMS Press, 1969.

39. Rose, C. E., and Doering, G. G.: "Stud tail" in cats. Fel. Pract. 6:28, 1976.
40. Rosenblatt, J. S.: Learning in newborn kittens. Sci. Am. 227:18, 1972.
41. Rosenblueth, A., and Bard, P.: The innervation and functions of the nictitating membrane in the cat. Am. J. Physiol. 100:537, 1932.
42. Sampson, S., and Eyzaguirre, C.: Some functional characteristics of mechanoreceptors in the larynx of the cat. J. Neurophysiol. 27:464, 1964.
43. Siegel, A., Edinger, H., and Dotto, M.: Effects of electrical stimulation of the lateral aspect of the prefrontal cortex upon attack behavior in cats. Brain Res. 93:473, 1975.
44. Stogdale, L., and Delack, J. B.: Feline purring. Compendium on Continuing Education 7:551, 1985.
45. Verberne, G., and DeBoer, J.: Chemocommunication among domestic cats, mediated by the olfactory and vomeronasal senses. I. Chemocommunication. Z. Tierpsychol. 42:86, 1976.
46. Weigel, I.: Small cats and clouded leopards. In Grzimek, H. C. B., ed.: Grzimek's Animal Life Encyclopedia. Vol. 12. New York: Van Nostrand Reinhold Co., 1975.
47. Wemmer, C., and Scow, K.: Communication in the Felidae with emphasis on scent marking and contact patterns. In Sebeok, T. A., ed.: How Animals Communicate. Bloomington: Indiana University Press, 1977.
48. Zanchetti, A., Baccelli, G., and Mancia, G.: Fighting, emotions, and exercise: Cardiovascular effects in the cat. In Onesti, G., Fernandes, M., and Kim, K. E., eds.: Regulation of Blood Pressure by the Central Nervous System. New York: Grune & Stratton, 1976.

ADDITIONAL READINGS

Blacklock, G. A. A cat's purr . . . on purpose? Cat Fancy 16:20, Aug. 1973.
Boudreau, J. C., and Tsuchitani, C. Sensory Neurophysiology. New York: Van Nostrand Reinhold Co., 1973.
Cannon, W. B. Bodily Changes in Pain, Hunger, Fear and Rage. 2nd ed. Boston: Charles T. Branford Co., 1953.
Darwin, C. R. The Expression of the Emotions in Man and Animals. New York: Greenwood Press, 1969.
De Molina, A. F., and Hunsperger, R. W. Organization of subcortical systems governing defence and flight reactions in the cat. J. Physiol. (Lond.) 160:200, 1962.
Eisenberg, J. F., and Kleiman, D. G. Olfactory communication in mammals. Annu. Rev. Ecol. System 3:1, 1972.
Eleftheriou, B. E., and Scott, J. P. The Physiology of Aggression and Defeat. New York: Plenum Publishing Corp., 1971.
Fried, P. A. The septum and hyper-reactivity: A review. Br. J. Psychol. 64:267, 1973.
Hart, B. L. Gonadal androgen and sociosexual behavior of male mammals: A comparative analysis. Psychol. Bull. 81:383, 1971.
Hart, B. L. Social interactions between cats and their owners. Fel. Pract. 6:6, Jan. 1976.
Hart, B. L. Behavioral aspects of selecting a new cat. Fel. Pract. 6:8, Sept. 1976.
Houpt, K. A. Animal behavior as a subject for veterinary students. Cornell Vet. 66:73, 1976.
Houpt, K. A. Domestic Animal Behavior for Veterinarians and Animal Scientists. Ames: Iowa State University Press, 1991.
Jenkins, T. W. Functional Mammalian Neuroanatomy. Philadelphia: Lea & Febiger, 1972.
Johansson, G. G., Kalimo, R., Niskanen, H., and Ruusunen, S. Effects of stimulation parameters on behavior elicited by stimulation of the hypothalamic defense area. J. Comp. Physiol. Psychol. 87:1100, 1974.
Kahn, B. Out of the frying pan—into the litter pan. Cat Fancy 15:18, Nov.-Dec. 1972.
Langworthy, O. R. Behavioral disturbances related to the decomposition of reflex activity caused by cerebral injury: An experimental study of the cat. J. Neuropathol. Exp. Neurol. 3:87, 1944.
Levinson, B. M. Forecast for the year 2000. In Anderson, R. S., ed. Pet Animals and Society. London: Baillière Tindall, 1974.
Leyhausen, P. Cat Behavior: The Predatory and Social Behavior of Domestic and Wild Cats. New York: Garland STPM Press, 1978.

McCuistiom, W. K. Feline purring and its dynamics. Vet. Med. Small Anim. Clin. 61:562, 1966.

Mykytowycz, R. Reproduction of mammals in relation to environmental odours. J. Reprod. Fertil. 19[Suppl.]:433, 1973.

Science probing why cats purr. Friskies Res. Dig. 10:16, Spring 1974.

Suehsdorf, A. The cats in our lives. National Geographic 125:508, 1964.

Ursin, H. Flight and defense behavior in cats. J. Comp. Physiol. Psychol. 58:180, 1964.

Verberne, G. Chemocommunications among domestic cats, mediated by the olfactory and vomeronasal senses. II. The relation between the function of Jacobson's organ (vomero-nasal organ) and flehmen behaviour. Z. Tierpsychol. 42:113, 1976.

Volokhov, A. A. The ontogenetic development of higher nervous activity in animals. In Himwich, W. A., ed. Developmental Neurobiology. Springfield, IL: Charles C Thomas, 1970.

Wada, J. A., and Sato, M. Directedness of defensive emotional behavior and motivation for aversive learning. Exp. Neurol. 40:445, 1973.

Worden, A. N. Abnormal behaviour in the dog and cat. Vet. Rec. 71:966, 1959.

Wynne-Edwards, V. C. Animal Dispersion in Relation to Social Behaviour. Edinburgh: Oliver & Boyd, 1962.

4

Feline Social Behavior

The social behavior patterns of animals are complex. Nine major social patterns can combine in 45 ways during the interaction of two or more cats.[85] Investigative, ingestive, eliminative, and sexual behaviors have some social adaptations but are considered in other more appropriate sections.

The social behavior of a species is of evolutionary importance in the survival of that species, and most behaviors are a direct reflection of social organization.

SOCIAL ORGANIZATION

Domestication involves selective breeding for several generations, but until recently, cat breeding has been uncontrolled. As a result, today's cats are organized socially much like their early ancestors, although these social patterns often are interspersed with patterns introduced by selective breeding.[93]

Intraspecies Relations

The cat usually is described as asocial. This implies that although it prefers solitude, the cat appears in small groups, demonstrating that allelomimetic (cooperative) behaviors do occur. Because cats are not seen in large groups, their exact behaviors are hard to study, and speculation often replaces fact. Thus the ancient Egyptians used a cat symbol to denote a false or deceitful friendship.[58] Communication, both by visual contact and by marking behaviors, helps to minimize the amount of close contact between individuals, so that feline social behavior is characterized by an avoidance of interactions.[41] Cats use an active spacing pattern and so are not randomly distributed within a space. They are more concentrated near food and shelter.[73]

Cats do make social contacts, and the primary one is between a female and her young. Specific epimeletic (care-giving) behavior is covered with maternal behavior, but the social development of the young can be significantly affected by this early experience. Early contact with the queen is significant to the kittens because when placed in a strange environment, they immediately display ectepimeletic (care-seeking) behavior.[80, 87] Particularly at 2 and 4 weeks of age, contact between littermates is important to calm them in strange surroundings.[80, 83]

Feline social relations usually are nonenduring: The queen weans her young and the sexual partners do not form bonds. Kittens are social, depending on the interactions of littermates and the queen to develop the skills and knowledge they will later need for a solitary existence. The family group disperses between 6 and 12 months.[97] There are individual exceptions to the solitary life-styles, in that some cats can become devoted and protective toward a social partner, and the longer these individuals are together, the stronger the bond becomes. Such a relationship is characterized by mutual grooming, hunting close to each other (about 50 yards apart), running together (about 6 feet apart), and sleeping together.[2, 21, 30, 60] Loss of one partner can produce some interesting behavior changes in the other, including anorexia and excessive vocalization.[48]

A modification of this semisocial relationship is the neighborhood meeting. In a neutral area in the early evening, local cats of both sexes may gather and sit in a loosely formed circle, usually within 5 yards of each other (Fig. 4–1). This quiet social gathering frequently lasts for several hours before the participants depart for their own home areas.[2, 22, 30]

Distribution of 237 cat colonies in Britain has been studied.[24] A high percentage of these cats are fed by people nearby or have access to food in waste bins. Food often is the common thread that keeps several cats in a specific area. About 45 per cent of the groups had fewer than ten cat members, as is typical, and 11 per cent had more than 50 members.[24, 63] Three-fourths of the British colonies were more than 5 years old and had been altered by human interactions in the past. Social densities of 2.5 to 3.3 cats per square kilometer or fewer have been reported.[63, 99] Distributions where cats must survive on natural prey only are not available.

Cat-Human Relations

The cat's reactions to environmental happenings reflect its lack of strong social bonds. When trapped in a dangerous situation, such as a

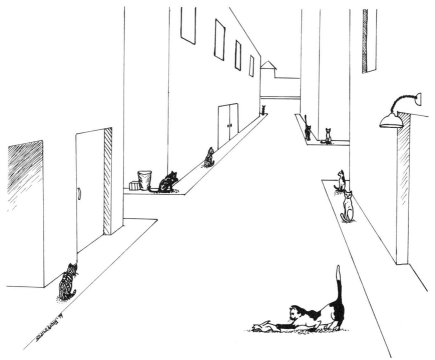

FIGURE 4–1. Social gatherings of neighborhood cats are one form of social contact between cats.

house fire, the cat's instinct for self-preservation dictates escape. Only if escape is blocked will the cat recruit assistance from a human and coincidentally save the human's life. Cats most frequently are honored with hero awards when using this behavior in a burning building. A cat occasionally does show more social consciousness in its heroics. Cats have been reported to serve as seeing-eye cats or hearing-ear cats, fight off snakes endangering a child, and call attention to a trapped cat or person.[76, 81]

Social Distances

Several distances and areas have social significance to the cat. The area traveled during normal activities is called the *home range*, and although it is considered circular, the shape is actually quite variable (Fig. 4–2). In addition to the central area, radiating paths often lead to secondary homesites for special purposes, such as hunting, elimination, and resting.[40, 61, 67, 92] Paths to commonly used locations are chosen for length and direction.[78] Both the paths and the special areas may be part

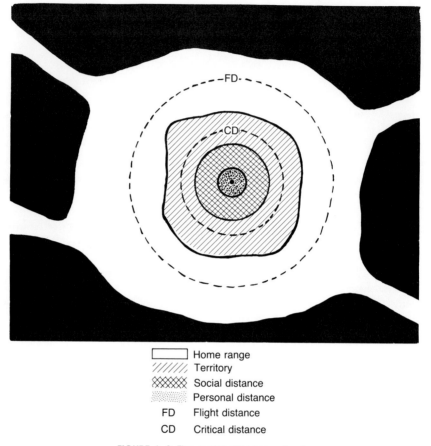

Home range
Territory
Social distance
Personal distance
FD   Flight distance
CD   Critical distance

FIGURE 4–2. The social distances of cats.

of the home range of several individuals.[40, 82] Usage of the paths is not based on dominance, but on a passive first-come, first-served basis. Scheduling can be important in a cat's routine, and feeding times or travel schedules determine when a cat is in a certain location. Sometimes cats that arrive at an intersection at the same time will sit for long periods, each waiting for the other to take the initiative (Fig. 4–3).[30, 61] One study indicated a home range of 800 × 300 m, which included the land close to the paths, although it was unused by the animal.[22] Other sources note home ranges of 0.2 acres where cats are well fed and up to 420 acres in the Australian bush.[2, 62–64, 66, 99] The home ranges of females do not overlap between groups. Specifics are inconsistent in free-ranging male cats because their home ranges may not have a specific outer boundary.[60] The home range size of males averages 3.5 times larger than

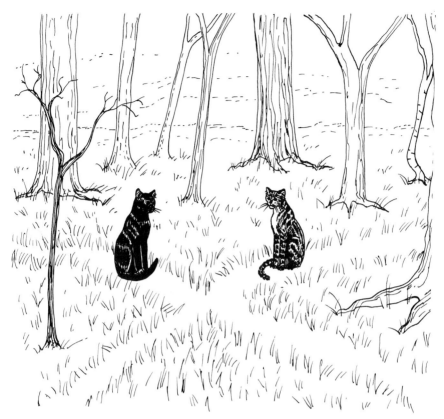

FIGURE 4–3. Cats meeting at an intersection of paths may wait for one another to proceed.

that of females in the same general area.[64] Cats are reported to travel 211 to 1578 m daily.[95]

A *territory* is an area that is actively defended against strangers of the same species (Fig. 4–2). A territory usually is smaller than a home range, but in the case of the house cat, territory and home range may be identical. The difficulty in obtaining more precise information about social distances is related to the cat's solitary nature, its agility, and its nocturnal patterns. In roaming cats, the minimal territorial size is estimated to be 0.1 square mile.[2, 61, 92] Males are more territorial, and form larger, more rigid, and more permanent territories.[92, 100] These areas are small enough to be observed by the resident male cat in toto, and are regularly patrolled and marked by him.[60] Seldom do territories overlap, and they are not contiguous with territories of other males.[2, 92] When population permits, cats spread out and make maximal use of the available space.[60]

The first-order home (the homesite, den, or resting area) is the prominent feature of the home range. Males will allow females into their territory but not in the immediate proximity of their homesite. In fact, the amount of aggression directed toward an intruder is inversely proportional to the distance from the homesite.[92]

When approached by a stranger of an unfamiliar species, a cat will flee when the stranger reaches a certain distance. That distance is called the *flight distance* (Fig. 4–2). A cat that cannot flee or that is unaware of the intruder will defend itself at a second, closer distance, known as the *critical distance* (Fig. 4–2). Unfortunately flight and critical distances have been used interchangeably, which causes some confusion to the reader. The flight distance for the cat is about 6 feet and probably somewhat longer for the kitten.[12, 71] Females with young have a greater critical distance than other cats, and some will aggressively meet an intruder from quite a distance.[100]

When the cat is approached by individuals of a species that it does not fear, two other distances become important. Special, well-accepted individuals are allowed an intimate approach, including physical contact, and thus may enter the cat's *personal distance* (Fig. 4–2). Other acquaintances will not be attacked, but are not allowed within the personal distance. Their accepted space is called the *social distance* (Fig. 4–2). Threat displays often serve to inhibit further approach by a violator of the personal distance.

Social distances are important to the cat because of its asocial nature. In fact, most cats form a much stronger bond with home range and territory than with any social being.

Social Orders

Social animal species have fairly well-defined dominance rankings to minimize agonistic behavior between individuals. A threat display by the dominant animal leads to a submissive display by the subordinate. Because the cat is not highly social, there are distinct differences in its social ordering. In groups of cats, such as in homes or colonies, the pattern of social orders is unique. One male assumes relative dominance based on territorial ownership.[63, 66, 97] For several days, this despot walks stiff-legged with raised back and tail, seizing each of the other cats, pushing their backs down with his hindquarters, and mounting each as if for copulation.[102] This mounting behavior is a sign of dominance in several other species, also without sexual connotations. The subordinate animal, male or female, responds with much vocalization and struggling and dashes away as soon as possible.[102] Aside from this dominant male, other cats do not differ in rank, which indicates the lack of a complete or stable hierarchy. The tendency to rub the face of another is the clearest single indicator of which individual might rank lower.[67] If the group is large enough and the area confining, there may be one or more pariahs.[2, 60, 97] Females treated with progestins temporarily lose social position.[50] Both social outcasts and progestin-treated females frequently are attacked by members of the group and become chronically wary of other cats. They display an almost constant growl and lowered body posture in the presence of the group. Cats may even choose a specific human to treat as a pariah, attacking him frequently.

Lack of a complete hierarchy between cats makes it difficult to predict the outcome of a confrontation. For social animals, size, weight, and sex factors can alter this agonistic behavior; however, for the cat, time of day, place, presence of food, past history, and the number of cats present are more significant.[2, 17, 22, 30, 58, 103] For example, if two cats meet on a path, the one that arrives at a different time than is usual frequently yields to the other cat. One cat does not take food away from another as a dominant would do from a subordinate in a rigid social hierarchy. Instead, each cat waits its turn or shares, if possible (Fig. 4–4). The addition of neutered animals to cat populations further complicates these relations because of behavior changes that result from changes in hormones.

Social Approaches

Two cats approaching each other use species-specific behaviors and investigate scent gland locations. The territorial cat smells first the nose

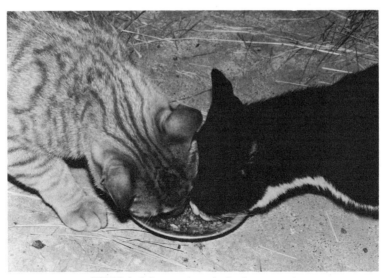

FIGURE 4–4. Two male cats sharing a meal.

and then the anal area of the intruder, who continues a slow exploration of the strange environment.[100, 103] The facial approach followed by the anogenital approach normally is used by cats that already know each other and have no reason for hostility (Fig. 4–5).[2] The facial approach is the most frequently used, and involves smelling the mouth and temporal regions, touching noses and areas of tactile hairs, and rubbing heads. The facial approach also is commonly used by a cat approaching a human, and even in this situation, it is followed by the anogenital posture as the cat presents its hindquarters to the human. The odor associated with the anogenital approach apparently has social significance to the cat because the scent of an anestrous female may actually have a repelling effect on a sexually mature male.[21, 101] Approaching cats usually align themselves in one of four ways, depending on the position of the cat being approached. Body-to-body contact, including that between nursing kittens, occurs in 79 per cent of the contacts; body-to-head–neck contact, 9 per cent; head–neck-to-head–neck contacts, 6 per cent; and head–neck-to-body contact, including the greeting sniff, 5 per cent.[101]

When confronted with its image in a mirror, a cat usually approaches with interest and frequently tries to locate the image behind the mirror. This indicates no self-identification.[33] If a threat reaction is initiated, it usually intensifies because of the continually increasing threat display by the image.

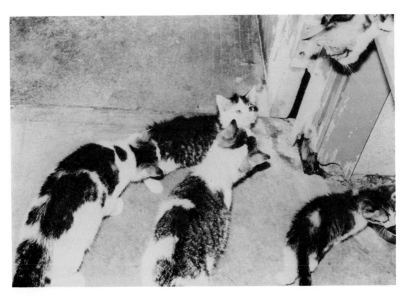

FIGURE 4–5. Adult cats showing a facial approach and an anogenital approach to a newly introduced kitten.

Breed Variations

Certain breeds and certain lines within certain breeds of cats that have been popular for a long time are known for their sociability. Selective breeding has allowed humans to alter the cat's appearance and, when the gene pool was diverse, to alter behavior as well. Rare breeds have small gene pools, which produce more asocial cats. In selecting a cat, it is important to evaluate relatives for sociability as well as for conformation.

Most Siamese cats are sociable, but certain lines do produce either extremely timid or aggressive cats.[25, 30] One of the most unusual breeds in this regard is the Kuiat because the females are notably more aggressive than the males, especially at shows. This unusual behavior has presented problems for more than one cat breeder.

SOCIALIZATION

Although every age is important in the normal development of a kitten, four periods are unique and particularly critical in behavioral development.[29, 84] The infantile or neonatal period is characterized by neonatal ingestive and sleep patterns. The transitional or intermediate period begins during the 2nd week with the appearance of adult patterns of eating and locomotion and of immature forms of social behavior. The socialization period is the time when all primary social bonds are formed and constitutes the single most important period during the cat's life. During this phase, striking behavioral changes occur because of growth and experience. The fourth period of kitten development, the adolescent or juvenile period, is primarily a time for maturation of motor skills.

Socialization is a process by which an individual forms an attachment to the other species it contacts during a limited time. (See Appendix D.) Early environments and social relations are definitely important in socialization. Because of the relatively asocial nature of the cat, the specific implications of this period are not fully understood. Socialization can occur between a kitten and humans or between a kitten and its "natural enemies," such as dogs, rats, mice, and birds. These attachments result in the "unusual," yet perfectly normal pictures often seen in newspapers (Fig. 4–6). Only after a great deal of training might a grown cat accept or tolerate a species with which it was not acquainted during its socialization phase.

The long process of domestication produces animals with a naturally reduced tendency to flee from humans. By working with a young animal, domesticated or not, one can reduce the flight distance to zero and thus environmentally effect a psychological change in an individual, which

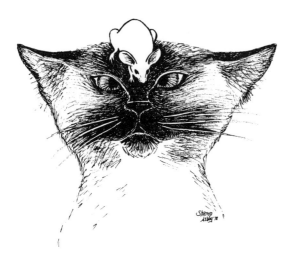

FIGURE 4–6. Kittens socialized to certain species accept that species as a normal part of their adult environment.

is called taming. Without this environmental contact, the kitten naturally tends to avoid humans, as often is the case with cats raised in a woodpile or hayloft. Much of a kitten's basic personality is inherited, with a distinct portion coming from the sire.[94] Queens that are friendly to humans do not necessarily have friendlier kittens.[94] Even when carefully raised in association with humans, kittens have a normal period of human avoidance, which gradually appears between 40 and 50 days of age, is strongly obvious shortly thereafter, and, if socialization to humans has occurred, ends sometime after the 70th day.

The kitten that generalizes taming to all members of a species is said to be *socialized* to that species. Because eyesight is still developing in the kitten, visual recognition probably is somewhat limited, as in the dog. Forms of young children do not look the same as those of adults to a kitten, so exposing it to both types of humans might be important to assure proper socialization. Rough play and handling during socialization result in the cat's becoming either wild and aggressive or timid and nervous with people.[13] Similar results occur if the kitten has little or no human contact during this early stage or if it is separated from its littermates and mother at 2 weeks of age.[33, 35, 96] The cat-human relationship may be more like an ectepimeletic, kitten-mother relationship than an adult nonspecific one. Behaviors such as rubbing against a person's leg, lying down to be petted, and kneading while being held, all behaviors for which cats have been selectively bred, illustrate this infant-maternal relationship.[38, 42] Vertical tail approaches to humans suggest a kitten approaching its queen rather than its littermates. Conversely, a cat licking a human is mimicking mutual grooming of contemporaries.

Species identification also occurs during the socialization period. Not only does this permit the cat to recognize other felines so that future matings are not a problem, but it also teaches the animal to tolerate, if not fully accept, other cats in social situations. Cats raised with members of other species in addition to their own accept both but form stronger attachments with their own species. If raised only with other species during socialization, the cat forms attachments only to the adopted species.[55] Future mate selection can then be a serious problem because the cat fails to identify with its own species.

The socialization process is faster if the kitten encounters stress or a strong emotional experience, such as hunger, pain, or loneliness.[86] This experience encourages rapid species identification. Once the socialization period passes, acquainting the cat with other species becomes virtually impossible.

The amount of time necessary for socialization of the cat is not known, and because the cat is asocial, a well-defined time may have never even developed. In other species, socialization begins with the appearance of behavioral mechanisms that maintain or prevent social contacts, and perhaps for the kitten, socialization starts with the development of emotional reactions.[86] The critical period ends with development of a fear response, which probably is associated with a particular stimulus causing the young to leave the vicinity.[86] The socialization period must then include the ages of 5 to 7 weeks and probably ranges from 3 to 9 weeks of age. Careful handling of the kitten may extend this period a few more weeks, and prolonged social exposure to certain individuals may even result in some form of attachment.[25, 30, 86]

The young kitten is imprinted to its mother within the first few days of life, as evidenced by its reaction to separation, and olfaction plays an important role in the formation of the bond. Early approach behaviors also ensure early socialization to cats. The end of this species identification period is signaled by an increased tendency to avoid the unfamiliar.[28] Secondary social relations can then be developed by means of socialization.

AGGRESSION

Agonistic behavior is a competitive interaction between two or more individuals that involves body postures and displays related to flight, defensive attack, and offensive attack. Aggression and the associated escape and passive postures are relatively common in the feline species because of its unique social behavior. Neutering does not dramatically decrease the amount of aggression between cats, even though it does increase the number of "friendly" interactions.[74]

Much of the confusion in the literature regarding aggression has resulted because several kinds of aggression are displayed by the cat. This fact often has been neglected, so that the reports of some aggression studies are confusing.

Affective Aggression

Eight types of aggressive behavior can be classified as affective aggression, but several behavioral characteristics appear in all types.[79] In affective aggression, cats show an intensive, patterned autonomic activation, which especially involves sympathoadrenal interactions. Although menacing vocalizations and threat postures may be only displays, they may progress to a full-rage attack with teeth and claws that is directed toward the provoking or threatening object, or to escape flight, or to tonic immobility.[19, 27, 96] These threats range from low intensity, in which the cat crouches and holds its ears slightly back; to middle intensity, in which the cat flattens its ears and hisses; and finally to high intensity, in which these displays are combined with arched back, piloerection, inverted U tail position, and lowered head. Submission is not considered part of a cat's behavioral repertoire because it retreats instead. Unlike the social species, a fleeing cat does not induce flight behavior in other cats. There is no "sympathetic induction of mood."[65]

Because it is not related to sexual or food-gathering behaviors, an act of affective aggression is not always goal-directed, and usually is initiated by either a somatic or an external stimulus that lowers the irritability threshold for the aggression.[79] It is known that a genetic factor is related to these behaviors. In certain cases, cats that are basically aggressive toward humans, other cats, or both have produced offspring that show these same behaviors, regardless of how they were raised. Visual and olfactory stimuli can elicit adultlike agonistic behavior patterns as early as 6 weeks of age.[54]

A cat that stands firm during an attack of affective aggression, rather than running away or submitting, has about a 65 per cent chance of inhibiting or avoiding the attack.[72]

Intermale Aggression. Fighting between tomcats probably is the most common form of feline aggression. The presence of testosterone in the prenatal and neonatal kitten masculinizes the young brain. Later production of testosterone potentiates the earlier presence of the hormone and produces male behaviors, including fighting. Castration usually eliminates this later facilitation of male aggression, so castrated cats commonly do not fight.[44] Testosterone plays a significant role in intermale aggressive behavior in the cat because it is selectively taken up by the portions of the brain that control aggressive behavior. In addition, it is responsible for the loose attachment and dermal thickness of the neck skin. Male aggression increases during periods of overcrowding and the mating season. The latter increase results from a greater number of encounters with young wandering males, called *floaters*, rather than from cyclic hormonal changes.[18] Aggressive behaviors of mating are more appropriately discussed with competitive, territorial, and sexual aggression.

Area males establish a "brotherhood" or "fraternity" by aggressive interactions. When a young male reaches puberty, one or two of the local tomcats begin to call in a soft vocalization similar to that of a tomcat calling an estrous female. When the young male approaches, severe fighting ensues.[60, 62] These encounters continue for about a year, and if the younger cat is still alive and has not become totally fearful, he is accepted into the group.[30, 60] Unlike other social groupings, the brotherhood has an absolute ranking order that holds regardless of whenever or wherever members meet.[60] The cats are of almost equal strength, so even a threat display rivalry can change the narrowly separated ranking positions.[30, 60, 61]

Any initial meeting between two males results in a similar behavior. An intense fight allowed to go to completion is followed by a situation in which threat displays adequately prevent further interactions.[2, 60]

Pain-induced Aggression. Pain effectively elicits defensive aggression, which frequently is seen when a cat's hair or tail is pulled or when its tail is stepped on. Continued application of pain eventually causes the cat to submit to the stimulus or try to escape it.[27] Early social play helps to teach the kitten what pain is as well as how much pain it can inflict on others. If slight oral pressure elicits a pain reaction from a littermate, then the kitten learns that this amount of oral pressure causes pain. Singly raised orphans are deprived of this learning experience. Those not getting several months to play with littermates also may not get the lesson of how not to bite hard.

Fear-induced Aggression. Frightened animals can react aggressively if escape is not possible when their critical distance is reached by an approaching animal or object. The cat that was not socialized to the approaching species or that has had only minimal contact with that species reacts with fear-induced aggression. In either case, the defensive attack lasts until escape is possible.

Maternal Aggression. A female's defense of her young is another form of affective aggression. Queens with litters are the least tolerant of approaches by other cats and intruders. This is one of the few times the female cat is truly an aggressor. Maternal aggression is regulated by hormonal influences on the appropriate hypothalamic centers of the brain and by environmental factors, particularly the presence of the kittens.[28, 39, 49]

Territorial Aggression. Defense of property is relatively common in the cat and probably was developed to aid in social spacing.[44] Both males and females can exhibit this aggression, but it is particularly noticeable in territorial males during the breeding season. Neighboring cats often are better tolerated than strange ones.[21] Encounters with the resident male usually involve fighting, but most strangers flee or submit much sooner than do residents.[21, 44] The resident male first tries to threaten the floater male but will fight to maintain his territory if intimidation is unsuccessful. Losing to the stranger can significantly affect the resident, who may even lose primary breeding status or undergo psychological castration.[18, 44] Territorial aggression is observed in female cats with young, who are very protective of the area near the kittens.[60]

An animal outside his own territory is less aggressive in inverse proportion to the distance from its homesite.[92]

Competitive Aggression. Competitive aggression normally is controlled by dominance status and associated threat-submission postures, but the cat lacks clear dominant-subordinate relations and dominance hierarchies. Animals that share a dominance position show frequent competition for a particular item, such as food. This competition can be solved by fighting during the encounter or by reacting in a compatible, first-come, first-served manner. The latter solution usually is seen in cats. Even in the groups with a dominant male, several nonspecifics, and pariahs, an early-arriving, low-ranking member usually finishes eating before the later-arriving dominant one begins if there is room for only one at a time.

Learned Aggression. Cats seldom are trained to attack but have, on occasion, learned that aggression can produce results. When a child pulls a cat's tail, the cat shows pain-induced aggression by scratching or biting, and the child responds by releasing the cat. Soon the cat acts aggressively toward the child even though the child applies no painful stimulus. Some cats even generalize to all humans from an experience with one.

Play Aggression. Kittens use social play to develop motor skills. If they do not have littermates to interact with, they may direct it toward the owner. Although most owners understand what to expect, a few kittens play-fight harder than most and some owners do not recognize it as normal. Even older cats occasionally play, and unintentional injuries do occur from sharp claws or teeth.

Sexual Aggression

Authorities disagree about the classification of sexual aggression. Some call it a type of affective aggression, whereas others believe that it deserves separate classification.[19, 20, 79] The confusion is understandable when the areas of the brain associated with sexual aggression are compared with those associated with other types of affective behaviors.[91] Because additional tracts within the central nervous system are involved, sexual aggression is considered to be somewhat different, and is covered in Chapters 5 and 6.

Predatory Aggression

Predatory aggression differs considerably from other forms for several reasons. These aggressive responses are not the result of fear or threat. The initiating factor is instead prey capture. Emotions are irrelevant. This type of aggression is more appropriately discussed with ingestive behavior in Chapter 7.

Neural Regulation of Aggression

Numerous studies have been conducted to determine the central nervous system components of aggression. Most of these studies fail to differentiate the specific types of aggression under study, so results must be carefully evaluated. The hypothalamus is the primary area involved with the threat reactions of affective aggression. With increasing electrical stimulation of the hypothalamus, characteristic components begin to appear sequentially: alerting, mydriasis, ear retraction, piloerection, hissing, and claw protrusion. Periventricular fibers into the central gray area of the midbrain probably also are related.[23, 89] The amygdala balances excitation and inhibition of external stimuli. The defense reactions can be elicited from the hypothalamus as early as 12 days of age and from the amygdala by 21 days.[31, 53] The neural substrate for escape in the hypothalamus and midbrain overlaps that for threat, and the amount of stimulation determines the resulting behavior.[1, 11, 16] Parts of the thalamus also can stimulate or inhibit a hypothalamic attack.[15, 69] In addition, the septum, lateral aspect of the prefrontal cortex, and hippocampus probably have some inhibitory actions on agonistic behaviors.[16, 69, 75, 89, 90] A ragelike syndrome has been associated with several neural areas but is not fully understood.

Certain neurotransmitters also have been shown to influence affective aggression. Dopamine, norepinephrine, and acetylcholine are enhancers of this behavior, whereas serotonin, termed the "civilizing hormone," has an inhibitory effect.[20, 79]

There are several explanations for the apparent inconsistency of threshold stimulus strength required to elicit aggression and other behaviors in various situations. Aggression may be easily evoked at times and only with great difficulty at other times. One theory describes an innate energy that is associated with each behavior and is constantly being generated. After a certain amount of this energy has been produced but not used, the excess is used to produce an alternate behavior.[72] Unused sexual energy can give rise to excessive territorial aggression or its threat displays.[60] A second theory holds that certain neurotransmitters, such as serotonin, are produced, and the excess not used for a specific behavior result in a different behavior.[72] In the third theory, aggressive behavior is held to be learned and, thus, does not originate internally.[72]

Other Aggressions

Epinephrine has the same metabolic pathway as the pigment melanin, and the same precursor is needed for the synthesis of both. Genetic manipulation of coat color could then be useful for breeding in or out certain behavioral characteristics, such as fear and aggression.[93]

Aggression evoked by any stimulus can be redirected to another target if the attack is prevented or if the primary target is no longer available. Once the cat has physically and psychologically been aroused to the point of attack, the accompanying emotion is not easily contained even though the target is no longer available. The threshold for the behavior's release is very low, and substitute targets are easily found. A tomcat that is threatening another quickly releases its aggression on a cat or human who interferes.

SOCIAL BEHAVIOR PROBLEMS

Social behavior, or its relative lack, has a profound effect on the behavior of the cat. Many changes in the environment as well as within the cat can result in abnormal behavior.

Restraint

Restraint of cats can be difficult because they may not recognize the person as an authority figure. In general, cats that are the least stressed are the most tolerant. Control of the dorsal neck initiates passive immobility, a remnant behavior from kittenhood. Thus an uncooperative animal often can be picked up by the back of the neck and held suspended. Subcutaneous injections also can take advantage of the passive immobility. While holding the cat by the loose skin just behind the head and sliding the cat slowly forward on the slippery examination table, the veterinarian can distract the cat's attention from the injection.

Intermuscular injections often will be tolerated if the cat can lean forward and away as the rear limb is held during the injection. In an alternate procedure, the rear limb is held by the same hand holding the dorsal cervical skin, allowing the second hand to give the injection into the caudal thigh muscles of the restrained limb.

Collecting a blood sample from a jugular vein often can be accomplished with minimal restraint. One hand covers the top of the head and holds the mandible to maneuver it to tip the head back, while the second hand lightly covers or holds the forepaws. As the needle penetrates the skin, the holder can lightly blow air on the cat's face for distraction.

Temporary immobilization is possible with two other procedures, giving enough time for basic examination procedures. Hands can be cupped over the cat's face so that the darkness and human smells provide some stress relief. A rubber band also can be gently applied across the cat's ears.[57]

Social Frustration

Social frustration in any of its numerous forms can create problems or aggravate an existing situation. A cat that is physically ill does not seek social relations with its peers, preferring instead the seclusion of a corner or isolated area. This behavioral tendency is useful in locating sick cats in a colony long before their illness would be obvious if they were housed individually.[26] Sick cats appear to have a lower pain threshold and a lower resistance to stress and other illnesses.[37, 59] Increased susceptibility is not unique to this situation, however, and chronic stress of any kind, including excessive attention by well-meaning humans, can result in immunosuppression. Stress can be minimized by eliminating unnecessary handling and providing a box or sack for security in strange surroundings.

Forced situations, such as restraint and the invasion of territory by a new cat or a human, also can be stressful. This is particularly true for intact males if there is crowding of the living space or reduced food sources. Signs of social stress vary from aggression to catalepsy. In the middle of this gamut of reactions are failure to bury feces, housesoiling, insufficient grooming, excessive grooming, overeating, anorexia, diarrhea, constipation, social withdrawal, vomition, and chronic piloerection (Fig. 4–7).

When introducing a new cat to a household that already has one or more cats, one should place the new cat in a separate room with food, water, and litter for a few days so that the resident cat or cats become familiar with the new cat's odors and sounds. The older the resident cat is, the longer this adjustment period can take; in fact, some older cats never learn to accept newcomers. After the olfactory adjustment period, the owner should partially open the door to allow the cats to meet each other on their own initiative but still maintain an area where the new cat feels secure. With time, the new cat will travel throughout the house. A cage or screen door between the cats also has been used for this introductory period.[13] A cat that has been away for a time—for example, while hospitalized—may have picked up additional odors and, therefore,

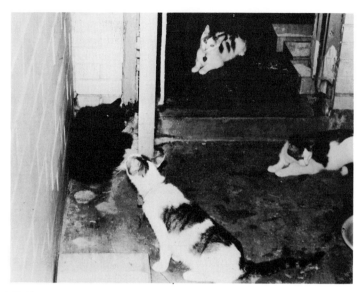

FIGURE 4–7. The resident male, forced into isolation by nonestrous females, shows both social withdrawal and insufficient grooming.

may need to be reintroduced to the household. The previously mentioned methods can be used under these circumstances.

People who have not had problems introducing several cats into a home although using no special precautions often find that at some point, the introduction of another cat results in behavioral changes in several of the resident cats. These changes occur when the point of overcrowding has been reached but can be altered by familiarizing the cats with one another. The new animal probably will be accepted after a period of confinement to a specific room, followed by introduction to the household as previously described. If the resident cats continue the undesirable behaviors, they, too, can be confined in small groups to various rooms and gradually be reintroduced to the rest of the house by the controlled opening of doors. In colonies, an arrangement of shelves or boxes allows individuals the desired privacy.

The signs of frustration associated with overcrowding are essentially the same as those associated with forced changes in routine and invasion of territory, whether by humans or by cats. In fact, the combination of overcrowding and territorial invasion creates many problem situations. Because of their strong territorial attachments, cats are best left at home when the owner is gone. There is less change in the animal's environment, and the isolation is not as disturbing to the cat as it would be to members of a social species.

Moving can seriously affect the cat because of its strong attachment to its home range. A cat taken to a new home all too often disappears and is never seen again by its owners. The homing instinct is so strong in most cats that new homeowners may find that an old cat is included with their new house. Cats have been reliably tracked over great distances in their efforts to reach their old homes. After being taken to a new home, the cat should be placed in an enclosed area with food, water, and litter and given as long as a week to adjust to the sounds and smells of the new location as well as to establish a feeling of security. Assurance and attention from the owner are helpful.[30] The door to that room or shed can then be left partially open so that the animal can explore and still use the room for security. Even these precautions may not help the older outdoor cat adjust.

Physical changes, including immunosuppression, may accompany the translocation of the cat. In addition, a prolonged fear reaction may occur, which leads to a chronic increase in gastrointestinal motility, whereas the opposite is true for a prolonged anger state.[27] It is undesirable to maintain the cat in this state of psychological and physical distress. The ideal solution is to remove the initiating factor and provide the quiet security desired by the cat. Unfortunately this option is not always possible, and the cat then must be desensitized to the environmental stimulus.

Tranquilization, particularly with the benzodiazepines, such as chlordiazepoxide (Librium; 0.5 to 5.0 mg P.O.) and diazepam (Valium; 0.5 to 2.0 mg P.O., I.V., or I.M.), can be useful in any frustration-caused problem, but the dosage must be carefully monitored to avoid heavy sedation.[36, 39] While under the influence of the drug, the cat is repeatedly exposed to the stimulus for varying durations, from 2 to 10 weeks, depending on the problem's severity and the cat's response. When a favorable response occurs, the dosage can be reduced by one-third and exposure to the stimulus can be repeated. In 1 to 2 weeks more, the dosage can again be reduced by a third and the exposure repeated. In another week or so, the drug is stopped. If signs of stress reappear, the tranquilizer may be used again until the signs are controlled. Then the procedure for desensitization is repeated and the drug dosage decreased more gradually.[36] The progestins also are described for use with behavior problems caused by frustration; however, their success probably is due more to their calming effect than to specific hormonal actions.[34]

Improper Socialization

Young kittens that do not experience normal socialization react in unusual ways later in life. Kittens obtained before 5 weeks of age may not socialize well to their own species and, as a result, become overly attached to humans. As they mature, these cats often become aggressive toward other cats or show an abnormal behavior, such as self-mutilation, to gain attention. Such extreme behavior could become learned if reinforced by attention.[44] Mating and maternal behaviors are affected because these cats do not recognize other cats or kittens as beings of the same species. A kitten raised without peers may not learn proper control of teeth or claws or may not learn to use them at all, since humans do not interact with the kitten as frequently as the mother would. Some of these youngsters develop timid or aggressive attitudes toward people and do not make suitable pets.[33, 35, 43] Orphans that do not mutilate one another by excessive sucking of one another can partially compensate for the lack of maternal care.[43]

The cat that is minimally socialized to other species by 8 weeks may direct aggressive actions toward members of these other species, such as adults, children, and dogs. This cat is suffering from the "isolated syndrome," and social stress on such an animal causes problems. The adoption of an adult cat or an older kitten is ill-advised unless its background is known. Sedation with a great deal of handling to desensitize the cat may be useful in some extreme situations.[25] A cat that is poorly socialized to humans may learn to accept one or two as part of its environment, but when confronted with strangers, it will crouch and growl in a pariahlike reaction. When extremely crowded, as when the owners give a party, the cat may even show aggression toward its friends. Putting the cat in a quiet room away from the social activities can eliminate a great deal of tension on both sides. The isolated syndrome handicaps the individual in social situations and gives it a marked preference for an environment relatively barren of other beings.[29]

Runts in a litter should be carefully evaluated before being accepted as a pet. Possible intimidation by littermates during this critical early period may have affected that animal's capacity for socialization.

Problem Aggression

Aggression is a commonly reported behavior problem for cats, representing up to 35 per cent of cases.[4, 7, 10] Because the claws and teeth of a cat are such formidable weapons, aggression by the cat can become a significant problem. Although figures vary, somewhere between 6 per cent and 20 per cent of the reported bites that animals inflict on humans are caused by cats, and most of those bitten are children.[32, 47, 51] Pain-induced aggression accounts for many of these incidents when young children, who may not understand the animal's warning signals, pull the hair or tail of the cat.

Petting-induced Aggression. Some cats, usually lying on a person's lap and being petted, suddenly claw and bite. The cat immediately jumps down, runs a short distance, and stops, perhaps to groom itself. Such cats usually are male. The reason for the action is unknown; however, two theories currently are used to explain its occurrence. One theory is that the cat initially enjoys the handling and petting, which finally become excessive and reach a threshold level. The cat bites and claws when the handling is no longer acceptable, since there is no other natural way to say, "Thanks, that is enough." The other theory holds that the petting and handling are so pleasurable that the cat falls into a light sleep, oblivious to its surroundings. The cat suddenly awakens and, while still not completely oriented, is aware only of "confinement" and fights its way to freedom. By the time it has jumped clear of the person, it is totally aware and, to dissociate from the situation, uses grooming as a displacement activity. Treatment of this cat with progestins may be successful in some problem cases.[44, 45]

Intermale Aggression. Because intermale aggression is related to testosterone, castration has been successful in minimizing 80 per cent to 90 per cent of the behavior in cats so treated.[44] In addition, various long-acting progestogens have been successfully used to control this aggression, including medroxyprogesterone acetate (Depo-Provera; 100 mg I.M.) and megestrol acetate (Ovaban; 1 mg/lb P.O. daily for 1 week, then 0.5 mg/lb daily for 1 week, followed by 0.5 mg/lb biweekly as needed). Several other drugs with similar actions also can be used. Specifics of male behaviors are discussed in Chapter 5.

Fear- and Frustration-induced Aggression. Fear or frustration can, if continued long enough, result in neurosis, and either can produce aggression. Cats that have not been well socialized to humans frequently are unable to escape an approaching individual, and become aggressive when the critical distance is reached. The most obvious method of relieving or preventing this form of aggression is to eliminate the source of fear or frustration, but that is not always possible. Tranquilizers of the benzodiazepine group can be used in a desensitizing program, as previously described. Some individuals never fully adapt, and must be maintained on low doses of the drugs; others need treatment only before exposure to the stimulus.

When initially confronting a cat that displays fear-induced aggression, one's primary problem may be getting close enough to the animal to work with it. In addition, the standard approaches, such as forced restraint, thick gloves, and a thrown blanket, only aggravate the situation. By spraying ketamine hydrochloride (10 mg/lb) or acepromazine maleate (1 mg/lb) into its mouth and waiting, one can safely create a workable situation, even though the full dose may not have been delivered.

Redirected Aggression. When a cat's aggression cannot be directed at the causative agent, it can be redirected at a person or animal close by. The initiating stress may be as subtle as the cat's not receiving a bedtime snack, resulting in an attack on the owners, noises, or unusual odors.[6, 9, 14]

Cats roaming near a favorite window also can trigger an attack by the confined cat when the owner comes home. Treatment mainly consists of eliminating the source of stress and punishing the attack.

Feline Dispersion Aggression. As kittens reach the age of 6 to 12 months, their social play bouts end with a fight. Over time, the length of the play gets shorter and the fight segment becomes more intense. The frequent aggressive interactions eventually result in the dispersion of the kittens into their solitary life-styles. It is the time of personality change from social kitten to asocial adult. If kittens have been separated from littermates previously, the aggressive interactions may still be expressed to owners or other animals. Many owners at least notice the personality change.

Feline Asocial Aggression. This is the type of aggression shown by older cats toward kittens. The usual situation in which feline asocial aggression shows up is when one of two older cats that had been "friends" dies. Both the owners and the remaining cat miss the animal, so a new kitten is brought in to become a replacement. The older cat becomes aggressive to the kitten whenever it approaches. The kitten is social and readily approaches the older cat, which really just wants to be left alone. The older cat responds aggressively to the kitten's approach. Management is difficult because it usually takes several months for the new kitten to become less social. Until then, the owner should keep the opportunities for interaction to a minimum.

Medically Related Aggression. Certain medical changes may be manifested clinically only as aggression. Not all these conditions are identified or understood. Treatments for certain conditions have been successfully used, but the mechanisms of action are still uncertain. The hypothyroid problem classically involves changes in a cat's appearance, but in one form of the disease, aggression is the clinical manifestation. The affected cat becomes "grumpy."[5] Although it may sleep on the bed with the owner at night, the cat might not allow the owner to sit on the sofa or walk past it. Thyroid hormone replacement is successful. Evaluations of T_4 values must be made; however, the fact that an excess of testosterone or estrogen in the circulating bloodstream also can decrease the normal levels must be considered.

Another medical condition that may cause aggression is epilepsy. The history often gives other clues of this condition. During these episodes, the cat may seem oblivious to its surroundings, stare into space for short periods, or suddenly start chasing its tail. Electroencephalographic (EEG) recordings show changes from normal patterns in fewer than 40 per cent of cases. In humans, alpha-chloralose is used to demonstrate EEG activation of a latent instability in the central nervous system and may become useful in veterinary medicine in making a diagnosis of epilepsy.[68] Although treatment with anticonvulsants is about 80 per cent successful, the drugs may have to be given at initially high doses, which are reduced according to clinical progress. Phenobarbital (0.5 to 1.0 mg/lb P.O. once or twice daily) usually is used but occasionally may require combination with other anticonvulsants. Because of the proximity of the hypothalamus and the hormone system, the success of adrenocorticotropin (ACTH; 1 unit/lb/wk I.M. or S.C. for 13 weeks, then half the dose weekly for 13 weeks) and medroxyprogesterone acetate (Depo-Provera; 100 mg I.M. for males and 50 mg I.M. for females) is not surprising. Frontal lobe epilepsy in humans does not always respond to anticonvulsants, but some cases have been successfully controlled by medroxyprogesterone acetate.[8]

Irritable aggression is the result of being less tolerant when the cat is not feeling well.[5] The animal can become irritable if forced to interact when it is ill. Impacted anal sacs, oral ulcers, and feline urologic syndrome are among many initiating problems that need to be ruled out.

Other medical abnormalities can affect the central nervous system cells or neurotransmitters. In addition to being caused by irritative brain lesions, such as encephalitis, aggression has been caused by tumors that bilaterally affect the hypothalamus.[27, 44, 46, 98] For certain predictable hypothalamically mediated aggressions, pretreatment with chlordiazepoxide hydrochloride (Librium; 0.5 to 1.0 mg P.O.) might be used for control.[52, 88] Occasional individuals recover spontaneously.[56]

Anesthetic drugs have been implicated in personality changes that involve aggression. Extremely vicious cats have had favorable personality changes after undergoing one or more episodes of prolonged deep barbiturate anesthesia.[70, 71, 77] In addition, personalities have been changed by withdrawing, during anesthesia, a third of the blood volume and then repeating the process 3 days later. Neural anoxia is the possible explanation for these occasional successes. The reduction of blood volume also might have been used occasionally on an individual with erythrocythemia, with resultant personality changes.[71]

Food additives, including meat preservatives, have been incriminated as causes of aggression.[3, 71] This condition is difficult to prove but should be considered whenever aggression begins or ceases after food brands or types are changed.

Extreme Timidity

The timid cat can be an undesirable pet and a difficult patient. Timidity can be inherited, although the specific behavior may not express itself until a later age.[3, 30] Timid kittens dislike restraint, do not relax when picked up, remain immobile instead of exploring a new area, do not follow people, are less playful, and fear noise.[3, 30] Stimulus desensitization, with decreasing dosages of tranquilizers and continuous stimulus exposure, can be useful for some of these cats. Some cats that have undergone anesthesia become extremely timid or aggressive, and require patient, careful handling to reverse the behavior. No correlation has yet been made between production of this behavior and handling techniques or use of a specific anesthetic agent. Care should be exercised, however, when using anesthetics, including ketamine hydrochloride, that are known to cause psychic phenomena in human patients.

CASE PRESENTATIONS

CASE 4–1. Six-year-old Siamese neutered female. The cat lived with two other cats and was fine until a fourth cat was added. In addition, the newcomer queened within a week after arriving. The Siamese cat began spraying all around the house within a few days of the fourth cat's arrival.

Diagnosis. Urine marking probably because of overcrowding.

Treatment. The newcomer was shut in a separate room with food, water, and litter. Because the Siamese cat did not continue spraying, it was not isolated. After 5 days, the door into the room was opened, and the newcomer gradually integrated with the residents without causing additional marking by the Siamese cat.

CASE 4–2. One-year-old domestic shorthair female. The cat got along fine with its female owner but was not especially friendly to other people, growling and crouching in the presence of the owner's boyfriend. Week-end guests were particularly upsetting for the animal. The animal was obtained as a kitten from an animal shelter.

Diagnosis. Stress reaction because of minimal human socialization and overcrowding.

Treatment. The cat was isolated in a separate room with food, water, and litter when guests were expected. Tranquilizers also could be used when isolation was not possible.

CASE 4–3. Three-year-old domestic shorthair neutered female. The cat lived with a neutered male littermate and a single woman owner. About 3 weeks ago the cat suddenly viciously attacked the male when he walked into a room. About a week later the cats were lying on either side of the owner being petted when the female again attacked the male. After the third attack, the cats were physically separated until the problem could be solved. Although the male was much larger than the female, he was more timid and less demanding.

Diagnosis. Territorial aggression.

Treatment. Medroxyprogesterone acetate (50 mg I.M.) controlled the behavior for 4 to 6 weeks before another injection was needed. The cat remained aggressive in one small area, but this caused no excessive problem and additional injections were not suggested.

CASE 4–4. Seven-and-one-half-year-old domestic shorthair neutered male. The cat lived with five other cats, a man, and a woman. Three weeks earlier the cat had been bathed to rid it of fleas, but 2 days later he began attacking the humans and the other cats. During an attack, his eyes appeared glazed, he growled excessively, and he walked with his head and shoulders low. After an attack, he calmed down in about 30 minutes. He was no problem as long as no other cats were around.

Diagnosis. Territorial aggression. The cat was displaying offensive threat followed by attack. The owners often gave reference to some event that happened about the same time, but it probably had no connection to the behavioral problem.

Treatment. Medroxyprogesterone acetate (100 mg I.M.) controlled the behavior for 4 to 8 weeks before another injection was needed. This cat usually did fine without treatment during the winter months.

CASE 4–5. Fourteen-month-old domestic shorthair neutered male. Ever since the cat was 5 or 6 months of age, it would bite any person. The frequency and intensity had intensified, so that it sought out humans. At first the interactions seemed to follow play, but that was no longer true.

Diagnosis. Feline dispersion aggression.

Treatment. Punishment for biting attacks by using a water pistol was enough to stop the problem. At first the cat avoided any person carrying a squirt gun, but as the behavior improved, there was less avoidance.

CASE 4–6. One-year-old domestic shorthair neutered female. This cat had recently been introduced into a home with two older cats. It immediately started hissing at the others and chased them aggressively. The cats could eat together, but this one would attack if the others moved.

Diagnosis. Feline asocial aggression, perhaps with some aspects of territorial aggression.

Treatment. This cat was separated from the other two and confined to a guest bedroom. After 2 weeks it was allowed controlled access to the rest of the house, with times out of the room gradually increasing in length. After 1 month there was a mutual tolerance of the other cats.

CASE 4–7. Eight-year-old domestic shorthair neutered male. For the past 2 years this cat had had recurring bouts of the feline urologic syndrome; during this time, it became progressively aggressive. The owners think that the problem was worse at the times when they knew it was sick.

Medical Workup. The physical examination was normal except that the urinary bladder wall felt thickened. A urinalysis showed that the cat had a urine pH of 7.6 with a trace of blood and protein.

Diagnosis. Irritable aggression as the result of the feline urologic syndrome.

Treatment. The cat's diet was changed to one that would acidify the urine; however, the cat would not eat the product. After experimenting with what the cat would eat, the urine pH was controlled with the addition of 2 tbsp of tomato juice placed on its regular food each day. The general disposition improved, but there continued to be occasional relapses.

CASE 4–9. One-year-old domestic shorthair neutered female. The kitten came into this home at 3 months of age and did some biting at that time. Most of the time it was a friendly, loving cat, but occasionally it would suddenly turn on the owners and start biting. Once it started, it did not stop easily. The referring veterinarian had tried megestrol acetate unsuccessfully.

Diagnosis. Feline dispersion aggression.

Treatment. When the biting attacks came, the owners tried punishing the cat with a squirt bottle and a rattle made from a soda can containing some rocks. This was somewhat successful, but the owners thought that the progress was not satisfactory and decided on euthanasia.

CASE 4–10. One-and-one-half-year-old domestic shorthair neutered male. Two weeks before presentation a 10-week-old kitten had been added to the household. This cat did not tolerate the kitten, hissing and swatting at it.

Diagnosis. Feline asocial aggression.

Treatment. The new kitten was put into a different area of the house, so that there was minimal interaction for 3 weeks. Gradual introduction over the next week resulted in the cats coexisting, but still with occasional aggressive interactions.

CASE 4–11. Six-month-old domestic shorthair female. The chief complaint was that over the previous month the kitten had started to bite hard in play.

Diagnosis. Feline dispersion aggression.

Treatment. The owners were advised to punish the kitten with a water sprayer, distract the kitten by picking it up by the scruff of the neck, or move away from it when the biting starts. By 9 months of age the kitten was showing less of a tendency to bite and the rough play was channeled into play with inanimate objects.

CASE 4–12. Four-month-old domestic shorthair female. The kitten was raised in a veterinary clinic, receiving lots of attention from people. By the time of presentation, it was biting a lot in play and had become the "terror of the clinic." The staff had tried squirting it with a water pistol, which it liked, and grabbing it by the scruff of the neck.

Diagnosis. Feline dispersion aggression.

Treatment. Different types of punishment were tried; a rattle (rocks in a soda can) seemed to work the best. In addition, the kitten was encouraged to chase objects such as toys on a string. After a month it went to the home of one of the staff members and gradually developed into an acceptable pet.

CASE 4–13. Three-year-old domestic shorthair neutered male. Three months before presentation the owner and two cats moved to the ground floor of an apartment building from a higher floor. The neutered female littermate would sit in a window and had started vocalizing, usually when it saw another cat. At that time the male would attack it.

Diagnosis. Redirected aggression.

Treatment. This cat was apparently stressed by the change in location and the perception of other cats threatening its territory. To control the redirected aggression, both cats were confined away from areas where they could see outside and this male was given diazepam (2 mg P.O. once a day) for 1 week. The problem was controlled, but the owners were warned that it could recur, especially in the spring of the next year.

CASE 4–14. Five-year-old domestic shorthair neutered male. The owner brought this cat in because of a concern about its health. Three months ago a new kitten was introduced into the home, and this cat hid from the kitten and fought it if approached. Even confining the kitten away from the resident cat did not help.

Medical Workup. The physical examination showed a cat that was 1 to 1.5 lb underweight. The only other findings were those consistent with a stress leukogram.

Diagnosis. Feline asocial aggression.

Treatment. Antianxiety tranquilizers (diazepam) helped to reduce the degree of reaction, especially when the cat was confined away from the kitten too. The owner thought that it was not good to keep the cat on tranquilizers and was not willing to wait for the kitten to get older, so he found a new home for the kitten.

CASE 4–15. Three-year-old domestic shorthair neutered male. This cat was one of several cats in this home. The last new cat was added 4 months ago, and at that time this cat started beating up all the others. The referring veterinarian had tried megestrol acetate without success.

Diagnosis. Redirected aggression that resulted from the stress of crowding.

Treatment. The owner was successfully able to keep all the cats by separating them into smaller groups and keeping each group in its own room.

CASE 4–16. Eight-month-old Persian female. This cat had been shown since 2 months of age, but in the past 2 months it had started hissing and growling at the judges. It also began to act as if it wanted to get away. The owners tried to fake a show situation, but the cat did not show the aggression then.

Diagnosis. Fear-induced aggression.

Treatment. It was suggested that the owners take the cat to small shows and try using Vicks Vaporub on the nose to try blocking odors that might be triggering the behavior. This technique was moderately successful, but the cat never showed to its full potential again and was retired to a pet home. Antianxiety tranquilizers could have been used if the owner had wanted to try other treatments.

CASE 4–17. One-year-old domestic shorthair neutered male. After seeing a strange cat through the living room window, this cat started fighting with a littermate neutered male. Since then the cats have fought whenever they have had the chance.

Medical Workup. This cat had a small abscess on the right forelimb.

Diagnosis. Redirected aggression.

Treatment. The stress of seeing another cat triggered aggression in this cat, but the only available outlet was the littermate, who retaliated in kind. Both cats were confined in separate areas of the house, away from the window. This allowed the cat to settle down, and both were successfully reintroduced gradually starting 1 week later.

CASE 4–18. Seven-year-old domestic shorthair neutered male. The night before presentation the cat had grabbed the back of the neck of the owner's baby as the infant lay on the floor crying. Its teeth did not puncture the skin.

Diagnosis. Territorial mounting.

Treatment. Keeping the baby and cat separate was not a workable solution. The cat continued to try to mount the child, so the owner found another home for the cat.

CASE 4–19. Five-year-old domestic longhair neutered male. The student owner got married to another cat owner. When the cats were introduced, the female would jump this one, causing it to hide constantly under the bed. If shut out of the bedroom, this cat hid under the sofa.

Diagnosis. Pariah behavior.

Treatment. Both cats were confined to different rooms and allowed to have the run of the house at separate times. Because the problem had been going on for 6 weeks, the cats stayed in separate rooms for about 1 month before they gradually were let out at the same times. The male became more outgoing and tolerant of the female and spent less time hiding under things.

CASE 4–20. Two-year-old domestic shorthair neutered male. The cat was castrated at 5 months of age because it was mounting another cat. That behavior had continued. When mounted, the other cat responded by assuming a crouched posture.

Diagnosis. Territorial mounting.

Treatment. The behavior is normal for a territorial cat and is not a sex behavior. The owner was accepting of the behavior once he understood this.

Also see cases 2–3, 2–4, 2–5, 2–6, 2–10, 5–3, and 10–7.

REFERENCES

1. Adams, D. B.: Cells related to fighting behavior recorded from midbrain central gray neuropil of cat. Science 159:894, 1968.
2. Beadle, M.: The Cat: History, Biology, and Behavior. New York: Simon and Schuster, 1977.
3. Beaver, B. V.: Feline behavioral problems. Vet. Clin. North Am. 6:333, 1976.
4. Beaver, B. V.: Feline behavioral problems other than housesoiling. J. Am. Anim. Hospital Assoc. 25:465, 1989.
5. Beaver, B. V.: Disorders of behavior. In Sherding, R. G., ed.: The Cat: Diseases and Clinical Management. New York: Churchill Livingstone, 1989.
6. Beaver, B. V.: Psychogenic manifestations of environmental disturbances. In August, J. R., ed.: Consultations in Feline Medicine. Philadelphia: W. B. Saunders Co., 1991.
7. Blackshaw, J. K.: Abnormal behaviour in cats. Australian Vet. J. 65:395, 1988.
8. Blumer, D., and Migeon, C.: Hormone and hormonal agents in the treatment of aggression. J. Nerv. Ment. Dis. 160:127, 1975.
9. Borchelt, P. L., and Voith, V. L.: Diagnosis and treatment of aggression problems in cats. Vet. Clin. North Am. [Small Anim. Pract.] 12:665, 1982.
10. Borchelt, P. L., and Voith, V. L.: Aggressive behavior in cats. Compendium on Continuing Education 9:49, 1987.
11. Brown, J. L., and Hunsperger, R. W.: Neuroethology and motivation of agonistic behaviour. Anim. Behav. 11:439, 1963.
12. Brunner, F.: The application of behavior studies in small animal practice. In Fox, M. W., ed.: Abnormal Behavior in Animals. Philadelphia: W. B. Saunders Co., 1968.
13. Bryant, D.: The Care and Handling of Cats. New York: Ives Washburn, 1944.
14. Chapman, B. L., and Voith, V. L.: Cat aggression redirected to people: 14 cases (1981–1987). J. Am. Vet. Med. Assoc. 196:947, 1990.
15. Chi, C. C., Bandler, R. J., and Flynn, J. P.: Neuroanatomic projections related to biting attack elicited from ventral midbrain in cats. Brain Behav. Evol. 13:91, 1976.
16. Clemente, C. D., and Chase, M. H.: Neurological substrates of aggressive behavior. Annu. Rev. Physiol. 35:329, 1973.
17. Cole, D. D., and Shafer, J. N.: A study of social dominance in cats. Behaviour 27:39, 1966.

18. Eaton, R. L.: The evolution of sociality in the Felidae. In Eaton, R. L., ed.: The World's Cats. 3rd ed. Seattle: Carnivore Research Institute, 1976.
19. Eleftheriou, B. E., and Scott, J. P.: The Physiology of Aggression and Defeat. New York: Plenum Publishing Corp., 1971.
20. Everett, G. M.: The pharmacology of aggressive behavior in animals and man. Psychopharmacol. Bull. 13:15, 1977.
21. Ewer, R. F.: Ethology of Mammals. London: Paul Elek, Ltd., 1968.
22. Ewer, R. F.: The Carnivores. Ithaca, NY: Cornell University Press, 1973.
23. Ewert, J. P.: Neuroethology. New York: Springer-Verlag, 1980.
24. Feral cat colonies in Great Britain. Bull. Inst. Study of Anim. Prob. 1:5, Mar.-Apr. 1979.
25. Fox, M. W.: New information on feline behavior. Mod. Vet. Pract. 56:50, 1965.
26. Fox, M. W.: Natural environment: Theoretical and practical aspects for breeding and rearing laboratory animals. Lab. Anim. Care 16:316, 1966.
27. Fox, M. W.: Aggression: Its adaptive and maladaptive significance in man and animals. In Fox, M. W., ed.: Abnormal Behavior in Animals. Philadelphia: W. B. Saunders Co., 1968.
28. Fox, M. W.: Ethology: An overview. In Fox, M. W., ed.: Abnormal Behavior in Animals. Philadelphia: W. B. Saunders Co., 1968.
29. Fox, M. W.: Neurobehavioral development and the genotype-environment interaction. Q. Rev. Biol. 45:131, 1970.
30. Fox, M. W.: Understanding Your Cat. New York: Coward, McCann & Geoghegan, 1974.
31. Fox, M. W.: The behaviour of cats. In Hafez, E. S. E., ed.: The Behaviour of Domestic Animals. 3rd ed. Baltimore: Williams & Wilkins Co., 1975.
32. Griffiths, A. O., and Silberberg, A.: Stray animals: Their impact on a community. Mod. Vet. Pract. 56:255, 1975.
33. Guyot, G. W., Cross, H. A., and Bennett, T. L.: The domestic cat. In Roy, M. A., ed.: Species Identity and Attachment: A Phylogenetic Evaluation. New York: Garland STPM Press, 1980.
34. Hart, B. L.: Gonadal hormones and behavior of the female cat. Fel. Pract. 2:6, July-Aug. 1972.
35. Hart, B. L.: Maternal behavior. II. The nursing-suckling relationship and the effects of maternal deprivation. Fel. Pract. 2:6, Nov.-Dec. 1972.
36. Hart, B. L.: Psychopharmacology in feline practice. Fel. Pract. 3:6, May-June 1973.
37. Hart, B. L.: Disease processes and behavior. Fel. Pract. 3:6, Nov.-Dec. 1973.
38. Hart, B. L.: Social interaction in cats. Fel. Pract. 4:12, May-June 1974.
39. Hart, B. L.: Types of aggressive behavior. Can. Pract. 1:6, May-June 1974.
40. Hart, B. L.: Behavioral patterns related to territoriality and social communication. Fel. Pract. 5:12, Jan.-Feb. 1975.
41. Hart, B. L.: A quiz on feline behavior. Fel. Pract. 5:12, May-June 1975.
42. Hart, B. L.: Social interactions between cats and their owners. Fel. Pract. 6:6, Jan. 1976.
43. Hart, B. L.: Behavioral aspects of selecting a new cat. Fel. Pract. 6:8, Sept. 1976.
44. Hart, B. L.: Aggression in cats. Fel. Pract. 7:22, Mar. 1977.
45. Hart, B. L., and Hart, L. A.: Canine and Feline Behavioral Therapy. Philadelphia: Lea & Febiger, 1985.
46. Henry, J. P.: Mechanisms of psychosomatic disease in animals. Adv. Vet. Sci. Comp. Med. 20:115, 1976.
47. Houpt, K. A.: Animal behavior as a subject for veterinary students. Cornell Vet. 66:73, Jan. 1976.
48. Houpt, K. A., and Beaver, B.: Behavioral problems of geriatric dogs and cats. Vet. Clin. North Am. [Small Anim. Pract.] 11:643, 1981.
49. Inselman-Temkin, B. R., and Flynn, J. P.: Sex-dependent effects of gonadal and gonadotropic hormones on centrally-elicited attack in cats. Brain Res. 60:393, 1973.
50. Jöchle, W., and Jöchle, M.: Reproductive and behavioral control in the male and female cat with progestins: Long-term field observations in individual animals. Theriogenology 3:179, May 1975.
51. Johnson, P. D., Pullen, M. M., and Cox, P. D.: The socio-economic implications of

animal bites—St. Paul, Minnesota 1976. Univ. Minn. Vet. Med. Reporter 114:1, May-June 1978.

52. Katz, R. J., and Thomas, E.: Effects of a novel anti-aggressive agent upon two types of brain stimulated emotional behavior. Psychopharmacology 48:79, July 9, 1976.
53. Kling, A., Kovach, J. K., and Tucker, T. J.: The behaviour of cats. In Hafez, E. S. E., ed.: The Behaviour of Domestic Animals. 2nd ed. Baltimore: Williams & Wilkins Co., 1969.
54. Kolb, B., and Nonneman, A. J.: The development of social responsiveness in kittens. Anim. Behav. 23:368, 1975.
55. Kuo, Z. Y.: Studies on the basic factors in animal fighting. VII. Inter-species coexistence in mammals. J. Genet. Psychol. 97:211, 1960.
56. Kydd, A. M., Boswood, B., and Watts, A. E.: A new syndrome in cats? Vet. Rec. 87:518, 1973.
57. Leedy, M. G., Fishelson, B. A., and Cooper, L. L.: A simple method of restraint for use with cats. Fel. Pract. 13:32, Sept.-Oct. 1983.
58. Lehman, H. C.: The child's attitude toward the dog versus the cat. J. Genet. Psychol. 35:62, 1928.
59. Levinson, B. M.: Man and his feline pet. Mod. Vet. Pract. 53:35, Nov. 1972.
60. Leyhausen, P.: Communal organization of solitary mammals. Symp. Zool. Soc. Lond. 14:249, 1965.
61. Leyhausen, P.: Cat Behavior: The Predatory and Social Behavior of Domestic and Wild Cats. New York: Garland STPM Press, 1978.
62. Leyhausen, P.: The tame and the wild—another just-so story? In Turner, D. C., and Bateson, P., eds.: The Domestic Cat: The Biology of its Behaviour. New York: Cambridge University Press, 1988.
63. Liberg, O.: Predation and social behaviour in a population of domestic cat. An evolutionary perspective. Ph.D. diss., Department of Animal Ecology, University of Lund, Sweden, 1981.
64. Liberg, O., and Sandell, M.: Spatial organisation and reproductive tactics in the domestic cat and other felids. In Turner, D. C., and Beteson, P., eds.: The Domestic Cat: The Biology of its Behaviour. New York: Cambridge University Press, 1988.
65. Lorenz, K., and Leyhausen, P.: Motivation of Human and Animal Behavior. New York: Van Nostrand Reinhold Co., 1973.
66. Macdonald, D. W.: The ecology of carnivore social behaviour. Nature [Lond.] 301:379, 1983.
67. Macdonald, D. W., Apps, P. J., Carr, G. M., and Kerby, G.: Social dynamics, nursing coalitions and infanticide among farm cats, *Felis catus*. Berlin: Paul Parey Scientific Publ., 1987.
68. Monroe, R. R.: Anticonvulsants in the treatment of aggression. J. Nerv. Ment. Dis. 160:119, 1975.
69. Morgenson, G. J., and Huang, Y. H.: The neurobiology of motivated behavior. Prog. Neurobiol. 1:55, 1973.
70. Mosier, J. E.: Common medical and behavioral problems in cats. Mod. Vet. Pract. 56:699, 1975.
71. Mosier, J. E.: Personal communication, 1970.
72. Moyer, K. E.: A model of aggression with implications for research. Psychopharmacol. Bull. 13:14, 1977.
73. Natoli, E.: Spacing pattern in a colony of urban stray cats (*Felis catus* L.) in the historic centre of Rome. Appl. Anim. Behav. Sci. 14:289, 1985.
74. Neville, P. F., and Remfry, J.: Effect of neutering on two groups of feral cats. Vet. Rec. 114:447, 1984.
75. Nonneman, A. J., and Kolb, B. E.: Lesions of hippocampus or prefrontal cortex alter species-typical behaviours in the cat. Behav. Biol. 12:41, 1974.
76. Patience pays off for hero cat. Friskies Res. Dig. 14:14, Spring 1978.
77. Personality change in a Siamese cat. Vet. Med. Small Anim. Clin. 59:144, 1964.
78. Poucet, B., Thinus-Blanc, C., and Chapus, N.: Route planning in cats, in relation to the visibility of the goal. Anim. Behav. 31:594, 1983.
79. Reis, D. J.: Central neurotransmitters in aggression. Res. Publ. Assoc. Res. Nerv. Ment. Dis. 52:119, 1974.

80. Rheingold, H. L., and Eckerman, C. O.: Familiar social and nonsocial stimuli and the kitten's response to a strange environment. Dev. Psychobiol. 4:71, 1971.
81. Romanes, G. J.: Mental Evolution in Animals. New York: AMS Press, 1969.
82. Rosenblatt, J. S.: Sucking and home orientation in the kitten: A comparative developmental study. In Tobach, E., Aronson, L. R., and Shaw, E., eds.: The Biopsychology of Development. New York: Academic Press, 1971.
83. Rosenblatt, J. S.: Learning in newborn kittens. Sci. Am. 227:18, 1972.
84. Rosenblatt, J. S., Turkewitz, G., and Schneirla, T. C.: Development of suckling and related behavior in neonate kittens. In Bliss, E. L., ed.: Roots of Behavior. New York: Harper & Row, 1962.
85. Scott, J. P.: The analysis of social organization in animals. Ecology 37:213, 1956.
86. Scott, J. P.: Critical periods in behavioral development. Science 138:949, 1962.
87. Seitz, P. F. D.: Infantile experience and adult behavior in animal subjects. Psychosom. Med. 21:353, 1959.
88. Sheard, M. H.: Lithium in the treatment of aggression. J. Nerv. Ment. Dis. 160:108, 1975.
89. Siegel, A., and Edinger, H.: Neural control of aggression and rage behavior. In Morgane, P. J., and Panksepp, J., eds.: Behavioral Studies of the Hypothalamus. Vol. 3, Pt. B. New York: Marcel Dekker, 1981.
90. Siegel, A., Edinger, H., and Dotto, M.: Effects of electrical stimulation of the lateral aspect of the prefrontal cortex upon attack behavior in cats. Brain Res. 93:473, 1975.
91. Sutin, J., Rose, J., Van Atta, L., and Thalmann, R.: Electrophysiological studies in an animal model of aggressive behavior. Res. Publ. Assoc. Res. Nerv. Ment. Dis. 52:93, 1974.
92. Todd, N. B.: Behavior and genetics of the domestic cat. Cornell Vet. 53:99, 1963.
93. Todd, N. B.: Cats and commerce. Sci. Am. 237:100, 1977.
94. Turner, D. C., Feaver, J., Mendl, M., and Bateson, P.: Variation in domestic cat behaviour towards humans: A paternal effect. Anim. Behav. 34:1890, 1986.
95. Turner, D. C., and Meister, O.: Hunting behaviour of the domestic cat. In Turner, D. C., and Bateson, P., eds.: The Domestic Cat: The Biology of its Behaviour. New York: Cambridge University Press, 1988.
96. Ursin, H.: Flight and defense behavior in cats. J. Comp. Physiol. Psychol. 58:180, 1964.
97. Voith, V. L., and Borchelt, P. L.: Social behavior of domestic cats. Compendium on Continuing Education 8:637, 1986.
98. Voith, V. L., and Marder, A. R.: Feline behavioral disorders. In Morgan, R. V., ed.: Handbook of Small Animal Practice. New York: Churchill Livingstone, 1988.
99. Warner, R. E.: Demography and movements of free-ranging domestic cats in rural Illinois. Journal of Wildlife Management 49:340, 1985.
100. Weigel, I.: Small cats and clouded leopards. In Grzimek, H. C. B., ed.: Grzimek's Animal Life Encyclopedia. Vol. 12. New York: Van Nostrand Reinhold Co., 1975.
101. Wemmer, C., and Scow, K.: Communication in the Felidae with emphasis on scent marking and contact patterns. In Sebeok, T. A., ed.: How Animals Communicate. Bloomington: Indiana University Press, 1977.
102. Winslow, C. N.: Observations of dominance-subordination in cats. J. Genet. Psychol. 52:425, 1938.
103. Worden, A. N.: Abnormal behaviour in the dog and cat. Vet. Rec. 71:966, 1959.

ADDITIONAL READINGS

Allen, R. P., Safer, D., and Covi, L. Effects of psychostimulants on aggression. J. Nerv. Ment. Dis. 160:137, 1975.
Allikmets, L. H. Cholinergic mechanisms in aggressive behaviour. Med. Biol. 52:19, Feb. 1974.
Andy, O. J., Giurintano, L., Giurintano, S., and McDonald, T. Thalamic modulation of aggression. Pav. J. Biol. Sci. 10:85, 1975.

August, J. R. Dog and cat bites. J. Am. Vet. Med. Assoc. 193:1394, 1988.

Baron, A., Stewart, C. M., and Warren, J. M. Patterns of social interaction in cats (*Felis domestica*). Behaviour 11:56, 1957.

Berntson, G. G., and Leibowitz, S. F. Biting attack in cats: Evidence for central muscarinic mediation. Brain Res. 51:366, 1973.

Blacklock, G. A. A cat's purr . . . on purpose? Cat Fancy 16:20, Aug. 1973.

Candland, D. K., and Milne, D. W. Species differences in approach—behavior as a function of developmental environment. Anim. Behav. 14:539, 1966.

Collard, R. R. Fear of strangers and play behavior in kittens with varied social experience. Child Dev. 38:877, 1967.

De Molina, A. F., and Hunsperger, R. W. Organization of subcortical systems governing defence and flight reactions in the cat. J. Physiol. [Lond.] 160:200, 1962.

Eichelman, B. Neurochemical studies of aggression in animals. Psychopharmacol. Bull. 13:17, 1977.

Fokin, v. F. Dynamics of active defensive reflex formation in cats. Zh. Vyssh. Nerv. Deiat. 25:752, 1975.

Fox, M. W. Psychomotor disturbances. In Fox, M. W., ed. Abnormal Behavior in Animals. Philadelphia: W. B. Saunders Co., 1968.

Fox, M. W. Behavioral effects of rearing dogs with cats during the "critical period of socialization." Behaviour 35:273, 1969.

Fox, M. W. Psychopathology in man and lower animals. J. Am. Vet. Med. Assoc. 159:66, 1971.

Glusman, M. The hypothalamic "savage" syndrome. Res. Publ. Assoc. Res. Nerv. Ment. Dis. 52:52, 1974.

Guyot, G. W., Cross, H. A., and Bennett, T. L. Early social isolation of the domestic cat: Responses during mechanical toy testing. Appl. Anim. Ethol. 10:109, 1983.

Hart, B. L. Gonadal hormones and behavior of the male cat. Fel. Pract. 2:7, May-June 1972.

Hart, B. L. Genetics and behavior. Fel. Pract. 3:5, Jan.-Feb. 1973.

Hart, B. L. The brain and behavior. Fel. Pract. 3:4, Sept.-Oct. 1973.

Hart, B. L. Gonadal androgen and sociosexual behavior of male mammals: A comparative analysis. Psychol. Bull. 81:383, 1974.

Hart, B. L. Behavioral aspects of raising kittens. Fel. Pract. 6:8, Nov. 1976.

Hart, B. L. Quiz on feline behavior. Fel. Pract. 7:20, May 1977.

Hart, B. L. Feline life-styles: Solitary versus communal living. Fel. Pract. 9:10, Sept.-Oct. 1979.

Hart, B. L. The behavior of domestic animals. New York: W. H. Freeman & Co., 1985.

Houpt, K. A., and Wolski, T. R. Domestic animal behavior for veterinarians and animal scientists. Ames: Iowa State University Press, 1982.

Hubbert, W. T., McCulloch, W. F., and Schnurrenberger, P. R., eds. Diseases Transmitted from Animals to Man. 6th ed. Springfield, IL: Charles C Thomas, 1975.

Jewell, P. A., and Loizos, C., eds. Play, Exploration, and Territory in Mammals. New York: Academic Press, 1966.

Joshua, J. O. Abnormal behavior in cats. In Fox, M. W., ed. Abnormal Behavior in Animals. Philadelphia: W. B. Saunders Co., 1968.

Kleiman, D. G., and Eisenberg, J. F. Comparisons of canid and felid social systems from an evolutionary perspective. Anim. Behav. 21:637, 1973.

Kršiak, M., and Steinberg, H. Psychopharmacological aspects of aggression: A review of the literature and some new experiments. J. Psychosom. Res. 13:243, 1969.

Langworthy, O. R. Behavioral disturbances related to the decomposition of reflex activity caused by cerebral injury: An experimental study of the cat. J. Neuropathol. Exp. Neurol. 3:87, 1944.

Laundré, J. The daytime behaviour of domestic cats in a free-roaming population. Anim. Behav. 25:990, 1977.

Macy, D. W., and Siwe, S. T. The use of ketamine as an oral anesthetic in cats. Fel. Pract. 7:44, Jan. 1977.

Mathews-Cameron, S., and Vogl, J. F. Diazepam treatment of fear-related aggression in a cat. Comp. Anim. Pract. 1:4, 1987.

McDougall, W., and McDougall, K. D. Notes on instinct and intelligence in rats and cats. J. Comp. Psychol. 7:145, 1927.

Mintz, N. L. Demand qualities and social development: Some experiments with puppies and kittens. Lab. Bull. Harv. Univ. 9:12, 1959.

Roldán, E., Alvarez-Pelaez, R., and de Molina, A. F. Electrographic study of the amygdaloid defense response. Physiol. Behav. 13:779, 1974.

Romaniuk, A., Brudzyński, S., and Grońska, J. Comparison of defensive behavior evoked by chemical and electrical stimulation of the hypothalamus in cats. Acta Physiol. Pol. 26:23, 1975.

Rosenblatt, J. S., Turkewitz, G., and Schneirla, T. C. Early socialization in the domestic cat as based on feeding and other relationships between female and young. In Foss, B. M., ed. Determinants of Infant Behavior. New York: John Wiley & Sons, 1961.

Rothfield, L., and Harman, P. J. On the relation of the hippocampal-fornix system to the control of rage responses in cats. J. Comp. Neurol. 101:265, 1954.

Schmidt, J. P. Psychosomatics in veterinary medicine. In Fox, M. W., ed. Abnormal Behavior in Animals. Philadelphia: W. B. Saunders Co., 1968.

Scott, J. P. Aggression. 2nd ed. Chicago: University of Chicago Press, 1975.

Spiegel, E. A., Miller, H. R., and Oppenheimer, M. J. Forebrain and rage reactions. J. Neurophysiol. 3:538, 1940.

Suehsdorf, A. The cats in our lives. National Geographic 125:508, 1964.

Thiessen, D. D., and Rodgers, D. A. Population density and endocrine function. Psychol. Bull. 58:441, 1961.

Tsai, L. S. Peace and cooperation among "natural enemies": Educating a rat-killing cat to cooperate with a hooded rat. Acta Psychol. Taiwan 5:1, 1963.

Wilson, M., Warren, J. M., and Abbott, L. Infantile stimulation, activity and learning by cats. Child Dev. 36:843, 1965.

Winslow, C. N. Patterns of competitive, aggressive, and altruistic behavior in the cat. Psychol. Bull. 38:564, 1941.

Wolski, T. R. Social behavior of the cat. Vet. Clin. North Am. [Small Anim. Pract.] 12:693, 1982.

5

Male Feline Sexual Behavior

Domestication has greatly altered the sexuality of animals, although probably less for cats than for other species. In domestic production, sexual behavior is intensified and controlled so that desired matings can be achieved.

SEXUAL MATURATION

Puberty

Near the time of birth, a surge of testosterone brings about masculinization of neurons that will later direct male feline sexual behavior; however, the Leydig cells remain inactive after this surge until the kitten is about 3 months of age.[73] By 3½ months of age there is sufficient testosterone to initiate the growth of penile spines, which reach full size between 6 and 7 months of age. Growth or recession of the spines has been positively correlated with androgen-dependent mating activity.[4] By 5 months the kitten's cells are mature enough for early spermatogenesis, but usually another 1 or 2 months must pass before spermatozoa can be found in the seminal tubules.[73]

Behavioral sexual maturity, as demonstrated by complete copulations, occurs sometime after sperm enter the seminal tubules, normally between 9 and 12 months. (See Appendix D.) In the wild, cats may not reach this degree of maturity until 18 months of age.[9, 54] Certain patterns associated with sexual behavior appear before true sexual maturity. Young kittens do not commonly mount or neck-grip in social play, but some males begin mounting, performing pelvic thrusts, and neck-gripping as early as 4 months of age (Fig. 5–1). They cannot yet achieve intromission,

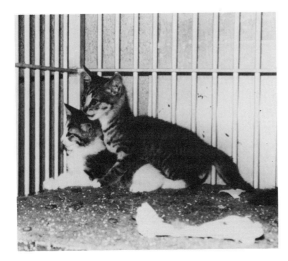

FIGURE 5–1. A 4-month-old male kitten mounting an uncooperative littermate in prepubertal play.

however. Owners frequently are aware of increased roaming, intermale aggression, and scent-marking with urine, all of which accompany the increase in testosterone at puberty.

Reproductive Cycle

Intact males typically leave the homes in which they were raised between 1½ and 3 years of age.[51, 59] They have been called "outcasts" if they settled away from other male cats, and "challengers" if they were peripheral to other toms.[59]

Male cats are regarded as polygamous, fertile, and sexually active throughout the year; however, studies indicate that males do cycle, although not obviously. The sexual activity cycle reaches a peak in the spring and a low point during the late fall in the northern hemisphere, when the female also is naturally nonreceptive.[3, 22, 65] This low point may be noticed behaviorally as only a decreased eagerness to mate, so that in a breeding operation, it is the most difficult time to keep males sufficiently vigorous.[65] Changes in sensory feedback from the penis also have been reported in association with reproductive cycles.[3]

Longevity

Mature male cats are likely not only to show sexual interests beyond their mating capabilities but also to maintain this desire even though reproductive functions may decrease with age.[71] Male behavior usually is evident throughout the animal's adult life and has been observed in cats that are 27 years old.[20, 79]

PREMATING BEHAVIOR

Territorial Effect

Territory is important in male sexual behavior. On arriving at a breeding area, the tomcat spends a variable amount of time investigating it; most toms will not breed in a strange place. The tomcat may require more than a month to become familiar with his new surroundings, although the insecurity usually lasts for only a few days. For the best results, breeders should bring the female to the area with which the male is familiar. If the territory is too small or the tomcat is confined to a small cage, reproductive capacity may be decreased.

Once an area is selected, the tomcat often sprays urine and expels anal sac accumulations. He backs up to objects that are about nose level, extends his pelvic limbs, raises his tail, and sprays (see Fig. 3–16). He may assume a front-end down, rear-end up posture, possibly to spray higher. As urine forcefully leaves the caudally directed penis, the tomcat usually wiggles his tail characteristically.[78] Other locations may be marked by cheek-rubbing.[10, 56, 58] The increased frequency of marking during the mating season may help to reassure the male of his surroundings as well as to attract estrous females, and to reinforce the resident's odor for the benefit of wandering males that seem oblivious to territories. Thus marking is associated with response to psychological disturbances, such as the invasion of territory.

Intermale Aggression

Territorial males become increasingly irritable and protective of their areas during mating season, partly because other males wander great distances, with less recognition of territories, to interact with several groups of females.[22, 59, 76] This increased contact between males results in increased intermale aggression, particularly during encounters between individuals sharing an area, such as in a laboratory. This aggression, which is controlled by testosterone, frequently is violent and even takes precedence over sexual behavior. In a home or laboratory setting, irritability is minimized if tomcats can neither see nor hear estrous females.

After the initial intermale encounter, subsequent meetings usually do not involve fights. This system allows all healthy males a chance to mate an estrous female, although territorial males have the best opportunity, especially for the first mating. Under controlled conditions, one tomcat usually is sufficient for 20 females.[28] Certain territorial males do not permit other males to mate within their area or in their presence, which causes the intruder to flee or become a psychological castrate. An occasional male does not leave home at sexual maturity but usually is restless in the presence of the resident tomcat.[54]

Courtship

For an individual tomcat, the amount of breeding experience and the familiarity with the breeding area are the primary influences on the duration and displays of courtship behavior. This period of mating usually lasts between 10 seconds and 5 minutes and primarily occurs at night. The tomcat initially calls with a loud, harsh vocalization, commonly termed *caterwauling*. This mating or courtship call serves to advertise the tomcat's availability to estrous females and to warn wandering males of his territoriality. Increased roaming and urine spraying also are part of the very early stages of mating.

One to five male cats follow a proestrous female, attracted by olfactory cues from her urine and vaginal secretions or by her vocalizations. One male, the "central male," stays much closer and performs most of the copulations with this female.[59, 60] At some point the male then takes the initiative, using either the facial or the anogenital approach (Fig. 5–2). Thus the chin- and face-rubbing of greeting may be more like courtship behavior than territorial marking.[25] Sniffing the genital area of proestrous and estrous females often results in flehmen, an extension of the head, neck, and upper lip (see Fig. 2–7). The male's flehmen behavior probably makes the female estrous odor more accessible to the openings of the vomeronasal organ. Lack of olfactory ability decreases the time spent smelling the environment and prolongs time used for mating.[5, 23] A softer mating call, which has been described as an imitation of the female's "heat cry," indicates readiness to mate.[75] The male usually circles the female before directly approaching her. More experienced tomcats may

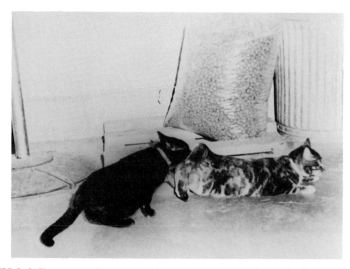

FIGURE 5–2. The anogenital approach of an estrous female by the territorial male.

follow the moderate mating call with running directly to the female and initiating mating behavior.[25, 29, 30] A trained tomcat may run directly to any cat presented in the breeding area and mount, whereas untrained ones may be partial to certain females and ignore others.[9] Only one in three healthy males becomes a vigorous, reliable breeder, and even testosterone is ineffective in increasing low sex drive.[65]

MATING BEHAVIOR

The Neck Grip

Although each tomcat has an individual style, there is a general pattern, and the neck grip is the most consistent behavior (Fig. 5–3). An experienced tomcat achieves the grip within 16 seconds.[77] Biting the skin of the dorsum of the neck is a remnant of behavior in lower animals, which use it to immobilize the female and provide proper orientation for mounting.[25, 79] The neck grip is not a form of male aggression. In fact, the male is extremely inhibited from showing aggression to an estrous female, and the mating neck bite may represent an inhibited form of the predatory neck bite.[27] Even being struck by a proestrous queen does not elicit retaliation. Seldom does the male's bite penetrate the skin, and his balance is shifted too far forward to indicate aggression.[27] The strong inhibition is probably due to the female's low posture, with more weight carried on the forelimbs, representing a signal to mount, not fight.[26, 65] The neck grip has been compared with the way a queen carries her kittens and to the lick-grooming behavior.[49, 57]

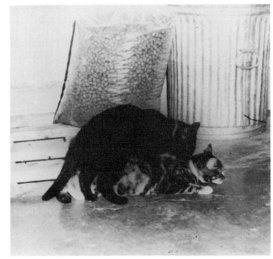

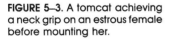

FIGURE 5–3. A tomcat achieving a neck grip on an estrous female before mounting her.

Copulation

The tomcat mounts the female, straddling her with first his forelimbs and then his hindlimbs (Fig. 5–4). The treading or stepping movements of the pelvic limbs help the male to arch his back and move caudally to position his perineal area for successful intromission. Pelvic thrusts, dorsoventral movements of the pelvic region, begin as he nears the proper posture, and the penis becomes erect. Intromission occurs after a final, slightly more forceful thrust, the pelvic lunge. These are followed by ejaculation. The neck grip is released, the penis withdrawn, and the female rapidly dismounted.

The entire mating behavior sequence lasts between 1 and 4 minutes, with experienced males achieving intromission in an average of 1.8 minutes.[77] Intromission-ejaculation-withdrawal takes only 5 to 15 seconds of this period (mean is 8.2 seconds).[65]

Repeated Matings

The pattern of repeated matings between a pair of cats varies considerably with the individuals. After each mating there is a postejaculatory refractory period before the male will mount again. The duration of this latent period varies from 5 to 15 minutes, increasing after each mating, so that the female must play a more active role in courtship. If the repeated matings continue long enough, the male may mount without using the neck grip.[26] The physiologic component of the postejaculatory refractory period is relatively constant because it has to do with the neural regulation of mating. The psychological portion is primarily responsible for the changes in refractory time.[37, 43] Mating enthusiasm can be renewed by introducing a new estrous female during the psycho-

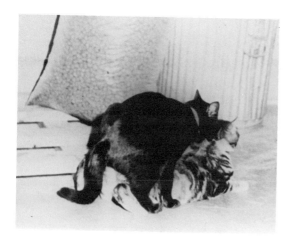

FIGURE 5–4. The breeding posture of the male cat.

logical phase. Otherwise, the fatigue will dissipate within 24 hours. The average number of intromissions per hour is 5.3, with 8.9 mounts during that time.[8] The frequency of copulations usually does not exceed 15 per 24 hours.[59, 60]

Miscellaneous Influences

Although experienced tomcats are eager to mate and may mount anything presented, rape is rare.[58] The female's presentation of an elevated perineum is almost physically essential for intromission to occur.

A male to be used as a stud can be trained through habituation to mount and mate an artificial vagina.[65] To condition a tomcat to mate quickly in a colony, one should bring receptive females to him in a special area, allow several matings, and then remove the female first.[49]

POSTMATING BEHAVIOR

Postmating behavior varies because of the latent period, but the tomcat begins by leaping away from the female's striking "after-reaction," which may be accompanied by her growling.[25] The male then licks his penis and forepaws before he goes to sit near the female, but out of her clawing distance.

Seldom is a pair bond of long duration formed. The tomcat often remains with the female only during a few matings, though some males extend that time for one estrous period. Seldom does a bond last between estrous cycles.

PATERNAL BEHAVIOR

Although most males show little interest in newborn kittens, there are some that do. This paternal behavior probably is seen more in the Siamese breed, where the tomcats lie with and groom the young.[9] At the other extreme are tomcats that indiscriminately kill the kittens. This behavior may be an inherited predisposition for bringing the female back into estrus so that the next litter would be sired by that male.[40] Infanticide is not common in domestic cats, possibly because the female does not return to estrus faster. This is in contrast to the large cats, to which domestic ones often are compared.[67] A more likely explanation is that the size and shape of the newborn approximate those of natural prey. This appearance, then, initiates the normal prey-killing instincts of the male, which does not have the hormonal inhibiting influence.

NEURAL REGULATION

The Brain

The relation of the brain to male sexual behavior has received a great deal of study. As expected, the limbic system, specifically the medial preoptic-rostral hypothalamic region, is primarily responsible. Bilateral ablation of these hypothalamic areas eliminates mounting and pelvic thrusts, a result that is not affected by testosterone.[33, 47] Bilateral removal of the neocortex produces variable results, which probably reflect disturbances in motor coordination rather than deficits in mating behavior. Because these motor capabilities are more important for male mating behavior than for female mating or maternal behavior, differences associated with neocortical control probably reflect the differences in motor needs rather than true sexual neurologic differences.[15]

Neural and Hormonal Interrelations

The complex interrelation between the brain and body hormones complicated many early reports. The late prenatal or neonatal kitten receives a surge of testosterone, which masculinizes the brain. Without this surge, the infant develops female behavior patterns and responds primarily to female hormones. The differences between males and females are relative for many behaviors, even though they are under hormonal control. At maturity there are three levels of hormonal control.[38] Certain hypothalamic nuclei produce gonadotropin-releasing factors that go to the pituitary gland. At the rostral lobe of the pituitary gland these releasing factors cause production of the gonadotropins: follicle-stimulating hormone (FSH) and luteinizing hormone (LH). FSH and LH work at the testes, where FSH stimulates the production of sperm cells and LH stimulates testosterone production by interstitial cells. Negative feedback mechanisms regulate hypothalamic production so that low FSH or LH levels are stimulatory. In castrates, these levels are therefore quite high.[38]

At puberty maturing interstitial cells begin producing adult levels of testosterone, which initiates male behaviors from the premasculinized brain. Regions of the hypothalamus contain and respond to concentrations of testosterone. Specific androgen-related behaviors include male sexual behavior, intermale aggression, and scent-marking patterns.

The Spinal Cord and Peripheral Nerves

Part of the male's sexual behavior is mediated by specific segments of the spinal cord. Spinal transection in the thoracic region may partially affect posturing but not the capacity for erection and ejaculation or associated caudosacral responses.[7, 19] Erection can be induced by stimulation of the second sacral nerve; ejaculation is mediated by the lumbosacral spinal cord at the internal pudendal nerves and triggered by tactile stimulation of the penile body by way of the dorsal nerve of the penis.[6, 37, 38, 69] Androgens intensify low spinal reflexes.[6]

Sympathetic fibers, by way of the hypogastric nerves, cause erection to subside and stop emission of prostatic fluids into the urethra, but the exact roles of the autonomic nervous system are not clearly defined.[6]

MALE SEXUAL BEHAVIOR PROBLEMS

Intact Male Behavior Problems

Much of the normal behavior of the intact male cat may be objectionable to the owner. The male sprays urine mainly to mark its territory, particularly during mating season, and its strong odor is offensive to humans. The increased activity associated with the mating season can result in a house cat that is difficult to live with or that is subject to injuries. Mating behavior also can be undesirable under a bedroom window at night.

Each of these behaviors is enhanced by postpubertal androgens, and castration is therefore the treatment of choice. Male cats castrated as adults may show a rapid decrease, a gradual decrease over about 3 months, or no decrease at all in sexually related fighting, roaming, and/or spraying, despite essentially undetectable blood testosterone levels by 6 hours after surgery.[35, 41, 44, 75]

Changes in mating behavior after castration can be divided into three types: rapid, gradual, and minimal decline. All three are characterized first by the disappearance of intromission, followed by increasingly longer mounts, and then by only short mounts without the neck bite, stepping, or pelvic thrusts. The first of the three types of changes involves disappearance of all sexual behavior shortly after castration.[68] The second type, gradual decline, is characterized by the cessation of intromissions within 2 to 3 months after surgery, although mounting persists for several more months.[37] In the third type of change, initial decrease in frequency of intromissions occurs, but sexual behavior persists for 8 months to 3½ years, while mounting continues indefinitely. Penile sensory thresholds are unaltered by castration.[21]

Sexual experience preceding castration has some influence on how long mating behavior is retained after surgery, indicating that a learning component is involved in sexual behavior. This is not a predictor of the success of surgery in stopping the behavior.[41, 45] Other male behaviors respond independently of age and sexual experience. Prepubertal castration usually prevents androgen-dependent behavior, and the cat does not ordinarily develop other secondary sexual characteristics, such as the thicker skin of the cheeks and neck. In addition, body weight may increase by the addition of a subcutaneous fat layer, especially in the inguinal region.[55]

Progestins usually can control such undesirable behaviors as roaming, fighting, and spraying in cats that do not change behaviors with castration or that cannot be castrated for some reason. As long as the initiating stimulus is present, the objectionable behavior resumes as soon as hormonal therapy is discontinued. Progestins counter male behaviors because they are both antiandrogenic and tranquilizing, possibly because of their suppression of neural components normally responsive to testosterone.[17, 36, 39] The antiandrogenic effect includes decreased spermatogenesis and a lowered social status; thus the use of progestins in a breeding tomcat should be discouraged.[17, 36, 53] Medroxyprogesterone acetate (Depo-Provera; 25 to 100 mg I.M. or S.C.) can remain effective up to 2 months, and is most effective when given at the higher dosage levels. Megestrol acetate (Ovaban, Megace; 0.5 to 1.0 mg/kg/day P.O. for 7 days; then either the same dose on alternate days P.O. for 7 days, or 0.25 to 0.5 mg/kg/day P.O. for 7 days; and finally 0.25 to 0.5 mg/kg P.O. every 2 to 3 days, as needed for maintenance) has been used instead of medroxyprogesterone acetate or if the cat is refractory to the former. These two progestins are successful in about one-third of the cases in which the problem is spraying or urine-marking, and are more successful in males and in animals from single-cat homes.[42] Administering delmadinone acetate (0.25 to 2.0 mg/kg P.O. for 7 to 14 days, or 10 to 20 mg/kg S.C.) results in similar changes, and normal male behaviors return within a few months.[31, 52, 53] Methyloestrenolone (Orgasteron; 5 to 10 mg per cat P.O. t.i.d. for 7 days, or 50 to 75 mg per cat for 5 days S.C., and then 5 mg per cat P.O. once daily as needed for maintenance for several days) is another drug that has been successful at controlling spraying.[32] In addition, chlormadinone acetate has been useful in doses similar to those of megestrol acetate, estopheral, and delmadinone acetate.[53, 72] Observed side effects of short-term use of progestins in the males are increased appetite and food intake. Long-term use has several potentially serious side effects and seldom is indicated.[13, 50]

Other factors also may affect a tomcat's sexual behavior. Experienced queens may show aggressive tendencies and inhibit a tomcat, whereas catnip may increase the male's sexual aggression.[18, 73] Population density also is known to affect reproduction. In addition to increased suprarenal (adrenal) activity, crowding negatively affects gonadal function.[74]

Tomcat urine is noted for its distinctive odor, which apparently is testosterone-dependent.[78] This odor, useful to mark territories and facilitate estrus in females, may be a pheromone or sulphur compound.[1, 16] It is present in bladder urine, and so may be the sulphur-containing amino acid felinine, which enters urine through the kidneys.[1] Castration minimizes the odor, and other products help to reduce it when surgery is not feasible. Cleaning compounds that contain ammonia should not be used to clean up areas with cat urine because the ammonia of the cleanser is the same as that of the urine. Newer products specifically made to break up the source of urine odors, such as Cat-Off, F.O.N., and Outright, work best, although a fine mist of Scope mouthwash, a scrubbing with Massengill's Douche Powder, or certain rug cleaners work just as well.[11]

Castrated Male Behavior Problems

Castrated male cats have been known to suddenly show male sexual behaviors, including spraying, fighting, mounting, neck grips, pelvic thrusting, and erection, after a period without them. There are several causal factors for each behavior, but all are based on neonatal masculinizing of the brain, which makes the cat neurologically male. Sexually dimorphous behaviors are primarily dependent on serum testosterone levels, but can be learned or activated by certain intense environmental stimuli such as invasion of territory. Notably, about 10 per cent of all cats castrated retain behaviors associated with intact tomcats.

Testosterone administration to castrated cats results in resumption of typical male behaviors, but there are individual differences, based primarily on the cat's precastration experience. Although testosterone is not likely to be administered clinically, anabolic steroids might be. These steroids can be metabolized into progesterone and into testosterone, which can produce male behaviors.[10] Because of the progesterone pathway, anabolic agents have been successfully used to limit typical male behaviors.[66] Results of this usage are not predictable.

Resumption of male behaviors by castrated individuals can be controlled by progestins. Provided the psychological frustration causing the male behavior is removed, the cat should continue normal behavior once the drug has worn off. Tension-relieving drugs, such as the benzodiazepine group of tranquilizers, may work as well or better because they reduce situational anxieties.[61]

Hypersexuality

Hypersexuality includes five feline behaviors: (1) male cats indiscriminately mounting male cats, (2) multiple mounting, (3) mounting of small kittens, (4) tenaciously clinging to females during copulation, and (5) masturbation.[64]

The mounting of male cats by male cats, although frequently observed, seldom represents true homosexual behavior because tomcats prefer female sexual partners if females are available. A dominant territorial male may mount any cat that enters his territory. The visiting cat, whether male or female, crouches with partial lordosis while the resident male mounts, treads, and neck-grips. The resident male that is placed in the visiting male's territory shows lordosis while the previously mounted cat mounts him.[65, 75] This activity is common between male kittens at about 3 months of age, but the presence of an estrous female usually stops it. Experimental depletion of serotonin from the feline brain has caused males to mount other males; however, pretreatment with chlordiazepoxide (Librium) at doses that do not interfere with muscle activity prevents this behavior.[70] Tomcats housed under a great deal of sexual stress might be managed by pretreatment with this drug.

The remaining four categories of hypersexual behavior usually are seen in confined tomcats that have no access to an estrous female. These behaviors have been linked to specific brain lesions, but all can be observed in situations of environmental deprivation. Cats that are not used as breeding animals can be spared much of this trauma by castration. The threshold stimulus to mate decreases under experimentally deprived conditions to the point that a minimal stimulus can elicit mating. Inappropriate mating can occur spontaneously if the tomcat does not mate for a prolonged time. As a result, a normal behavior is expressed in atypical situations. Multiple mountings of males by males, the mounting of young kittens, which normally do not initiate the mating response, the mounting of other species, the clinging to females during copulation to the point that attempts to pull them apart result in both being suspended in midair, masturbation, and the mounting of inanimate objects are expressions of this depressed threshold stimulus. Each aberrant mounting can be self-perpetuating, and erection, occasionally with ejaculation, can result.

Masturbation and the mounting of inanimate objects usually develop in young, isolated males or when young males are housed in pairs.[64, 65] As complaints, they are more common in castrated males.[12] A house cat usually chooses to mount a furry toy. Masturbation is more common in laboratory animals, and frequently is accomplished by rubbing the perineal area on the cage floor in a pendulum manner or rubbing the area against the front feet.[56]

Although spontaneous emissions are uncommon, a case has been reported.[2, 9]

Genetic Problems

Three genetically determined conditions are known to affect the tomcat's ability to mate. Male tortoiseshell and calico cats are almost always sterile, and show no interest in estrous females. These XXY individuals may be treated like kittens by their peers.[24] A few males of these colors are fertile, however, and express normal libido.

The dominant autosomal W gene associated with the blue-eyed white cat produces semisterility. This effect is natural selection against this gene, which produces deaf, semisterile, poorly sighted cats that also have a lowered disease resistance.[14]

Cryptorchidism is rare in the cat, and thus has not been well studied. Strong evidence exists, especially in other species, that the condition may be heritable.[63] Retained testicles produce testosterone but not sperm cells, so that a bilaterally affected male acts like an intact tomcat but cannot produce offspring. A unilaterally affected tomcat can produce male offspring that may or may not have the trait and female offspring that may be carriers of the trait.

Other Problems

Some males show persistent mounting with intense, prolonged pelvic thrusting but no intromission. In some cases that is due to the formation of a hair ring around the base of the glans penis.[34, 37, 46, 48] Sometimes the caudally directed penile spines collect hair from the female's perineum, which may not have been removed by normal grooming. In other tomcats the problem might be due to improper pelvic orientation, which usually results from lack of experience.

Feminizing syndromes are rare in male cats but have been reported.[62] In male cats so affected several possibilities should be considered: a genetic XXY male, a true hermaphrodite, a female pseudohermaphrodite, a cat with a Sertoli cell tumor, especially if it has a retained testicle, and a cat that has had massive female hormonal therapy in the past.

Unusually low testosterone levels might play a role in lack of libido, but once the brain has been masculinized in the kitten, very low concentrations are necessary to activate libido and other male behaviors in the adult.[49]

CASE PRESENTATIONS

CASE 5–1. Six-year-old Siamese neutered male. The cat was part of the family since it was a kitten, and stayed outdoors about 50 per cent of the time. There were two other cats, one of which came after the problem started. Although the male cat occasionally used the litter box, he usually sprayed the house. The owners thought that the problem had started when a stray tomcat sprayed outside the window. Other than an occasional forelimb lameness, the cat had had no health problems.

Medical Workup. The physical examination and laboratory data were normal; however, the urine was noted to have a particularly strong odor. Subsequently his serum testosterone level was found to be almost that expected from intact tomcats.

Diagnosis. Territorial marking.

Treatment. Either medroxyprogesterone acetate (100 mg I.M.) or megestrol acetate (5 mg P.O.) controls the behavior, although it returns if medication is discontinued. In this case the owners chose to continue the hormonal therapy, knowing the long-term complications, so the megestrol acetate was reduced to the lowest dose that will control the cat's behavior. For these owners the only alternative to the hormones was euthanasia.

CASE 5–2. Six-year-old Persian male. The cat was odd-eyed, deaf, and white, with questionable olfactory abilities. This tomcat knew when a female was in estrus, but much of its mating behavior was abnormal. It did not mount and did not get a good neck grip. In addition, during courtship, it used both its fore paws and its teeth roughly, almost to the point of "beating up" the female. It had been caged so that it could observe normal matings and had been paired with experienced females.

Diagnosis. Abnormal mating behavior possibly related to genetic factors.

Treatment. None. Tranquilizers had no effect on the courtship or mating behaviors.

CASE 5–3. Three-and-one-half-year-old Persian male. The cat was kept in a house with three females and another male cat. The second tomcat was much older and the dominant animal in the territory. Because the owners were small-scale Persian breeders, estrous females occasionally were brought into the group, but at no time had the younger tomcat shown any male sexual behaviors, not even spraying.

Diagnosis. Psychological castration.

Treatment. The cat was given to another owner who had no cats, and within a year normal male behaviors had appeared, including mating with strange estrous females.

CASE 5–4. Eight-month-old Siamese-cross neutered male. Castration was done 3 months earlier, and since the surgery, this cat had started jumping on the legs of the owners and riding them. According to the owners, the cat also had started mounting stuffed toys and ended up urinating on them.

Diagnosis. Masturbation with ejaculation.

Treatment. Because the behavior had its own measure of reward for the animal, the degree of dissatisfaction must become greater than the reward. The cat was kept in an environment without things that seemed to trigger the masturbation except under controlled situations. The owners kept a water squirt bottle handy for punishment. In addition, the cat was given a 3-week reducing-dose treatment of megestrol acetate. Within 1 month the owners reported a gradual reduction of the behavior to their satisfaction.

CASE 5–5. Three-year-old domestic shorthair neutered male. During 2 weeks the owners noticed this cat masturbating on a pillow at least once a day. After they took the pillow away, the cat continued the behavior on the owner's leg whenever possible.

Diagnosis. Masturbation.

Treatment. Megestrol acetate (5 mg P.O. once daily) did not produce any change in the frequency of the behavior within 5 days, and the cat was becoming afraid of the owners because they carried a water squirt bottle for punishment. These results were not desirable to the owners, so it was decided to let the cat have access to the pillow again in an area where the owners were not likely to have to watch the behavior.

Also see cases 3–1, 4–4, 4–18, and 4–20.

REFERENCES

1. Albone, E. S.: Mammalian Semiochemistry: The Investigation of Chemical Signals between Mammals. New York: John Wiley & Sons, 1984.
2. Aronson, L. R.: Behavior resembling spontaneous emission in the domestic cat. J. Comp. Physiol. Psychol. 42:226, 1949.
3. Aronson, L. R., and Cooper, M. L.: Seasonal changes in mating behavior in cats after desensitization of glans penis. Science 152:226, 1966.
4. Aronson, L. R., and Cooper, M. L.: Penile spines of the domestic cat: Their endocrine-behavior relations. Anat. Rec. 157:71, 1967.
5. Aronson, L. R., and Cooper, M. L.: Olfactory deprivation and mating behavior in sexually experienced male cats. Behav. Biol. 11:459, 1974.
6. Beach, F. A.: Hormones and Behavior. New York: Cooper Square Publishers, 1961.
7. Beach, F. A.: Cerebral and hormonal control of reflexive mechanisms involved in copulatory behavior. Physiol. Rev. 47:289, 1967.
8. Beach, F. A., Zitrin, A., and Jaynes, J.: Neural mediation of mating in male cats. I. Effects of unilateral and bilateral removal of the neocortex. J. Comp. Physiol. Psychol. 49:321, 1956.
9. Beadle, M.: The Cat: History, Biology, and Behavior. New York: Simon & Schuster, 1977.
10. Beaver, B. V.: Mating behavior in the cat. Vet. Clin. North Am. 7:729, 1977.
11. Beaver, B. V.: The marking behavior of cats. Vet. Med./Small Anim. Clinician 76:792, 1981.
12. Beaver, B. V.: Feline behavioral problems other than housesoiling. J. Am. Anim. Hosp. Assoc. 25:465, 1989.
13. Beaver, B. V.: Disorders of behavior. In Sherding, R. G., ed.: The Cat: Diseases and Clinical Management. New York: Churchill Livingstone, 1989.
14. Bigbee, H. G.: Personal communication, 1977.
15. Bjursten, L. M., Norrsell, K., and Norrsell, U.: Behavioural repertory of cats without cerebral cortex from infancy. Exp. Brain Res. 25:115, 1976.

16. Bland, K. P.: Tom-cat odour and other pheromones in feline reproduction. Vet. Sci. Commun. 3:125, 1979.
17. Blumer, D., and Migeon, C.: Hormone and hormonal agents in the treatment of aggression. J. Nerv. Ment. Dis. 160:127, 1975.
18. Bryant, D.: The Care and Handling of Cats. New York: Ives Washburn, 1944.
19. Campbell, B., Good, C. A., and Kitchell, R. L.: Neural mechanisms in sexual behavior. I. Reflexology of sacral segments of cat. Proc. Soc. Exp. Biol. Med. 86:423, 1954.
20. Comfort, A.: Maximum ages reached by domestic cats. J. Mammal. 37:118, 1956.
21. Cooper, K. K., and Arnson, L. R.: Effects of castration on neural afferent responses from the penis of the domestic cat. Physiol. Behav. 12:93, 1974.
22. Dards, J. L.: The behaviour of dockyard cats: Interactions of adult males. Appl. Anim. Ethol. 10:133, 1983.
23. Doty, R. L.: Mammalian Olfaction, Reproductive Processes, and Behavior. New York: Academic Press, 1976.
24. Ehrman, L., and Parons, P. A.: The Genetics of Behavior. Sunderland, MA: Sinauer Associates, 1976.
25. Ewer, R. F.: Ethology of Mammals. London: Paul Elek, Ltd., 1968.
26. Ewer, R. F.: The Carnivores. Ithaca, NY: Cornell University Press, 1973.
27. Ewer, R. F.: Viverrid behavior and the evolution of reproductive behavior in the Felidae. In Eaton, R. L., ed.: The World's Cats. Seattle: Feline Research Group, 1974.
28. Fox, M. W.: Natural environment: Theoretical and practical aspects for breeding and rearing laboratory animals. Lab. Anim. Care 16:316, 1966.
29. Fox, M. W.: Understanding Your Cat. New York: Coward, McCann & Geoghegan, 1974.
30. Fox, M. W.: The behaviour of cats. In Hafez, E. S. E., ed.: The Behaviour of Domestic Animals. 3rd ed. Baltimore: Williams & Wilkins, 1975.
31. Gerber, H. A., Jöchle, W., and Sulman, F. G.: Control of reproduction and of undesirable social and sexual behaviour in dogs and cats. J. Small Anim. Pract. 14:151, 1973.
32. Gerber, H. A., and Sulman, F. G.: The effect of methyloestrenolone on oestrus, pseudopregnancy, vagrancy, satyriasis, and squirting in dogs and cats. Vet. Rec. 76:1089, 1964.
33. Hart, B. L.: Abolition of mating behavior in male cats with lesions in the medial preoptic-anterior hypothalamic region. Am. Zool. 10:296, 1970.
34. Hart, B. L.: Gonadal hormones and behavior of the male cat. Fel. Pract. 2:7, May-June 1972.
35. Hart, B. L.: Behavioral effects of castration. Fel. Pract. 3:10, Mar.-Apr. 1973.
36. Hart, B. L.: Behavioral effects of long-acting progestins. Fel. Pract. 4:8, July-Aug. 1974.
37. Hart, B. L.: Normal behavior and behavioral problems associated with sexual function, urination, and defecation. Vet. Clin. North Am. 4:589, 1974.
38. Hart, B. L.: Physiology of sexual function. Vet. Clin. North Am. 4:557, 1974.
39. Hart, B. L.: Medication for control of spraying. Fel. Pract. 7:16, May 1977.
40. Hart, B. L.: The client asks you: A quiz on feline behavior. Fel. Pract. 8:10, Mar. 1978.
41. Hart, B. L.: Problems with objectionable sociosexual behavior of dogs and cats: Therapeutic use of castration and progestins. Comp. Cont. Educ. Small Anim. Pract. 1:461, 1979.
42. Hart, B. L.: Objectionable urine spraying and urine marking in cats: Evaluation of progestin treatment in gonadectomized males and females. J. Am. Vet. Med. Assoc. 177:529, 1980.
43. Hart, B. L.: The Behavior of Domestic Animals. New York: W. H. Freeman & Co., 1985.
44. Hart, B. L., and Barrett, R. E.: Effects of castration on fighting, roaming, and urine spraying in adult male cats. J. Am. Vet. Med. Assoc. 163:290, 1973.
45. Hart, B. L., and Cooper, L.: Factors relating to urine spraying and fighting in prepubertally gonadectomized cats. J. Am. Vet. Med. Assoc. 184:1255, 1984.
46. Hart, B. L., and Hart, L. A.: Canine and Feline Behavioral Therapy. Philadelphia: Lea & Febiger, 1985.
47. Hart, B. L., Haugen, C. M., and Peterson, D. M.: Effects of medial preoptic-anterior hypothalamic lesions on mating behavior of male cats. Brain Res. 54:177, 1973.
48. Hart, B. L., and Peterson, D. M.: Penile hair rings in male cats may prevent mating. Lab. Anim. Sci. 21:422, 1971.

49. Hart, B. L., and Voith, V. L.: Sexual behavior and breeding problems in cats. Fel. Pract. 7:9, Jan. 1977.
50. Henik, R. A., Olson, P. N., and Rosychuk, R. A.: Progestogen therapy in cats. Comp. Cont. Educ. 7:132, 1985.
51. Houpt, K. A., and Wolski, T. R.: Domestic Animal Behavior for Veterinarians and Animal Scientists. Ames: Iowa State University Press, 1982.
52. Jöchle, W.: Progress in small animal reproductive physiology, therapy of reproductive disorders, and pet population control. Folia Vet. Lat. 4:706, 1974.
53. Jöchle, W., and Jöchle, M.: Reproductive and behavioral control in the male and female cats with progestins: Long-term field observations in individual animals. Theriogenology 3:179, 1975.
54. Joshua, J. O.: Abnormal behavior in cats. In Fox, M. W., ed.: Abnormal Behavior in Animals. Philadelphia: W. B. Saunders Co., 1968.
55. Joshua, J. O.: Some conditions seen in feline practice attributable to hormonal causes. Vet. Rec. 88:511, 1971.
56. Kling, A., Kovach, J. K., and Tucker, T. J.: The behaviour of cats. In Hafez, E. S. E., ed.: The Behaviour of Domestic Animals. 2nd ed. Baltimore: Williams & Wilkins Co., 1969.
57. Langworthy, O. R.: Behavioral disturbances related to the decomposition of reflex activity caused by cerebral injury: An experimental study of the cat. J. Neuropathol. Exp. Neurol. 3:87, 1944.
58. Leyhausen, P.: Cat Behavior: The Predatory and Social Behavior of Domestic and Wild Cats. New York: Garland STPM Press, 1978.
59. Liberg, O.: Predation and social behaviour in a population of domestic cat. An evolutionary perspective. Ph.D. diss., Department of Animal Ecology, University of Lund, Sweden, 1981.
60. Liberg, O.: Courtship behaviour and sexual selection in the domestic cat. Appl. Anim. Ethol. 10:117, 1983.
61. Marder, A. R.: Personal communication, 1985.
62. Mason, K. V.: Oestral behaviour in a bilaterally cryptorchid cat. Vet. Rec. 99:296, 1976.
63. McFarland, C., Herron, M., Burke, R. J., and Richkind, M.: Cryptorchidism and fertility. Fel. Pract. 8:14, 1978.
64. Michael, R. P.: "Hypersexuality" in male cats without brain damage. Science 134:553, 1961.
65. Michael, R. P.: Observations upon the sexual behavior in the domestic cat (*Felis catus* L.) under laboratory conditions. Behaviour 18:1, 1961.
66. Mosier, J. E.: Common medical and behavioral problems in cats. Mod. Vet. Pract. 56:699, 1975.
67. Natoli, E.: Mating strategies in cats: A comparison of the role and importance of infanticide in domestic cats, *Felis catus* L., and lions, *Panthera leo* L. Anim. Behav. 40:183, 1990.
68. Rosenblatt, J. S., and Aronson, L. R.: The decline of sexual behavior in male cats after castration with special reference to the role of prior sexual experience. Behaviour 12:285, 1958.
69. Semans, J. H., and Langworthy, O. R.: Observations on the neurophysiology of sexual function in the male cat. J. Urol. 40:836, 1938.
70. Sheard, M. H.: Lithium in the treatment of aggression. J. Nerv. Ment. Dis. 160:108, 1975.
71. Smithcors, J. F.: Sexual capacity of males. Mod. Vet. Pract. 58:579, 1977.
72. Stansbury, R. L.: Altered behavior in castrated male cats. Mod. Vet. Pract. 46:68, July 1965.
73. Stein, B. S.: The genital system. In Catcott, E. J., ed.: Feline Medicine and Surgery. 2nd ed. Santa Barbara, CA: American Veterinary Publications, 1975.
74. Thiessen, D. D., and Rodgers, D. A.: Population density and endocrine function. Psychol. Bull. 58:441, 1961.
75. Todd, N. B.: Behavior and genetics of the domestic cat. Cornell Vet. 53:99, 1963.
76. Weigel, I.: Small cats and clouded leopards. In Grzimek, H. C. B., ed.: Grzimek's Animal Life Encyclopedia. Vol. 12. New York: Van Nostrand Reinhold Co., 1975.
77. Whalen, R. E.: Sexual behavior of cats. Behaviour 20:321, 1963.
78. Whitehead, J. E.: Tomcat spraying. Mod. Vet. Pract. 46:68, Feb. 1965.

79. Worden, A. N.: Abnormal behaviour in the dog and cat. Vet. Rec. 71:966, 1959.

ADDITIONAL READINGS

Andy, O. J. Catecholamine effects on limbic induced hypersexuality. Anat. Rec. 187:525, 1977.

Bard, P., and Macht, M. B. The behaviour of chronically decerebrate cats. In Wolstenholme, G. E. W., and O'Connor, C. M., eds. Neurological Basis of Behaviour. Boston: Little, Brown & Co., 1952.

Barton, A. Sexual inversion and homosexuality in dogs and cats. Vet. Med. (Praha) 54:155, 1959.

Beach, F. A., Zitrin, A., and Jaynes, J. Neural mediation of mating in male cats. II. Contributions of the frontal cortex. J. Exp. Zool. 130:381, 1956.

Beaver, B. V. Feline behavioral problems. Vet. Clin. North Am. 6:333, 1976.

Beaver, B. V., Terry, M. L., and LaSagna, C. L. Effectiveness of products in eliminating cat urine odors from carpet. J. Am. Vet. Med. Assoc. 194:1589, 1989.

Bergsma, D. R., and Brown, K. S. White fur, blue eyes, and deafness in the domestic cat. J. Hered. 62:171, 1971.

Boudreau, J. C., and Tsuchitani, C. Sensory Neurophysiology. New York: Van Nostrand Reinhold Co., 1973.

Brunner, F. The application of behavior studies in small animal practice. In Fox, M. W., ed. Abnormal Behavior in Animals. Philadelphia: W. B. Saunders Co., 1968.

Burke, T. J. Feline reproduction. Vet. Clin. North Am. 6:317, 1976.

Chalifoux, A., and Gosselin, Y. The use of megestrol acetate to stop urine spraying in castrated male cats. Can. Vet. J. 22:211, 1981.

Cooper, K. K. Cutaneous mechanoreceptors of the glans penis of the cat. Physiol. Behav. 8:793, 1972.

Dunbar, I. F. Behaviour of castrated animals. Vet. Rec. 96:92, 1975.

Eleftheriou, B. E., and Scott, J. P. The Physiology of Aggression and Defeat. New York: Plenum Publishing Corp., 1971.

Fox, M. W. Ethology: An overview. In Fox, M. W., ed. Abnormal Behavior in Animals. Philadelphia: W. B. Saunders Co., 1968.

Fox, M. W. The veterinarian: Mercenary, Saint Francis—or humanist? J. Am. Vet. Med. Assoc. 166:276, 1975.

Gessa, G. L., and Tagliamonte, A. Role of brain monoamines in male sexual behavior. Life Sci. 14:425, 1974.

Green, J. D., Clemente, C. D., and DeGroot, J. Rhinencephalic lesions and behavior in cats. J. Comp. Neurol. 108:505, 1957.

Hagamen, W. D., Zitzmann, E. K., and Reeves, A. G. Sexual mounting of diverse objects in a group of randomly selected, unoperated male cats. J. Comp. Physiol. Psychol. 56:298, 1963.

Hart, B. L. The brain and behavior. Fel. Pract. 3:4, Sept.-Oct. 1973.

Hart, B. L. Types of aggressive behavior. Can. Pract. 1:6, May-June 1974.

Hart, B. L. Gonadal androgen and sociosexual behavior of male mammals: A comparative analysis. Psychol. Bull. 81:383, 1974.

Hart, B. L. Behavioral patterns related to territoriality and social communication. Fel. Pract. 5:12, Jan.-Feb. 1975.

Hart, B. L. Spraying behavior. Fel. Pract. 5:11, July-Aug. 1975.

Hart, B. L. Quiz on feline behavior. Fel. Pract. 6:10, May 1976.

Hart, B. L. Behavioral aspects of raising kittens. Fel. Pract. 6:8, Nov. 1976.

Hart, B. L. Aggression in cats. Fel. Pract. 7:22, Mar. 1977.

Hart, B. L. Olfaction and feline behavior. Fel. Pract. 7:8, Sept. 1977.

Kleiman, D. G., and Eisenberg, J. F. Comparisons of canid and felid social systems from an evolutionary perspective. Anim. Behav. 21:637, 1973.

Kuo, Z. Y. Studies on the basic factors in animal fighting. VII. Interspecies coexistence in mammals. J. Genet. Psychol. 97:211, 1960.

Levinson, B. M. Man and his feline pet. Mod. Vet. Pract. 53:35, Nov. 1972.

Leyhausen, P. The communal organization of solitary mammals. Sump. Zool. Soc. Lond. 14:249, 1965.

Marvin, C. Hormonal influences on the development and expression of sexual behavior in animals. In Fox, M. W., ed. Abnormal Behavior in Animals. Philadelphia: W. B. Saunders Co., 1968.

Michael, R. P. Sexual behaviour and the vaginal cycle in the cat. Nature 181:567, 1958.

Mykytowycz, R. Reproduction of mammals in relation to environmental odours. J. Reprod. Fertil. 19 (Suppl.):433, 1973.

Pfaff, D. W. Interactions of steroid sex hormones with brain tissue: Studies of uptake and physiological effects. In Segal, S. J., ed. The Regulation of Mammalian Reproduction. Springfield, IL: Charles C Thomas, 1973.

Romatowski, J. Use of megestrol acetate in cats. J. Am. Vet. Med. Assoc. 194:700, 1989.

Rosenblatt, J. S. Effects of experience on sexual behavior in male cats. In Beach, F. A., ed. Sex and Behavior. New York: John Wiley & Sons, 1965.

Rosenblatt, J. S., and Aronson, L. R. The influence of experience on the behavioural effects of androgen in prepubertally castrated male cats. Anim. Behav. 6:171, 1958.

Schwartz, A. S., and Whalen, R. E. Amygdala activity during sexual behavior in the male cat. Life Sci. 4:1359, 1965.

Scott, P. P. The domestic cat as a laboratory animal for the study of reproduction. J. Physiol. (Lond.) 130:47P, 1955.

Smith, R. C. The Complete Cat Book. New York: Walker & Co., 1963.

Spraying by castrated tomcats. Mod. Vet. Pract. 56:729, 1975.

West, M. Social play in the domestic cat. Am. Zool. 14:427, 1974.

Zitrin, A., Jaynes, J., and Beach, F. A.: Neural mediation of mating in male cats. III. Contributions of occipital, parietal and temporal cortex. J. Comp. Neurol. 105:111, 1956.

6

Female Feline Sexual Behavior

Variability is a normal feature in all phases of female sexual behavior of *Felis catus*, especially among purebreds. Selective breeding for both domestication and breed development has tended to intensify feline sexuality and enhance the diversity of female sexual behaviors.

SEXUAL MATURATION

The developing prenatal or early neonatal kitten that is not exposed to a testosterone surge develops the female nervous system, and at puberty the female behavior characteristics become apparent. The onset of puberty in the cat varies considerably, depending on several factors. For the tame domestic cat, the first signs of estrus appear between 3½ and 12 months of age, usually at 5 to 9 months. (See Appendix D.) Burmese cats are the youngest cycling breed, whereas Persian and free-ranging cats are apt to reach puberty at an older age, even as late as 15 to 18 months.[23, 37] Behavioral signs of the first estrus usually are associated with the physiologic ability to conceive.[6]

Environmental factors can affect the onset of puberty. Most young females that are born early in the season or that are exposed to tomcats, cycling females, or increasing amounts of light show signs of first estrus before similar individuals born later or not exposed to these factors.

REPRODUCTIVE CYCLES

Seasonal Variations

The female cat is seasonally polyestrous and has several estrous cycles during each of its two or three seasons per year. In the latitudes of the

141

United States and Europe, most cats are anestrous from late September through late December or January and may show reduced sexual activity for a few months preceding this period. Seasonal cycle peaks occur between mid-January and early March and between May and June, although they tend to be delayed in the northern latitudes and hastened in the southern. There is a great deal of individual variation, and some cats—particularly short-haired varieties—cycle all year.[12, 36, 37] At the other extreme, a wild cat may have only one seasonal cycle each year, so that more time can be spent teaching skills to the young.[5, 12]

The use of artificial light from September to March to lengthen "daylight" hours has been successful in many colonies to get females to cycle year round.

Estrous Cycle

Anestrus. The anestrous female may rebuff an approaching tomcat by hissing and striking out. If she accepts the tomcat with relative indifference, she flexes her spine when he mounts and covers the perineum tightly with her tail, almost achieving a sitting position instead of the lordosis seen during estrus. The same behavior is exhibited by prepubertal kittens that weigh more than 1500 g, when mounted by a male. Kittens that weigh less than 1000 g remain passive to the neck grip because it resembles the carrying grip used by the queen.[50] The anestrous female also exhibits aggressive behaviors in attempting to free herself from an undesired mounting. Olfactory signals from her vulvar area are repulsive to some tomcats, which quickly turn away after smelling her perineum.[50]

Proestrus. The onset of estrous behavior may seem rather sudden to the owner because of a relatively short proestrous phase. Proestrus lasts between 1 and 3 days, and the associated behavior is highly variable among individuals. It typically begins as a subtle increase in general activity and progresses to increased rubbing against objects, especially with the head and neck. This behavior may prompt owners to report that their cat has become friendlier. Urine spraying may occur.[8] A tomcat's approach no longer results in immediate sexual aggression by the female. Although the male cat's neck grip and mount initially may cause the female to crouch partially and tread temporarily, his advances eventually initiate her aggression. Her rubbing the chin and cheek on objects, including the tomcat, becomes marked within 36 hours of the onset of proestrus, and when done to a person, it may be related to courtship rather than to marking.[19] Rubbing progresses to rolling, either gentle or violent, that usually is associated with purring, rhythmic opening and closing of the claws, squirming, and stretching (Fig. 6–1).[50, 70] Catnip may evoke a similar behavior.

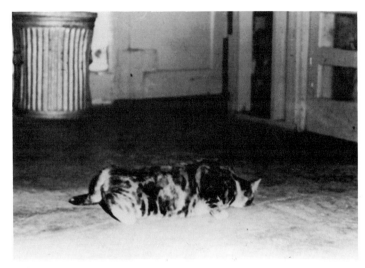

FIGURE 6–1. The characteristic rolling behavior of proestrus and estrus.

The female begins calling to a male, using the "heat cry," a vocalization unique to proestrus and estrus. This sound is a monotone howling that lasts up to 3 minutes at one time. About 12 per cent of the females eventually call continuously, although this behavior is more prevalent in Siamese females. Another 14 per cent vary considerably in the frequency of the call.[37] This cry is mimicked by the tomcat, answered by the female, and again mimicked by the male. The female may spray urine, so that both the urine and the sebaceous secretions left by rubbing serve to attract males, particularly in areas where cats live relatively close together.[19, 75]

Estrus. As the female enters estrus a dramatic change occurs in her behavior toward the male. She still rolls and rubs, but no longer does she aggressively refuse the male's attempts to mount. Instead, she exhibits a crouching lordosis. In this position the ventral thorax and abdomen touch the floor, and the perineum is elevated because the hindlimbs are positioned caudal to the body and extended perpendicular to the ground (Fig. 6–2). This copulatory stance can be induced by stroking the queen's back, thighs, or neck. Her tail is laterally displaced, and there may be a slight amount of sanguineous discharge on the vulva.[70]

The behavioral events of mating begin with appetitive sexual behavior, or courtship. The elaborate courtship behaviors are important because of the basically asocial nature of the animal. To ensure that males will be available and can succeed in intermale competition—although the winner may not be the one she eventually chooses—the female starts advertising before she is fully receptive. This courtship period also helps

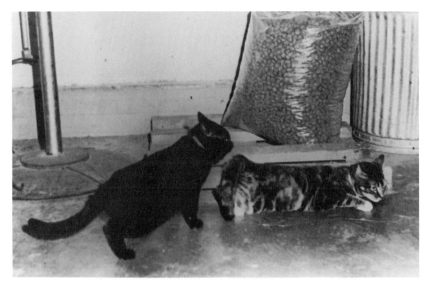

FIGURE 6–2. The natural lordosis posture of an estrous cat.

to give the greatest number of healthy males an equal chance at repro-duction.[42] The female usually sits some distance away from the compe-tition. She may show preference or dislike for an interested male. This choice probably has an olfactory basis, as changes in the nasal mucosa occur in association with the estrous cycle.[52] Evidence indicates that odors affect reproduction in several mammals by means of the nervous and endocrine systems, and theories to the contrary fail to take the learning process into account.[52, 73]

Lordosis, which is necessary if intromission is to occur, can be stimulated by the treading of the mounted male. While the male performs copulatory thrusts, the female adjusts her position slightly by alternate treading with her hindlimbs. During estrus this rhythmic step, as well as the tail deviation, can be initiated by gently tapping the female's peri-neum or flank. During mating behavior the facial expression often is intense, similar to that seen in aggressive cats and some that are fearful. Additionally, the ears are positioned rostrolaterally. The crouching, rubbing, rolling, and treading portions of courtship last between 10 seconds and 5 minutes and are shorter in duration with repeated breedings.[5, 24]

The female's postmating behavior is characteristically dramatic. As the male starts to withdraw his penis after ejaculation, the female's pupils suddenly dilate. As she is freed she utters the copulatory cry, a shrill, piercing vocalization, and then turns aggressively on the male. To a familiar male, the female may be less aggressive and might instead proceed directly into the "after-reaction." During after-reaction, the consummatory portion of the female's sexual behavior, she again rolls on the floor and licks her vulva (Fig. 6–3).

Typical estrous mating behavior resumes in 11 to 95 minutes (mean is 19 minutes). Experienced pairs may mate as frequently as eight times in 20 minutes, or ten times per hour.[5, 23, 24] As mating continues over the next few days, the time between these behaviors becomes longer. The female mating interval decreases, and she becomes more active in encouraging the male to mount. This is particularly true of naive females.[77] Thus the male is primarily responsible for the increased time lapse between breedings. An estrous female can be conditioned to assume the estrous posture whenever she is placed in the mating area, even in the absence of a male.[50, 77]

A mutual attraction between tomcat and queen can last for extended periods. A female usually accepts a number of males during her estrous period, and many litters have multiple sires.[19, 21, 23] Females in proximity to related males are more likely to leave their home areas during estrus than are those without related males nearby.[45] If there is a central tomcat,

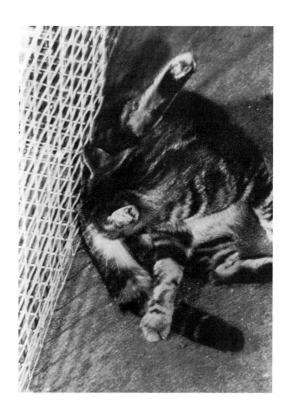

FIGURE 6–3. The female licks her external genitalia after mating.

he is the primary breeder of that female group, even if other peripheral males are courting the females.[44]

Another useful feature in reproduction management of this asocial species is the fact that the cat is an induced ovulator. The estrous female does not ovulate unless mating occurs. Ovulation probably is induced by vaginal stimulation with the male's penile spines or by artificial means, such as with a glass rod. Artificial stimulation requires several insertions of about 10 seconds' duration each, 5 to 10 minutes apart over a 48-hour period. Successful stimulation causes the aggressive after-reaction; however, more than one natural mating may be necessary for conception.[67] The number of ovulation sites on the ovary varies directly with the number of matings, and all follicles leave the ovary at the same time.[21]

Ovulation has been prevented by a systemic shock factor from abdominal surgeries, but only if it occurs within 55 minutes after mating.[2]

The female remains in estrus for 4 to 6 days, a period that may include proestrus and metestrus, and she is most receptive on the 3rd and 4th days if mated during that time. Estrus ends rather abruptly, within 24 hours after coitus. If the cat is pregnant, she usually will not return to estrus again until the next seasonal peak or the next year. However, about 10 per cent of the pregnant queens display estrous behavior and produce a vaginal smear typical of estrus, possibly because of estrogen secretion by the placenta during the 3rd to 6th week of gestation.[3, 65, 69] Mating at this time can result in superfetation.[69] Nursing queens also have been known to exhibit estrus 7 to 10 days after parturition; however, this usually does not occur during lactation, thus not until 6 to 8 weeks after a queen gives birth. It can be delayed as long as 21 weeks.[37, 65] Postpartum estrus has a shorter duration than the initial estrus, averaging 3.8 days.[62]

When no tomcat is present, the female remains in estrus for 10 to 14 days and returns to estrus in 2 to 3 weeks. Although the average estrous cycle is 21 to 29 days, it can vary from 5 to 73 days. Young females exhibit minimal signs, become hyperexcitable, anorectic, or withdrawn and have a shorter estrous period. In contrast, older females continue to cycle, although the interval between estrous periods might increase and duration and intensity of estrous behavior decrease.

Because some of the environmental factors that can affect the onset of puberty in the female also can affect the onset of estrus, the nonpregnant female has been described as being in "potential" estrus during the mating season.[23, 24, 38] The result of exposure to certain factors, such as a tomcat or other cycling females, is the appearance of proestrus and estrus within a few hours to 3 to 4 days and a synchronization with female groups.[44, 45] Valeric acid is plentiful in vaginal secretions during estrus and may be associated with synchronization.[11] Other factors, such as a colony relocation can result in coordinating estrous cycles for 42 per cent to 77 per cent of the females.[78]

Estrous behavior has been controlled with vasectomized male cats. In females mated to such tomcats, estrus lasts for approximately 7 days and is followed by a 36- to 44-day interestrous period of pseudopregnancy.[24, 53, 58] This type of luteinization is rare in the cat without vaginal stimulation.[24]

The behavior of a female cat, her vaginal smear, and her phase in the reproductive cycle are closely correlated. Of the cats exhibiting estrous behavior in one study, 78 per cent had a fully cornified estrous vaginal smear and another 18 per cent were in proestrus.[50]

Metestrus. With the appearance of leukocytes in the vaginal smear, the behavior of metestrus begins.[49] This phase seldom lasts for more than 24 hours and is included in time ranges given for estrus because all of the postural responses continue and mounting is allowed. During this phase the female aggressively rejects the male only when he attempts intromission.

INTERSPECIES MATINGS

Periodically newspaper articles appear about the offspring of cats that have mated with other animals, but most of those articles are not substantiated. A reported cat-rabbit cross that hopped around one town was, in reality, a manx cat with a spinal cord problem. *Felis catus* has 38 diploid chromosomes, as do most of the large cats in the Felidae family.[20, 76] Ocelots are the noted exception, with 36 chromosome pairs. Crosses of domestic cats with larger cats that have 38 chromosome pairs have been reported, but the fertility of the offspring is variable.[26]

PREGNANCY

The uncontrolled female cat is always pregnant, nursing, or both, except possibly in the late fall, and her entire body is geared for these conditions. Thus a female in a home environment where she is not allowed to breed probably is healthier physiologically and psychologically if she is ovariohysterectomized.

Gestation

The duration of gestation in the cat ranges from 60 to 68 days; the average length is 65 to 66 days. Gestation periods of 52 to 71 days have been reported; however, births before 60 days should be regarded as premature because they often are accompanied by a higher than normal rate of stillbirths and early postnatal deaths.[55, 67]

During the last third of pregnancy, obvious behavioral changes occur, although some queens have already been showing increased docility. Along with rapid weight gain, caused primarily by fetal growth, there is an increase in appetite and a decrease in activity and agility. Distention of the mammae also may occur.

In the week immediately preceding parturition, the queen seeks a dark, dry area in which she can remain relatively undisturbed. Ideally, this place also provides shelter from the elements and contains a soft bedding material; it may be a communal nest.[47] Early selection of the nesting area allows time for the area to take on the female's odor, so that she can relax in a familiar environment. This is somewhat similar to the function of sprayed urine in the tomcat's environment. The amount of seclusion preferred by a female during parturition is highly individual. Some seek out human companionship at this time and may choose the owner's bed as the queening area; most prefer seclusion, finding the hayloft of a barn more acceptable. Also during this week the queen drives off kittens from the previous litter that are still with her. After queening, she may accept them back to nurse with her new offspring. During this period before delivery, the queen usually spends an increasing amount of time on self-grooming, particularly of the mammary and perineal areas. This may be due to increased cutaneous sensitivity in those regions.[5, 19, 63] She also may become more irritable or defensive, possibly as a result of the extreme stress associated with this time of pregnancy.

As parturition becomes imminent, the female becomes increasingly restless, digs at the floor or nesting material, and assumes a defecation posture without defecating. There may be calling vocalizations, especially by Siamese cats, and a few queens become excessively anxious and even hysterical.[23]

Parturition

Most births occur at night, often in isolated locations, so parturition is not always observed. Because the cat is multiparous, the four phases normally associated with parturition—contraction, emergence, delivery, and expulsion of the placenta—are repeated several times. A kitten birth terminates at the onset of contractions for the next. With multiparous animals, the delivery of a placenta does not necessarily mark the end of parturition.

Each phase of parturition is highly variable, although the order holds true for most births. The initiation of each phase usually is marked by an abrupt behavioral change, from contractions that trigger genitoabdominal licking to placental delivery that results in the placenta's consumption.

Contraction Phase. During the first phase, contraction, the queen spends a great deal of time licking herself or the newborns already delivered. Contractions of the abdominal musculature are obvious, and probably accompany uterine contractions. Pelvic limb movements by the queen should help to distinguish these abdominal contractions from fetal movements.[63] Other signs of restlessness are present. In addition to squatting and scratching, the queen may circle, rearrange bedding, roll, or rub. She appears uncomfortable and seems to be constantly trying to adjust for some disturbance at the caudal portion of her body, even bracing her body against various objects. The duration of the contraction phase is variable, ranging from 12 seconds to 1½ hours.[16, 63]

Emergence Phase. During the emergence phase, uterine contractions cause the kitten to pass through the birth canal and pause in the vulva (Fig. 6–4). The amniotic sac normally has been broken by uterine contractions, but if not, the queen's licking soon breaks it. The release of fluids from the amniotic sac causes the queen to spend additional time licking the fluids and, coincidentally, herself and the newborn.[31, 36, 63] Experienced queens may direct more attention to the newborn, but other behaviors are similar to those of the contraction phase.

Delivery Phase. In the third phase, delivery, the fetus emerges from

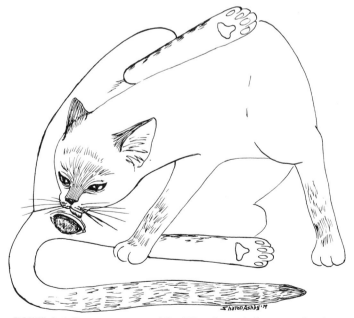

FIGURE 6–4. The emergence of the kitten through the queen's vulva.

the vulva (Fig. 6–5).[63] Licking directed specifically at the newborn increases, although the queen may not begin immediately after the delivery. The licking supplies the stimulus for starting the newborn's respiration. Initially in lateral recumbency, the queen may try to reposition herself after the delivery and may coincidentally drag the kitten around by the still-attached umbilical cord, perhaps even stepping or sitting on it. Distress cries from this newborn or others may be ignored by the queen at this time, perhaps because of the excitement associated with parturition or because of incomprehension of the vocal cue, or both.[63] Kittens can be injured during this period. Shortly after parturition—usually 1 to 4 minutes later—the queen becomes responsive to the kittens.[16, 63] In about one-third of the births a queen severs the umbilical cord soon after the delivery (Fig. 6–6).

The length of the interval between kitten births varies widely, ranging from 32 seconds to more than 50 minutes.[36, 63] Most kittens are born within 15 to 30 minutes of one another, with a total delivery time of 1 to 2 hours.[12, 13] Some normal queens occasionally require as long as 33 hours to complete the deliveries, but external disturbances, such as the owner's absence or the moving of a nesting area, usually precipitate this extreme delay. Uterine inertia is relatively rare in cats.[39] There is no

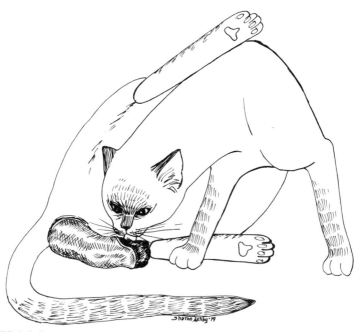

FIGURE 6–5. The delivery of the neonate, still partially covered by the amniotic sac.

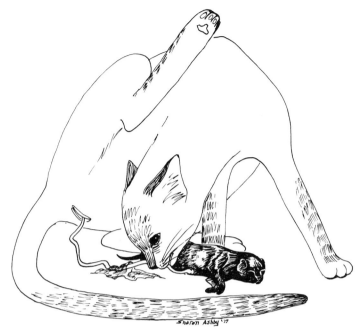

FIGURE 6–6. The queen severs the umbilical cord with her teeth.

relation between the sequence of a kitten's birth and the interval between its birth and that of its littermates.

Placental Phase. During the last phase of parturition the placenta is expelled from the genital tract. Immediately before this expulsion the queen becomes restless, again focusing her attention on the caudal part of her body. She promptly responds to the emergence of the placenta, sometimes eating it before it has completely emerged (Fig. 6–7).[63] No relationship has been shown between the sequence of the births and either the interval of response to the placentas or the rate and completeness of their consumption.[63] At times a second or even third kitten is born before the umbilical cord of the first is severed or the placenta passed, but each is attended to as time permits. Nutritive value from the afterbirth is considerable and allows the queen to spend more time with her offspring for the first few days than if she had to seek food as usual. In addition, this behavior minimizes the soiling of the nest area. The queen continues genital and neonatal licking and, usually during the placental phase, severs the umbilical cord with her carnassial teeth. Their crushing action, the stretching of the vessels, or both prevent fatal umbilical hemorrhage.[29, 63] The queen's care during this phase makes cannibalism a rare consequence of overzealous eating of the placenta and cord.

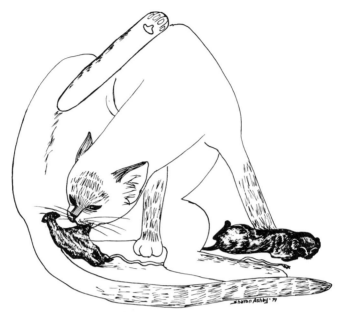

FIGURE 6–7. The queen responds to placental emergence by consuming the tissue.

Litter Size

The number of kittens in a single litter varies considerably; the usual range is from one to nine births. Record litters of 13 kittens and one unusual incidence of a queen carrying 18 fetuses have been reported.[9, 79] Of the kittens born alive, between 72 per cent and 87 per cent will be successfully raised to weaning.[37, 54, 64] Three to five kittens, then, is an average litter, even for artificially induced pregnancies, and the male-female ratio of these kittens varies from 1:1 to 4:3. Although 7 per cent of older queens litter three times a year, the mean is 2.5 litters.[45, 59] Most litters result from matings on 3 consecutive days, but litter size is not affected by the number of days the queen mates.[55] Most queens bear between 50 and 150 kittens in a breeding life of about 10 years if allowed to mate naturally.[81] Although some may produce for 13 or more years, peak productivity is between the ages of 2 and 8 years.[5, 38] One cat is known to have produced 420 kittens in 17 years, and another is said to have been pregnant at 26 years of age.[15, 79]

Normal birth weight varies between 80 and 120 g; the average weight is about 113 g.[25, 33] The total birth weight relative to the queen's weight is significantly greater for kittens born to smaller queens than for kittens born to larger queens, despite the fact that larger queens produce more kittens in each litter.[25]

In cats, the incidence of aborted fetuses and stillbirths is one or two per litter.[37, 64] These events may be difficult to observe because the queen normally eats these fetuses. The stillborn rate is higher in older queens and in the Persian, Maine coon cat, Himalayan, and Manx.[46, 54, 55, 64]

MATERNAL BEHAVIOR

Maternal-Young Interactions

The primary social pattern exhibited by the female cat is maternal behavior. This behavior involves exaggerated licking of self and young as well as the care of the young.[63] For the first few days after parturition, the queen remains almost continuously with the kittens, seldom leaving for more than 2 hours at a time, and then mainly to eat and exercise. Much of this early time is spent nursing the offspring, although the kittens may not nurse for as long as 2 hours postpartum. For nursing, the queen "presents," assuming lateral recumbency with her legs and body completely enclosing the kittens (Fig. 6–8). She may even twist her body to expose more of the mammary region. To stimulate the young to begin nursing, the queen licks and often awakens them. The direction of licking initially helps to orient the blind kittens to the mammary region,

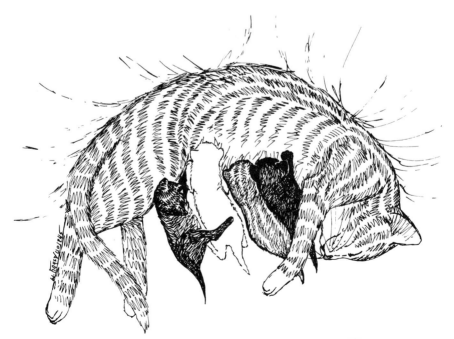

FIGURE 6–8. The "presenting" posture of a queen to her kittens.

but later, licking is concentrated on the kitten's anogenital region to stimulate eliminations. The queen's ingestion of this waste also helps to keep the home area unsoiled. On presentation by the queen, the entire litter usually nurses, although only one or two individuals may nurse at once. During the first week about 90 per cent of the queen's time is spent with her kittens; as much as 70 per cent is spent nursing them. By the fifth week her time with the kittens has decreased to 16 per cent.[57, 63] Each kitten initially spends about 25 per cent of its time nursing; this decreases to about 20 per cent by the 5th week.[40] Kittens spend almost all their time in contact with one another or the queen for the first 3 weeks; contact time only decreases to 85 per cent over the next few weeks.[57] Cooperative nursing between queens has been reported without preference to which kittens belong to which mother.[47]

The queen's nursing relationship to her young changes with time.[41] During the first 4 weeks she initiates and stimulates their interest in nursing, but she eventually runs away from their advances. Maternal-young feeding relations are discussed in more detail in Chapter 7.

The queen-kitten interaction continues to change as the young gain mobility and independence. They may include the queen in their play, although she increasingly avoids interaction with the kittens as they get older, paralleling her changes in nursing behavior. To control their biting and chewing of her, she may bat the kittens on the nose, drag them away, or turn and move away from them if a growl warning does not work. The same discipline technique—a bat on the nose and a "no"—can be used by a human. Experimental evidence indicates that this training must be initiated before 6 weeks of age if it is to be retained in adulthood.[23]

Kitten Relocation

Kittens that wander from the home area usually are retrieved by the queen, who carries them back to the nest by the dorsum of the neck (Fig. 6–9). Retrieval probably is initiated by the kitten's distress vocalizations of a certain minimal intensity. It is not known whether the queen can differentiate individuals by their distress vocalizations or whether her response is generalized.[5, 63] Because all queens in a colony show anxiety on hearing the wails of kittens from other litters, the general response probably is the case. The kittens' distress cries are a necessary signal to alert the queen of trouble, and deaf queens may totally ignore their misplaced young. This anxiety production in the queen is of significant survival value for the kittens and explains why the female becomes so concerned when one of the kittens is removed from the nest, vocalizing as it is moved. The queen usually approaches whomever or whatever is holding the youngster, retrieves it from the intruder, and carries it back

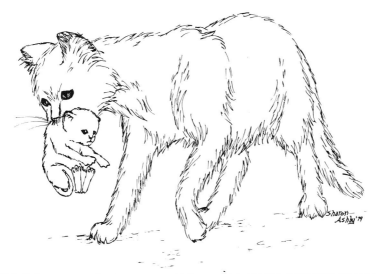

FIGURE 6–9. A queen carries her young, which assumes reflexive immobility, by the dorsum of its neck.

to the nest. The latency between kitten retrievals dramatically increases after the behavior has been used several times in succession.[43] The retrieval behavior peaks at about 1 week postpartum, possibly reflecting decreasing vocalization by kittens as they grow older.[63]

Distressing situations, created by such things as loud noises or overcrowding, can cause the queen to move her young, again carrying them by the dorsum of the neck, although a few inexperienced females may hold other portions of a kitten, such as its leg. Some cats can be so nervous in an environment that they will move their litter four or five times a night. Whenever all the kittens have been transferred to the new location, the mother returns at least one more time to the old nest, indicating that she is not aware the move has been completed.[5, 43] It is common for a female to move her litter sometime around the 3rd or 4th week postpartum.[5]

Maternal Aggression

Maternal aggression in defense of young can be one of the fiercest forms of aggression shown by a cat. The female may attack humans or other cats without a threat display, almost eagerly.[19] Even a placid, human-loving cat can become highly aggressive toward people she knows if they try to remove her very young kittens from the home area. Because this probably is a function of her hormonal state, caution should be exercised in any attempt to handle young kittens. Another factor that may contribute to the ferocity of maternal behavior is that in the effort to keep her group together, the queen must block her own flight response to danger. Thus she is more excitable and reactive to situations within her reach.[5] Because the domestic cat normally is not allowed to release her aggressions, when maternity lowers the aggression threshold, all the repressed energy of hostility is released at once.[19] Maternal aggression may be expressed as intolerance of other queens and their kittens, but selective breeding has helped to reduce this undesirable behavior, as well as other forms of maternal aggression.[22]

Infant Adoption

When two or more females give birth at about the same time and are housed in the same area, they may take turns nursing each other's kittens. At other times the more forward of the females, whether or not she has queened or will do so soon, may take kittens from the more timid queen. It also is common, if one of the two females is the daughter of the other, for the daughter to nurse her own kittens while she and her half-siblings nurse the older female.[23]

The early contact between mother and young forms a bond that continues their successful relationship until the time of the kittens' final dispersal. Much of this bond probably is formed because of licking. For about the first week, especially immediately after birth, while the bond is forming, most queens readily accept any kitten. A queen's fostering of kittens is most successful before the maternal bond is established with her own kittens and when the foster kittens are about the same age as her own. Care must be taken if the kittens to be fostered are more than 1 week of age because females are known to react to young according to their size and not according to the age of the female's own young; therefore, the foster kittens may be ignored or attacked rather than accepted. Another factor that influences a queen's acceptance of foster kittens is the view the kitten presents to the approaching queen. If the female approaches the caudal area of a kitten, she may respond with anogenital licking. But if a cranial view of the same kitten is presented, she may display aggression.[5, 19]

During the first week after littering, the queen may accept the young of other species, so pictures of cats nursing bunnies, rats, and puppies often are seen. Despite raising young of another species, a queen can still be a hunter of that species, even bringing the prey home to feed her "offspring."

Another time when the female may accept kittens other than her own is when hers start leaving the home area. At this time the maternal bond decreases sharply, and the queen ceases to differentiate between her young and other kittens.[20] That also is a common time for young housed together to begin sharing mothers. Ingestive patterns of the kittens are changing, in that the female starts bringing solid food to the kittens. In certain situations other cats also bring food to kittens, indicating that this behavior may be initiated by kitten size or activity patterns.[20]

Miscellaneous Influences

The queen serves several functions during kitten development, but during the latter portions of her contact with the young, she teaches them that in dangerous situations, a specific growl signals a "run for cover" message.[5] She also demonstrates hunting skills and other fundamentals necessary for an independent existence, so that her offspring may learn by observation.

Early care, as well as the health of both neonate and mother, can have a profound effect on clinical entities in the older kitten. For example, most Himalayan queens are poor milk producers, and supplements may be necessary to prevent neonatal starvation and poor nervous system development.[46]

Although domestication often prolongs maternal-young interactions, evidence suggests that feral queens and kittens normally separate about 4 months postpartum.

NEUROLOGIC AND HORMONAL CONTROLS

Female sexual behavior in the cat primarily is governed by the central nervous system, either directly or through hormonal influence.

Spinal Cord

The lumbar spinal cord contains short reflex arcs associated with certain portions of estrous behavior, even in anestrous females and in males.[40, 80] Stimulation of the perineum causes reflex elevation of the pelvis, treading, and lateral deviation of the tail, although facilitation of these reflexes in normal cats is strictly associated with the hormonal state of that animal.[48]

Peripheral Nerves

Connection by sensory portions of peripheral nerves to the lumbar spinal area also is regulated by hormones because estrogens facilitate posturing by the female.[30] Although the role of the clitoris is uncertain in the cat, deep pressure and tactile sensations to the vaginal walls result in the copulatory cry.[30] Removal of the pelvic nerve plexus, which supplies both the uterus and the vagina, results in fewer copulatory cries, less postcoital rolling, and fewer ovulations.[17] The afferent fibers that carry this information centrally are believed to be associated with the hypogastric nerves, which are more active during estrus.[74]

The sympathetic portion of the nervous system controls the smooth muscle around the ovary and uterine tube in particular. With emotional stress these muscles can be forced into a prolonged contraction, which can block ovulation or result in a tubal pregnancy, although the latter has not been documented in the cat to date. Clitoral engorgement is under parasympathetic control, and sensation is by means of the pudendal nerve.

If the genitalia of the estrous cat are denervated, mating behavior remains the same, but postmating activity is eliminated.[1] This suggests that the peripheral nervous system initiates the postmating response in the central nervous system.

The Brain

Several areas of the brain regulate sexual behavior in the cat. Within the hypothalamus the supraoptic region controls sexual responses, especially those mediated by estrogen, and lesions of this rostral hypothalamus result in permanent anestrus. The caudal hypothalamic region and the caudal brainstem are responsible for reflexes essential to copulation.[40] Ovarian function also is maintained by a normal caudal hypothalamus, probably because of its interrelation with the gonadotropic activities of the pituitary, and ovulation can be induced in hormonally primed cats by stimulation of the hypothalamus.[40, 60] By contrast, lesions of the rostral tuberal or caudal portions of the hypothalamus block ovulation.[60]

The ventromedial hypothalamus demonstrates a generalized response to vaginal stimulation, whereas portions of the lateral reticular nucleus and medullary reticular formation show a more specific response and are influenced by hormonal variations.[71] Stilbestrol placed directly in the caudal hypothalamus results in estrous behavior but without the normal vaginal cellular changes.[28] The highest amount of peripheral hormone uptake by selected brain sites occurs in the preoptic and ventromedial hypothalamus. The greatest effects from vaginal electrical stimulation are seen in the rostral hypothalamus, whereas the caudal cell response is influenced by estrogen. This suggests that the caudal hypothalamus plays a role in the regulation of postcopulatory behavior as well as in ovulation.[56] After coitus, electrical activity in the arcuate nucleus of the caudal hypothalamus increases norepinephrine levels, which leads to the release of luteinizing hormone releasing factor (LHRF) to stimulate the pituitary to produce luteinizing hormone (LH). Ovulation then occurs 1 to 3 days after coitus, after the LH peak.[58] These data are from a study that indicates no relation exists between either the cortical or hypothalamic electroencephalographic activity and the behavioral or hormonal status of the animals.[70]

The hypothalamus also is the reception area from the retina, pineal gland, or both for environmental light. When the amounts of orange and red intensities in daylight fall below a certain level, the anestrous portion of the reproductive cycle begins.[68] Input from this light to the hypothalamus releases follicle-stimulating (gonadotropic) releasing hormone (GN-RH), a neurohumoral factor that regulates the pituitary gland.[30, 68] The pituitary responds by producing follicle-stimulating hormone (FSH), which, with ovarian estrogens, affects the genital system. It, in turn, feeds back to the hypothalamus. Timed lighting can eliminate this anestrous season, and the lighting conditions of a home may be sufficient to keep the cat cycling year round.

Control of the estrous behaviors of rolling and vocalization is exerted by the amygdaloid nuclei and the pyriform cortex.[40] In addition, the amygdala shows electroencephalographic changes during the postcoital reaction, suggesting that it may be involved in ovulation.[30] Lesions of the lateral medulla or lateral midbrain stop the copulatory cry and after-reaction of an estrous female, although she will tolerate being mounted and exhibit lordosis, pelvic elevation, and lateral tail deviation, even when anestrous.[4, 71]

The hypophysis regulates the ingestion of placentas for a short period postpartum.[19]

Brain and hormonal interactions are so closely related that it is almost impossible to separate one from the other. Without estrogen, the behaviors of a normal, intact female do not occur. It can be concluded, then, that estrogen has its primary effect on specific, complex brain areas and results in specific behaviors.

Hormones

Without the influence of estrogens, as after ovariectomy, the cat will not display the behaviors associated with estrus, pregnancy, parturition, or motherhood but will increase the size of her territory. Even the aggressive component of anestrous behavior gradually decreases after surgery, so that after 5 or 6 months, the cat will passively tolerate mounting. This passivity may be due to the removal of progesterone, which also is eliminated by an ovariectomy. If the ovaries are removed during estrus, blood levels of estrogen and behaviors typical of anestrus return within 24 hours.[50] Later external supplementation of estrogens to this female results in the return of estrous behavior, with both onset of action and duration of action being closely dependent. Vaginal epithelial changes also occur, even at dosage levels lower than those necessary for behavioral changes.[51] Estrous behavior continues in these treated, ovariectomized animals as long as supplementation is continuous; once the animal no longer receives the exogenous gonadal hormone and is allowed to return to the anestrous state, she proves highly refractive to additional estrogen.[2]

During pregnancy, hormone production is taken over by the placenta. The ovarian luteal function decreases after day 16, and by day 45 the ovaries can be removed and the pregnancy still maintained.[58, 66] Progesterone is produced by the placenta after 21 days, indicating an interaction between the fetus and the placenta, which governs hormone production.[58, 66]

Another hormone that affects estrus is oxytocin released by vaginal cells. Oxytocin functions to increase mobility of uterine and uterine tube smooth muscle, and thus facilitates sperm transport.[30]

Certain drugs have been used to control estrus in the cat over the years, but they have not been too successful. Regulation of endogenous hormones with exogenous hormones must be carefully controlled, and real success probably requires more sophisticated knowledge of the neural-hormonal interactions. Anabolic steroids and hormones may suppress the release of FSH to affect the queen or act directly on the fetal kittens.[18]

FEMALE SEXUAL BEHAVIOR PROBLEMS

Stress-Related Problems

Stress on the female cat can create a number of behavior problems, depending on the individual and her hormonal state. Inhibition of innate releasing mechanisms, as for prey killing, can result in some unusual reactions, particularly in queens. Such stress as noise, malnutrition, or moving can result in varied reactions, including anestrus, lack of milk production, failure to deliver, extreme fearfulness, frantic running, increased restlessness, abandonment of young, chronic diarrhea, epileptic-like seizures, excessive moving of kittens, excessive neonatal grooming, urine spraying, and redirected aggression or cannibalism. Work in several species has shown that high population density has a negative effect on gonadal and mammary activity, with concurrent adrenal hypertrophy.[72] This decrease in reproductive activity is potentially serious in the cat because of its asocial nature. To some individuals, small numbers may constitute overcrowding.

For stressful situations, removal of the inducing factors is necessary to eliminate the problem. Progesterone (1 mg/lb), medroxyprogesterone acetate (Depo-Provera; 25 to 50 mg I.M. or S.C.), or megestrol acetate

(Ovaban; 10 mg P.O. for 1 day, 5 mg P.O. for 1 day, and then 2.5 mg P.O. for 1 day) also may help the queen return to normal. In addition to supplying the hormone whose level has suddenly fallen at parturition, progesterone has a calming effect by suppressing the dorsomedial hypothalamic center, which is related to rage.[34] Tranquilizers also may be successful.

Maternal Neglect. Maternal neglect has several causes, but the results are the same: Without proper care, the kittens die. Many of these queens are excessively human-oriented and neglect their kittens in favor of human attention. Necropsies of the neglected young usually reveal empty stomachs and full urinary bladders, implying failure of the queen to nurse the kittens and to stimulate elimination by anogenital licking. Of neonatal deaths, 8 per cent to 19 per cent result from maternal neglect.[31, 82]

Relocation of the kittens by the queen can be affected by stress. The desire to move kittens is strongest within the first few hours after parturition and again at 25 to 35 days after queening, but stress factors can increase the incidence of this moving behavior. On rare occasions a queen forgets where she moved her kittens and becomes highly vocal and restless.

Cannibalism. Eating of the young occurs frequently in cat colonies, and certain forms of it are normal. Queens routinely consume aborted fetuses and stillborn kittens, probably to keep the nest unsoiled and to prevent attracting predators to the area. When one queen in an open colony gives birth, others that are not pregnant or near term may consume the neonates. It is theorized that the infant's size and shape closely resemble those of natural prey and may initiate a normal prey-killing instinct. An increased incidence of cannibalism has been associated with a large litter, the second pregnancy, and illness in the kittens.[31] Other situations can provoke cannibalism, such as stress produced by the queen's inability to find an appropriate queening area.[23] Also, if extremely malnourished, a queen may cannibalize her young. This situation represents one in which self-preservation overrules maternalism. Still another type of cannibalism is hormonal cannibalism, which results from incomplete hormonal inhibition of the prey-killing instinct in a female cat. The same hormones that are responsible for maternal behavior are probably responsible for inhibition of the prey-killing instinct. Cannibalism accounts for 12.5 per cent of preweaning kitten losses.[82] Eviscerating and ingesting a kitten while chewing the umbilical cord too closely are not true cannibalism, and although this does occur, especially with the nervous cat, it is rare.

The correction of problem cannibalism depends on the initiating factors. At least 2 weeks before the expected littering date, the minimization of stress is highly desirable, as is the provision of an isolated queening area, or even a separate cage in a colony situation. Progestins are successful in preventing hormonal cannibalism.

Delayed Parturition. The interruption or prolongation of parturition is a frequent sequela to stress. Human-dependent cats commonly have a prolonged labor, and when a kitten is first presented with its head protruding from the vulva, this type of queen may make no attempt to complete the delivery or to clean the kitten after delivery is completed. This behavior may be repeated with each kitten. Disturbances to a delivering queen can delay further births, but normal parturition usually resumes within 12 to 24 hours. Mild tranquilization, particularly with acepromazine (0.125 to 0.25 mg/lb I.M. or S.C.), is helpful in initiating resumption of normal parturition. It is best that one dispense the medication rather than cause a disturbance to the queen by bringing her to a veterinary clinic. Delays in parturition caused by uterine inertia are rare in the cat.[39]

Pseudocyesis

Pseudocyesis is another condition that seldom occurs in felids.[7] Because corpora lutea start regressing around 21 days postovulation in the nonpregnant animal, after peak luteal production at 16 to 17 days, false pregnancy seldom lasts more than 45 days. Signs of the condition, although typically mild in the cat, may range from physical signs of pregnancy to "kitten-tending," the adoption of other animals or soft toys. Milk production and labor also can occur. Nonfertilized ovulation is necessary to induce pseudopregnancy, and merely petting an estrous female has, on rare occasions, induced ovulation.[35] When this physiologic situation occurs, it produces psychological manifestations and illustrates the extent to which the cat's body is adapted for a pregnant state. Pseudocyesis is self-limiting, so drug therapy usually is unnecessary. Tranquilizers, repositol testosterone (1 mg/lb), or repositol stilbestrol (0.25 mg/lb) have been used in extreme cases.[69] The cat typically is in estrus again within 44 days.[58]

Hypersexuality

Nymphomania is a relatively common variation of female sexual behavior, especially in Siamese and Persian cats.[24, 61] This prolonged, exaggerated, easily aroused estrous behavior often accompanies cystic ovaries.[23] The caudate nucleus of the brain also has been implicated with this form of feline hypersexuality, which, along with other personality extremes induced by excitement, has been classified as a hysterical disorder.[14, 58]

True homosexual behavior in female cats is unusual. Although females may mount other females, this is a consequence of sexual energy not released during estrus rather than preference for the same sex. As a result of tension and frustration, an estrous female may suddenly mount another female or even a passive male. Prepubertal kittens may engage in play behavior that partially resembles sexual patterns, with indiscriminate mounting between sexes. (See Fig. 5–1.)

Masturbation is unusual, except in cats with high estrogen levels or prolonged estrogen exposure, and is accomplished mainly by rubbing the anogenital region against the floor while suspending the body with the forelimbs. In addition, the cat usually vocalizes and licks her genital area.[40]

Other Problems

Pseudohermaphroditism does occur in felids. The male pseudohermaphrodite has testicles, but the external genitalia appears feminine, perhaps slightly modified. The female pseudohermaphrodite has male external genitalia with female internal organs and gonads, but this condition is extremely uncommon because testosterone influence, which would be responsible for the external appearance, is rare without gonads.[27]

Removal of the genital tract of the female cat in general and ovariectomy in particular can be associated with certain changes. Weight gain often is the first change cited, but this usually is attributed to decreased roaming and increased accessibility of food. In addition to generalized subcutaneous layering, a characteristic fat deposit in the inguinal skin folds is associated with neutering.[39] It is highly controversial whether the lack of activity normally associated with estrogen can have such a marked effect on fat deposition, since estrogens are influential only two or three times a year. This is perhaps another area that involves the lack of progesterones instead.

Lactation can follow an ovariohysterectomy performed near the regression or termination of the life of a corpus luteum. In the cat this regression probably is between 20 and 35 days postovulation.

An estrous female may not mate with a particular tomcat for several reasons, including environmental stress, invasion of her territory, and undesirability of the tomcat. Time together for such individuals eventually may result in successful copulations, although owners may not be aware of them. Physical restraint of an objecting female can permit an experienced tomcat to mate her.[32] In addition, tranquilizers and catnip have been successfully used to calm nervous female cats.[13] The cat subjected to controlled but infrequent matings may undergo endometrial as well as psychosomatic changes. If prolonged, this situation can lead to chronic diarrhea, aggression, or seizures.[38]

Blue-eyed, deaf white cats are perpetuated primarily by selective breeding. Females with this genetic makeup are semisterile, in addition to having other problems, discussed in Chapter 2.[10]

Hormonal therapy for any of a variety of clinical entities, from treatment of skin conditions to estrus prevention, has been accompanied by a myriad of complications. Some female cats fail to start cycling once drug therapy has been terminated; others develop endometrial hyperplasia and pyometra. These conditions can occur in ovariohysterectomized females if any uterine tissue remains, as when the uterus is severed proximal to the cervix. In addition, neutered cats have exhibited mild estrous signs after hormonal therapy.

CASE PRESENTATIONS

CASE 6–1. One-and-one-half-year-old Siamese neutered female. An ovariohysterectomy was performed when the cat was 6 months old, but during the past month the cat began showing typical signs of estrus. In addition to rolling and heat crying, the cat has postured for and accepted mounting by two males.

Medical Workup. The physical examination and routine laboratory data were within normal limits, but the vaginal smear and serum estrogen levels were typical of an estrous female.

Diagnosis. Estrus.

Treatment. An exploratory laparotomy revealed cystic ovarian tissue in the usual position of the right ovary, indicating that some ovarian tissue was left during the initial surgery.

CASE 6–2. Four-year-old domestic shorthair female. The cat is housed with four other females and a male. The female queened earlier than the owners expected and so was not isolated from the other cats. Shortly after giving birth the queen abandoned the young, and the other cats were found eating the newborns. One kitten was still alive.

Diagnosis. Lack of maternal instinct owing to hormonal imbalance, environmental stress, or both.

Treatment. The queen and surviving kitten were immediately isolated, and the queen was injected with 10 mg progesterone. Although the queen then accepted the neonate, it died within 24 hours, apparently from the earlier chill during the initial abandonment.

CASE 6–3. Four-and-one-half-month-old Persian female. The cat is owned by a breeder who sought consultation because of an unusual rolling behavior. Although the presenting signs were typical of estrus, the breeder insisted that she had never owned a cat that came into heat before 8 months of age.

Medical Workup. The vaginal smear was typical of estrus, and vaginal stimulation with a moist cotton swab produced the typical after-reaction.

Diagnosis. Estrus.

Also see case 8–5.

REFERENCES

1. Bard, P.: Effects of denervation of the genitalia on the oestrous behavior of cats. Am. J. Physiol. 113:5, Sept. 1935.
2. Beach, F. A.: Hormones and Behavior. New York: Cooper Square Publishers, 1961.
3. Beach, F. A., ed.: Sex and Behavior. New York: John Wiley & Sons, 1965.
4. Beach, F. A.: Cerebral and hormonal control of reflexive mechanisms involved in copulatory behavior. Physiol. Rev. 47:289, 1967.
5. Beadle, M.: The Cat: History, Biology, and Behavior. New York: Simon & Schuster, 1977.
6. Beaver, B. V.: Mating behavior in the cat. Vet. Clin. North Am. 7:729, 1977.
7. Beaver, B. V.: Feline behavioral problems other than housesoiling. J. Am. Anim. Hosp. Assoc. 25:465, 1989.
8. Beaver, B. V.: Psychogenic manifestations of environmental disturbances. In August, J. R., ed.: Consultations in Feline Medicine, Philadelphia: W. B. Saunders Co., 1991.
9. Beaver, B. V. G.: Supernumerary fetation in the cat. Fel. Pract. 3:24, May-June 1973.
10. Bergsma, D. R., and Brown, K. S.: White fur, blue eyes, and deafness in the domestic cat. J. Hered. 62:171, 1971.
11. Bland, K. P.: Tom-cat odour and other pheromones in feline reproduction. Vet. Sci. Commun 3:125, 1979.
12. Boudreau, J. C., and Tsuchitani, C.: Sensory Neurophysiology. New York: Van Nostrand Reinhold Co., 1973.
13. Bryant, D.: The Care and Handling of Cats. New York: Ives Washburn, 1944.
14. Chertok, L., and Fontaine, M.: Psychosomatics in veterinary medicine. J. Psychosom. Res. 7:229, 1963.
15. Comfort, A.: Maximum ages reached by domestic cats. J. Mammal. 37:118, 1956.
16. Cooper, J. B.: A description of parturition in the domestic cat. J. Comp. Psychol. 37:71, 1944.
17. Diakow, C.: Effects of genital desensitization on mating behavior and ovulation in the female cat. Physiol. Behav. 7:47, July 1971.
18. Davis, L. E.: Adverse effects of drugs on reproduction in dogs and cats. Mod. Vet. Pract. 64:969, 1983.
19. Ewer, R. F.: Ethology of Mammals. London: Paul Elek, Ltd., 1968.
20. Ewer, R. F.: The Carnivores. Ithaca, N.Y.: Cornell University Press, 1973.
21. Ewer, R. F.: The evolution of mating systems in the Felidae. In Eaton, R. L., ed.: The World's Cats. Seattle: Feline Research Group, 1974.
22. Fox, M. W.: Aggression: Its adaptive and maladaptive significance in man and animals. In Fox, M. W., ed.: Abnormal behavior in animals. Philadelphia: W. B. Saunders Co., 1968.
23. Fox, M. W.: Understanding Your Cat. New York: Coward, McCann & Geoghegan, 1974.
24. Fox, M. W.: The behaviour of cats. In Hafez, E. S. E., ed.: The Behavior of Domestic Animals. 3rd ed. Baltimore: Williams & Wilkins, 1975.
25. Hall, V. E., and Pierce, G. N.: Litter size, birth weight, and growth to weaning in the cat. Anat. Rec. 60:111, 1934.
26. Halsema, L. J.: Living room leopard cat. Friskies Res. Dig. 11:6, Summer 1975.
27. Hare, W. C. D.: Female pseudohermaphroditism. Fel. Pract. 9:4, Jan.-Feb. 1979.
28. Harris, G. W., Michael, R. P., and Scott, P. P.: Neurological site of action of stilboestrol

in eliciting sexual behavior. In Wolstenholme, G. E. W., and O'Connor, C. M., eds.: Neurological Basis of Behaviour. Boston: Little, Brown & Co., 1952.

29. Hart, B. L.: Maternal behavior. I. Parturient and postparturient behavior. Fel. Pract. 2:6, Sept.-Oct. 1972.
30. Hart, B. L.: Physiology of sexual function. Vet. Clin. North Am. 4:557, 1974.
31. Hart, B. L., and Hart, L. A.: Canine and feline behavioral therapy. Philadelphia: Lea & Febiger, 1985.
32. Hart, B. L., and Voith, V. L.: Sexual behavior and breeding problems in cats. Fel. Pract. 7:9, Jan. 1977.
33. Hemmer, H.: Gestation period and postnatal development in felids. In Eaton, R. L., ed.: The World's Cats. 3rd ed. Seattle: Carnivore Research Institute, 1976.
34. Henik, R. A., Olson, P. N., and Rosychuk, R. A.: Progestogen therapy in cats. Comp. Cont. Educ. 7:132, 1985.
35. Histochemistry 43:191, 1975.
36. Houpt, K. A., and Wolski, R. R.: Domestic animal behavior for veterinarians and animal scientists. Ames: Iowa State University Press, 1982.
37. Jemmett, J. E., and Evans, J. M.: A survey of sexual behaviour and reproduction of female cats. J. Small Anim. Pract. 18:31, 1977.
38. Joshua, J. O.: Abnormal behavior in cats. In Fox, M. W., ed.: Abnormal Behavior in Animals. Philadelphia: W. B. Saunders Co., 1968.
39. Joshua, J. O.: Some conditions seen in feline practice attributable to hormonal causes. Vet. Rec. 88:511, 1971.
40. Kling, A., Kovach, J. K., and Tucker, T. J.: The behaviour of cats. In Hafez, E. S. E., ed.: The behaviour of domestic animals. 2nd ed. Baltimore: Williams & Wilkins, 1969.
41. Lawrence, C.: Individual differences in maternal behaviour in the domestic cat. Appl. Anim. Ethol. 6:387, 1980.
42. Leyhausen, P.: Communal organization of solitary mammals. Symp. Zool. Soc. Lond. 14:249, 1965.
43. Leyhausen, P.: Cat Behavior: The Predatory and Social Behavior of Domestic and Wild Cats. New York: Garland STPM Press, 1978.
44. Liberg, O.: Predation and social behaviour in a population of domestic cat. An evolutionary perspective. Ph. D. diss., Department of Animal Ecology, University of Lund, Sweden, 1981.
45. Liberg, O.: Courtship behaviour and sexual selection in the domestic cat. Appl. Anim. Ethol. 10:117, 1983.
46. Lott, J. N., and Herron, M.: Sudden death syndrome in kittens. Fel. Pract. 7:16, May 1977.
47. Macdonald, D. W., Apps, P. J., Curr, G. M., and Kerby, G.: Social Dynamics, Nursing Coalitions, and Infanticide Among Farm Cats, Felis catus. Berlin: Paul Parey Scientific Publishers, 1987.
48. Maes, J. P.: Neural mechanism of sexual behaviour in the female cat. Nature 144:598, 1939.
49. Michael, R. P.: Sexual behaviour and the vaginal cycle in the cat. Nature 181:567, 1958.
50. Michael, R. P.: Observations upon the sexual behavior of the domestic cat (Felis catus L.) under laboratory conditions. Behaviour 18:1, 1961.
51. Michael, R. P., and Scott, P. P.: The activation of sexual behaviour in cats by the subcutaneous administration of oestrogen. J. Physiol. (Lond.) 171:254, 1964.
52. Mykytowycz, R.: Reproduction of mammals in relation to environmental odours. J. Reprod. Fertil. 19 (Suppl.):433, 1973.
53. Paape, S. R., Shille, V. M., Seto, H., and Stabenfeldt, G. H.: Luteal activity in the pseudopregnant cat. Biol. Reprod. 13:470, 1975.
54. Povey, R. C.: Reproduction in the pedigree female cat. A survey of breeders. Can. Vet. J. 19:207, 1978.
55. Prescott, C. W.: Reproduction patterns in the domestic cat. Aust. Vet. J. 49:126, 1973.
56. Ratner, A., Koenig, J. Q., and Frazier, D. T.: Hypothalamic unit activity in the cat: Effects of estrogen and vaginal stimulation. Proc. Soc. Exp. Biol. Med. 137:321, 1971.
57. Rheingold, H. L., and Eckerman, C. O.: Familiar social and nonsocial stimuli and the kitten's response to a strange environment. Dev. Psychobiol. 4:71, 1971.

58. Richkind, M.: The reproductive endocrinology of the domestic cat. Fel. Pract. 8:28, Sept. 1978.
59. Robison, R., and Cox, H. W.: Reproductive performance in a cat colony over a 10-year period. Lab. Anim. 4:99, 1970.
60. Sawyer, C. J., and Robison, B.: Separate hypothalamic areas controlling pituitary gonadotropic function and mating behavior in female cats and rabbits. J. Clin. Endocrinol. Metab. 16:914, 1956.
61. Schmidt, J. P.: Psychosomatics in veterinary medicine. In Fox, M. W., ed.: Abnormal Behavior in Animals. Philadelphia: W. B. Saunders Co., 1968.
62. Schmidt, P. M., Chakraborty, P. K., and Wildt, D. E.: Ovarian activity, circulating hormones and sexual behavior in the cat. II. Relationships during pregnancy, parturition, lactation and the postpartum estrus. Biol. Reprod. 28:657, 1983.
63. Schneirla, T. C., Rosenblatt, J. S., and Tobach, E.: Maternal behavior in the cat. In Rheingold, H. L., ed.: Maternal Behavior in Mammals. New York: John Wiley & Sons, 1963.
64. Scott, F. W., Geissinger, C., and Peltz, R.: Kitten mortality survey. Fel. Pract. 8:31, Nov. 1978.
65. Scott, P. P.: The domestic cat as a laboratory animal for the study of reproduction. J. Physiol. (Lond.) 130:47P, 1955.
66. Scott, P. P.: Diet and other factors affecting the development of young felids. In Eaton, R. L., ed.: The World's Cats. 3rd ed. Seattle: Carnivore Research Institute, 1976.
67. Scott, P. P., and Lloyd-Jacob, M. A.: Some interesting features in the reproductive cycle of the cat. Stud. Fert. 7:123, 1955.
68. Stapley, R.: Factors affecting the reproductive behavior of the feline. I. Photoperiodicity and controlled exposure to light. Friskies Res. Dig. 14:8, Spring 1978.
69. Stein, B. S.: The genital system. In Catcott, E. J., ed.: Feline Medicine and Surgery. 2nd ed. Santa Barbara, CA: American Veterinary Publications, 1975.
70. Sutin, J., and Michael, R. P.: Changes in brain electrical activity following vaginal stimulation in estrous and anestrous cats. Physiol. Behav. 5:1043, 1970.
71. Sutin, J., Rose, J., Van Atta, L., and Thalmann, R.: Electrophysiological studies in an animal model of aggressive behavior. Res. Publ. Assoc. Rec. Nerv. Ment. Dis. 52:93, 1974.
72. Thiessen, D. D., and Rodgers, D. A.: Population density and endocrine function. Psychol. Bull. 58:441, 1961.
73. Todd, N. B.: Behavior and genetics of the domestic cat. Cornell Vet. 53:99, 1963.
74. Varbanova, A., Doneshka, P., and Vassileva-Popova, J. G.: Changes in EEG and in the activity of the whole cervical vagus upon application of sex hormones. In Vassileva-Popova, J. G., ed.: Physical and Chemical Bases of Biological Information Transfer. New York: Plenum Publishing Corp., 1975.
75. Verberne, G., and DeBoer, J.: Chemocommunication among domestic cats, mediated by the olfactory and vomeronasal senses. I. Chemocommunication. Z. Tierpsychol. 42:86, Sept. 1976.
76. Weigel, I.: Small cats and clouded leopards. In Grzimek, H. C. B., ed.: Grzimek's Animal Life Encyclopedia. Vol. 12. New York: Van Nostrand Reinhold Co., 1975.
77. Whalen, R. E.: The initiation of mating in naive female cats. Anim. Behav. 11:461, 1963.
78. Wildt, D. E.: Effect of transportation on sexual behavior of cats. Lab. Anim. Sci. 30:910, 1980.
79. Wood, G. L.: Animal Facts and Feats. New York: Doubleday & Co., 1972.
80. Worden, A. N.: Abnormal behaviour in the dog and cat. Vet. Rec. 71:966, 1959.
81. Wynne-Edwards, V. C.: Animal Dispersion in Relation to Social Behaviour. Edinburgh: Oliver & Boyd, 1962.
82. Young, C.: Preweaning mortality in specific pathogen-free kittens. J. Small Anim. Pract. 14:391, 1973.

ADDITIONAL READINGS

Bard, P., and Macht, M. B. The behaviour of chronically decerebrate cats. In Wolstendholme, G. E. W., and O'Connor, C. M., eds. Neurological Basis of Behaviour. Boston: Little, Brown & Co., 1952.

Barton, A. Sexual inversion and homosexuality in dogs and cats. Vet. Med. 54:155, 1959.

Beaver, B. V. Feline behavioral problems. Vet. Clin. North Am. 6:33, Aug. 1976.

Beaver, B. V. Disorders of behavior. In Sherding, R. G., ed. The Cat: Diseases and Clinical Management. New York: Churchill Livingstone, 1989.

Beyer, C. Effect of estrogen on brain stem neuronal responsivity in the cat. In Sawyer, C. H., and Gorski, R. A., eds. Steroid Hormones and Brain Function. Berkeley: University of California Press, 1971.

Brunner, F. The application of behavior studies in small animal practice. In Fox, M. W., ed. Abnormal Behavior in Animals. Philadelphia: W. B. Saunders Co., 1968.

Burke, T. J. Feline reproduction. Vet. Clin. North Am. 6:317, Aug. 1976.

Cerny, V. A. Failure of dihydrotestosterone to elicit sexual behavior in the female cat. J. Endocrinol. 75:173, 1977.

Chesler, P. Maternal influence in learning by observation in kittens. Science 166:901, 1969.

Cline, E. M., Jennings, L. L., and Sojka, N. J. Breeding laboratory cats during artificially induced estrus. Lab. Anim. Sci. 30:1003, 1980.

Colby, E. D. Induced estrus and timed pregnancies in cats. Lab. Anim. Care 20:1075, 1970.

Dawson, A. B. Early estrus in the cat following increased illumination. Endocrinology 28:907, 1941.

Diegmann, F. G., Loo, B. J., and Grom, P. A. Female pseudohermaphroditism in the cat. Fel. Pract. 8:45, Sept. 1978.

Eleftheriou, B. E., and Scott J. P. The physiology of aggression and defeat. New York: Plenum Publishing Corp., 1971.

Evans, I. Suppression of estrus in cats. Fel. Pract. 2:10, Dec. 1972.

Ewer, R. F. Viverrid behavior and the evolution of reproductive behavior in the Felidae. In Eaton, R. L., ed. The World's Cats. Seattle: Feline Research Group, 1974.

Failla, M. L., Tobach, E., and Frank, A. A study of parturition in the domestic cat. Anat. Rec. 111:482, 1951.

Fox, M. W. New information on feline behavior. Mod. Vet. Pract. 56:50, Apr. 1965.

Fox, M. W. Natural environment: Theoretical and practical aspects for breeding and rearing laboratory animals. Lab. Anim. Care 16:316, 1966.

Fox, M. W. The veterinarian: Mercenary, Saint Francis or humanist? J. Am. Vet. Med. Assoc. 166:276, 1975.

Fraser, A. F. Behavior disorders in domestic animals. In Fox, M. W., ed. Abnormal Behavior in Animals. Philadelphia: W. B. Saunders Co., 1968.

Friedgood, H. B. Induction of estrous behavior in anestrous cats with the FSH and LH of the anterior pituitary gland. Am. J. Physiol. 126:229, 1939.

Gerber, H. A., Jöchle, W., and Sulman, F. G. Control of reproduction and of undesirable social and sexual behaviour in dogs and cats. J. Small Anim. Pract. 14:151, 1973.

Gottlieb, G. Ontogenesis of sensory function in birds and mammals. In Tobach, E., Aronson, L. R., and Shaw, E., eds. The Biopsychology of Development. New York: Academic Press, 1971.

Green, J. D., Clemente, C. D., and DeGroot, J. Rhinencephalic lesions and behavior in cats. J. Comp. Neurol. 108:505, 1957.

Hart, B. L. Facilitation by estrogen of sexual reflexes in female cats. Physiol. Behav. 7:675, 1971.

Hart, B. L. Gonadal hormones and behavior of the female cat. Fel. Pract. 2:6, July-Aug. 1972.

Hart, B. L. Types of aggressive behavior. Can. Pract. 1:6, May-June 1974.

Hart, B. L. Normal behavior and behavioral problems associated with sexual function, urination, and defecation. Vet. Clin. North Am. 4:589, Aug. 1974.

Hart, B. L. The catnip response. Fel. Pract. 4:8, Nov.-Dec. 1974.

Hart, B. L. Spraying behavior. Fel. Pract. 5:11, July-Aug. 1974.

Hart, B. L. Aggression in cats. Fel. Pract. 7:22, July-Aug. 1977.

Hart, B. L. Objectionable urine spraying and urine marking in cats: Evaluation of progestin treatment in gonadectomized males and females. J. Am. Vet. Med. Assoc. 177:529, 1980.

Hart, B. L. The Behavior of Domestic Animals. New York: W. H. Freeman & Co., 1985.

Hart, B. L., and Cooper, L. Factors related to urine spraying and fighting in prepubertally gonadectomized male and female cats. J. Am. Vet. Med. Assoc. 184:1255, 1984.

Houdeshell, J. W., and Hennessey, P. W. Megestrol acetate for control of estrus in the cat. Vet. Med. Small Anim. Clin. 72:1013, 1977.

Houpt, K. A. Animal behavior as a subject for veterinary students. Cornell Vet. 66:73, 1976.

Jöchle, W. Progress in small animal reproductive physiology, therapy of reproductive disorders, and pet population control. Folia Vet. Lat 4:706, 1974.

Jöchle, W., and Jöchle, M. Reproductive and behavioral control in the male and female cat with progestins: Long-term field observations in individual animals. Theriology 3:179, 1975.

Kavanagh, A. J. The reticulo-cortical evoked response: Changes correlated with behaviour and estrogen in female cats. Diss. Abstr. Int. 30:995B, 1969.

Kleiman, D. G., and Eisenberg, J. F. Comparisons of canid and felid social systems from an evolutionary perspective. Anim. Behav. 21:637, 1973.

Marvin, C. Hormonal influences on the development and expression of sexual behavior in animals. In Fox, M. W., ed. Abnormal Behavior in Animals. Philadelphia: W. B. Saunders Co., 1968.

Michael, R. P. Neurological mechanisms and the control of sexual behaviour. Sci. Basis Med., 1965, p. 316.

Mosier, J. E. Common medical and behavioral problems in cats. Mod. Vet. Pract. 56:699, 1975.

O'Connor, P., and Herron, M. A. Estrus after ovariohysterectomy. Fel. Pract. 6:28, Sept. 1976.

Palen, G. F., and Goddard, G. V. Catnip and oestrous behaviour in the cat. Anim. Behav. 14:372, 1966.

Peretz, E. Estrogen dose and the duration of mating period in cats. Physiol. Behav. 3:41, 1968.

Pfaff, D. W. Interactions of steroid sex hormones with brain tissue: Studies of uptake and physiological effects. In Segal, S. J., ed. The Regulation of Mammalian Reproduction. Springfield, IL: Charles C Thomas, 1973.

Porter, R. W., Cavanaugh, E. B., Critchlow, B. V., and Sawyer, C. H. Localized changes in electrical activity of the hypothalamus in estrous cats following vaginal stimulation. Am. J. Physiol. 189:145, 1957.

Romanes, G. J. Mental Evolution in Animals. New York: AMS Press, 1969.

Scott, J. P. The analysis of social organization in animals. Ecology 37:213, 1956.

Scott, P. P., and Lloyd-Jacob, M. A. Reduction in the anoestrus period of laboratory cats by increased illumination. Nature 184:2022, 1959.

Smith, B. A., and Jansen, G. R. Early undernutrition and subsequent behavior patterns in cat. J. Nutr. 103:xxix, 1973.

Smith, R. C. The Complete Cat Book. New York: Walker & Co., 1963.

Stewart, M. F. Maternal behaviour in cats. Br. Vet. J. 127:397, 1971.

Stover, D. G., and Sokolowski, J. H. Estrous behavior of the domestic cat. Fel. Pract. 8:54, July 1978.

Sulman, F. G. Suppression of estrus in cats. Vet. Med. 56:513, 1961.

Thornton, D. A. K., and Kear, M. Uterine cystic hyperplasia in a Siamese cat following treatment with medroxyprogesterone. Vet. Rec. 80:380, 1967.

West, M. Social play in the domestic cat. Am. Zool. 14:427, 1974.

Wilkins, D. B. Pyometritis in a spayed cat. Vet. Rec. 91:24, July 1972.

Windle, W. F. Induction of mating and ovulation in the cat with pregnancy urine and seminal extracts. Endocrinology 25:365, 1939.

7

Feline Ingestive Behavior

The neonate initiates ingestive behavior within an hour after birth, usually after the completion of parturition. As maturation of the kitten progresses, numerous modifications are made in the behavior associated with eating.

SUCKLING INGESTIVE BEHAVIOR

Early Phase

During the first 3 weeks of life, feeding sessions are initiated primarily by the queen. She arouses the usually sleeping kittens by her movements and licking, and positions herself around the young, almost enclosing them with her limbs and ventrum. The rooting reflex causes the kitten to burrow into a warm object, usually its queen or littermates, and may be present up to 11 days. (See Fig. 2–8.) Maturation of the senses, particularly vision, and of homeostatic mechanisms alters all neonatal reflexes. During the appetitive searching component of nursing behavior, the kitten's movements toward the queen are awkward, but they become progressively more coordinated as the kitten's control of its muscular and nervous systems increases with age. Communal nests allow some queens to have nursing coalitions.[84]

The sucking reflex is present at birth and can be tactilely stimulated over a large perioral area.[78] Such stimulation results in a head turn in the direction of the stimulus and accompanying sucking movements. (See Fig. 2–9.) Small objects in the mouth also stimulate the reflex, which is strongest immediately after awakening. Within a few days the sucking reflex is limited to lip contact, and foreign objects in the mouth are rejected.[78] This is probably when olfactory cues become more important in teat location than trial and error, which is the initial method the kitten uses. Kittens whose olfactory bulbs are destroyed experimentally cannot initiate sucking, even with previous experience, but such damage does not interfere with their ability to learn how to suck from a bottle.[73] The sucking reflex normally disappears by day 23.[71, 73] Taste and texture can be discriminated shortly after birth but are of minor significance in normal sucking.[97]

The kitten's initial contact with the teat results in a withdrawal motion of the head, followed by a downward motion and perhaps another withdrawal before the teat finally is enclosed by the mouth. This random head bob decreases as the kitten's ability to discriminate the teat increases. By day 4 kittens are relatively proficient at suckling the queen, and by 1 week little nuzzling is necessary.

Before the end of the 3rd day, and sometimes as early as the 1st day, a form of teat preference develops, which may be rigid. As many as 80 per cent of individuals nurse only from a specific nipple.[37, 102, 107] When preferences are more loosely defined, a kitten nurses from a pair of teats, usually near each other, or from a general region of the mammary surface.[102, 103] Some individuals do not develop any preference and nurse randomly.[101, 107, 108] The incidence of teat preference is independent of litter size.[102] The development of teat preference may minimize claw injuries among littermates, provide optimal stimulation to ensure milk production, and allow more rapid completion of nursing. Variability has developed with domestication because the behavior has not been considered in selective breeding.

If a specific teat is not sucked for about 3 days, milk production by that mammary gland stops.[41] The appearance of the mammary region of a nursing queen makes it obvious that only certain nipples are used.

Nursing positions are identified by olfactory means, and kittens seldom nurse strange teats after the first few days if normal nursing is allowed.[38, 46] A kitten that takes the wrong nipple may leave it immediately or may continue to suckle until the rightful "owner" nuzzles at it. Only when nursing the preferred teat will a kitten tenaciously cling when challenged for it.[102] Unlike pigs, kittens nursing from the cranially positioned teats do not necessarily become larger than their littermates.[37] Teat positions are maintained for about 1 month, at which time the preference becomes less rigid. At about the same time, kittens show less discrimination in nursing foster queens.[38, 41] In cat colonies in which multiple litters are housed together, kittens commonly suckle queens indiscriminately, with little or no teat preference development. When bottle feeding is necessary, repeated use of the same bottle and nipple and avoidance of noxious or unfamiliar odors on human hands are desirable.

The "milk tread," considered part of the nursing behavior of kittens, consists of rhythmic alternate movements of the forepaws against the mammary gland. A similar pattern is observed as the neonate tries to steady its suckling position. Functionally the milk tread may serve to push the queen's skin away from the neonate's nose, but soon it becomes more important to help stimulate milk flow.[39, 40] The behavior is primarily used when milk is not coming as fast as the kitten can drink and usually is alternated with nonrhythmic sucking.

Purring by both the queen and kittens often accompanies nursing.[20]

The neonate initially spends a great deal of time nursing. Each session may last up to 45 minutes, totaling about 8 hours per day.[10, 104] This amount of nursing allows most kittens to double their birth weight in 1 week, triple it in the 2nd week, and quadruple it by the end of the 3rd week.[10, 117] In addition, there is as much as a tenfold increase in subcutaneous body fat for insulation to aid in homeostasis.[117]

Intermediate Phase

During the second phase of nursing behavior, suckling is initiated by the queen, although the kittens play an increasing role. In the beginning, 40 per cent of the feedings are kitten-initiated, with marked increases later.[101] The intermediate phase usually lasts from the 2nd to 3rd week of life to the end of the 4th to 5th week, when development of vision and use of visual cues, as well as coordination of motor abilities, allow the kittens to actively approach the queen even when she is not in the nest area. She, in turn, lies in lateral recumbency to present the mammary region for the young to nurse. (See Fig. 6–8.) Toward the end of this phase the kittens may initiate sucking with the queen in a standing position, but she will then respond by lying down.

Avoidance Phase

Near the end of the 1st month, kittens are very active in initiating nursing, and the queen becomes increasingly evasive of them. At first the queen avoids some of the advances of the young by jumping onto objects they cannot reach, but as the kittens' motor skills develop, they become increasingly difficult to avoid. Avoidance is made even more difficult because their efforts usually are individualized rather than coordinated. The queen may lie in sternal recumbency to prevent access to the teats, and if the kittens become too persistent, she bats at them or gets up and moves away. When she does allow nursing, the queen usually is sitting or standing, with the kittens contorted into several postures. If she has only one kitten in the litter, she may not show this avoidance phase.

Weaning Phase

Weaning is a gradual, variable process that results from inaccessibility of the queen and increasing ability of the kittens to hunt. In the wild, cats do not wean their young, but if the queen is still lactating, the milk is of little nutritional value after 12 weeks.[24, 109] When this decreased value is coupled with normal dispersion necessary to obtain prey, weaning simply happens. Even without increased avoidance by the queen, there is a natural tendency for the young to decrease their nursing at about the time of normal weaning.[54] When kittens are confined with the queen or have ready access to her, nursing may continue for several months, although 8 to 10 weeks is most common.[46, 72, 102] There is an inverse correlation between litter size and length of time the queen allows nursing.[10] Smaller litters nurse longer. Some queens will let their kittens nurse until just before the birth of the next litter, as much as a year later, and then aggressively chase them away. The older offspring may return shortly after the queen gives birth and continue nursing, lying among the neonates.

TRANSITIONAL INGESTIVE BEHAVIOR

The transitional stage of ingestive behavior occurs while the kitten is both nursing and eating solid food. Starting near the end of the 4th week of age, this mixed nutritional period lasts until the kitten is weaned, at about 8 weeks. Domestic kittens begin eating solid food between 28 and 50 days of age (mean is 32 days), often by following the queen to the food bowl or accidentally stepping in the food.[14, 102, 109] Immediately preceding the transition to solid food, kittens eat dirt or litter.

If the queen is a hunter, she introduces her young to solid food in the form of small, dead prey. When the kittens are around 35 days old she eats the prey in their presence, but by 6 weeks some of the kittens start eating with her on their own. This ensures that solid food will be available to the young when they are ready. The queen apparently brings prey to the nest in response to the characteristics of kittens of an appropriate age, since a nonlactating queen may bring prey to another queen's kittens of the appropriate age.[10, 39]

HUNTING BEHAVIOR

Felis catus has been described as the most perfect carnivore because its entire body is geared to predatory life. In addition to sensory and locomotor adaptations, the cat has laterally flattened canine teeth, which permit it to sever the spinal cord of its prey without damaging the vertebral bodies. The lever action of the jaw and the scissor action of the premolars also hasten the killing and eating of prey because no molar grinding action is necessary. Thus the cat has rudimentary molars and almost no lateral jaw motion. The cat eats from the side of its mouth, using the premolars to tear flesh, rather than from the front like a grazing animal. While the cat is chewing, the ear and vibrissae on the side nearer the prey are noticeably flattened to the head.[50] Sharpened claws on the thoracic limbs aid in catching prey, and their retractability by means of specialized ligaments helps to maintain their extreme sharpness. Padded feet allow attack by ambush, and the shortened alimentary canal permits rapid digestion so that the cat does not have to carry excess weight.

Developmental Hunting

Prey recognition begins toward the end of the 1st month, when the queen brings home dead prey for her offspring to smell and eventually taste. In another 3 to 4 weeks the queen brings weak or wounded prey so that the young can begin acquiring their own hunting skills. For each of these behaviors, the queen's own prey-killing and eating instincts must be inhibited, primarily in response to kitten-related cues.

Hunting techniques are developed by practice during play and during prey sessions with the queen. The chase and catch aspects of hunting are thought to be innate, whereas the manipulative and positive contact responses are acquired behaviors.[10, 47, 100] The chasing, catching, and killing aspects of hunting also may be learned, but this fact is controversial. The nape bite is the prey-killing behavior that usually does not appear in play and must be perfected with practice on actual prey. When the kitten's hunting style fails and the mouse or other prey escapes, the kitten is given another opportunity because the queen recaptures the mouse and drags it back to the young. Kittens follow the queen on hunting trips to perfect their skills as they approach self-sufficiency. By 15 to 18 weeks exploration and hunting take up to 68 per cent of the young cat's time.[116]

Predatory tendencies are inherited and probably have been modified by domestication, so that prey-killing cats usually are less defensive and more aggressive than nonhunters.[1] These tendencies are influenced by early experience. Competency in predation is related to the presence of the queen during the kitten's exposure to prey and to experience as an adult.[18, 25, 26, 62] Kittens hunt the same prey they observed their mother kill and bring home. Of the young that never observe this process, about half will learn hunting skills on their own. Learning to kill prey is limited to the 6th to about the 20th week, but for the few cats that learn after that age, the process appears almost laborious.[83] Even though a kitten is never exposed to hunting, at an appropriate age the cat responds to the squeak of a mouse by attacking it.[49] The way a kitten is raised also is important in future hunting behavior. A young kitten raised only with a mouse or a rat seldom becomes a hunter, but the approximately 17 per cent that become hunters do not hunt the type of prey with which they were raised. If the kitten is raised with a mouse or a rat in addition to other kittens, socialization to the natural prey is minimal.[74, 75]

The Hunt

Prey Capture. Although rustlings or squeakings may attract the cat's attention, the sight of moving prey is the primary factor that initiates hunting behavior. With experience a cat can learn to recognize immobile prey.[112] Kittens can visually orient to prey as early as 9 days of age.[100] Hunger and prey-killing are independent, although the former can lower the threshold for the latter.[16, 82] After being alerted to potential prey, even prey as large as itself, a cat approaches the prey in a stalking ambush. The cat initially heads to a particular area. When it arrives the gait changes to a slow walk as it looks over the area.[112] Once prey has been spotted, the cat crouches close to the ground and uses a slinking trot, stopping periodically behind cover. It lies there temporarily, with fore legs under and elbows protruding. The entire pes is on the ground under the cat. The head is stretched forward, as are the ears. Whiskers are spread. As its eyes follow the prey, the cat usually twitches its tail.[10] The stalking continues periodically until the cat nears striking range. At that time it again stops and lowers its body, proceeding at a cautious, low-profile walk (Fig. 7–1). At the last available cover there is a final pause, during which its tail twitches with great intensity and the caudally positioned pelvic limbs tread so as to swing its entire hindquarters to and fro.[10] Then, after a short run, if necessary, the cat springs forward to seize the prey. In this pouncing attack its pelvic limbs remain on the

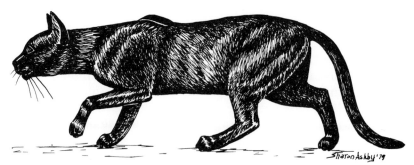

FIGURE 7–1. The stalking walk of prey hunting.

ground and only its forefeet are used in the capture (Fig. 7–2). As soon as its forelimbs leave the ground, its hindlimbs spread apart to stabilize the cat and help it brake. In this way the cat can change direction to accommodate changes made by the fleeing prey. If instead both thoracic and pelvic limbs were off the ground during the lunge, the cat would be committed in its direction of travel. The cat that misses its intended prey makes no attempt to correct the error. Instead it temporarily withdraws and then, if conditions are still favorable, renews its attack.[83] Cats have been known to leave one mouse in favor of another, more active one.[10]

The Nape Bite. Captured prey are restrained and positioned for the kill with the forepaws and killed by the nape bite. The accomplished hunter aims this bite at the dorsal aspect of the neck, directing its canine teeth between adjacent cervical vertebrae to sever the spinal cord or into the atlanto-occipital joint to pierce the medulla oblongata.[70, 83] The innate directing force is governed visually by the constriction of the prey's neck and tactilely by the direction of the prey's hair. The canine teeth of *F. catus* are flattened laterally so that they serve as a wedge.[40, 83] In addition, there are numerous nerve receptors at the base of these teeth, probably to help direct the killing bite. Rapid contraction time for the muscles of mastication permits a rapid bite after correct placing is achieved.[40, 47] A

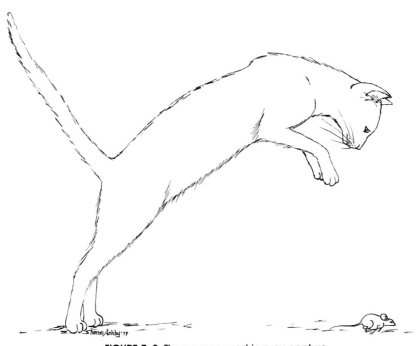

FIGURE 7–2. The pounce used in prey capture.

young, inexperienced kitten, especially a timid one, initially may not use enough strength to kill the prey, but competition with littermates and repeated attacks increase the excitement until it eventually makes the kill. A few kittens never reach that point, and for older cats the necessary amount of excitement is difficult to achieve. After a few successful kills kittens appear to become less skillful as they individualize and perfect their techniques in more difficult situations, such as when the mouse is not running directly away. Killing of prey is related to size and hunger. The probability of a kill increases with hunger and decreases with larger prey size.[16] When these factors are in conflict, the cat is more apt to play with the prey first.[16]

The learning process associated with the nape bite involves several interesting features. When the bite is not directed correctly, the kitten may secure another portion of the prey's body. The prey may turn around and bite the kitten's nose.[10] The initial kill usually is unexpected by the kitten, and it tries to continue playing with the now motionless prey. The kitten must make several kills before it associates the nape bite with its ability to transform live prey into food, and only then does hunger initiate prey-catching actions.[10, 39, 83] If the prey is killed by a method other than the nape bite, the cat may perform a nape bite on the dead animal, usually before eating it but occasionally after the initial stages of ingestion.[83] When not used for awhile, the skills associated with killing tend to atrophy.[83]

Prey Ingestion. Eating killed prey is another behavior based on experience. If the kitten learns from the queen to eat dead prey, it will eat the prey it catches. The kitten that has eaten raw meat but not fresh prey will eat the prey it catches if the prey is cut open to release the smell of fresh tissue or if it accidentally draws blood or tears muscle during the kill. Cats raised as vegetarians will kill, but they usually do not eat the prey.[10]

After the kill a cat often grooms itself and then take its dead prey to a quiet area before eating it. When eating a mouse even a young cat begins with the head and works caudally while crouching over it. This orientation is tactile, based on the lie of the prey's hair. Some cats may try to bite the abdomen first but soon move to the head. The entire animal usually is consumed except, occasionally, for the tail.

Catching, killing, and eating prey are behaviors along a continuous gradient of activation.[96] Each has its own threshold level for performance. To get close enough to kill some mice, a cat must attempt to catch more than it can eat. Some mice escape—perhaps two out of three.[80] A cat that is introduced to a limitless number of mice one at a time first catches, kills, and eats the prey. In time the animal catches and kills but does not eat the mice. With continued introduction of mice the cat catches them but does not kill or eat. Finally, with physical fatigue, the mice are ignored.[115] Cats catch an average of 15 mice per test.[90]

The environment probably necessitated that early felids use high-search, low-pursuit hunting techniques. Because of this evolutionary development and because the prey is small, cats normally are solitary hunters. On occasion two or three individuals hunt within 50 to 75 yards of one another; however, true cooperative hunting is rare and mainly restricted to courting pairs.[33, 76]

As a means of rodent control, the cat is unsurpassed. Although cats are important in this control, the emigration of cats into an area without resident cats lags the increase in rodent populations.[94, 95] Cats cannot completely depopulate an area of rodents, but they can prevent a population increase.[84] Other control methods depopulate a specific area only, but spaces within 50 yards of homes with hunting cats do not become reinfested.[35, 82] In a study of recently killed cats, most had one or two mice in their stomachs. One animal had 12.[112] Records that have been kept concerning ingestion of rodents show that one cat killed 22,000 mice in 23 years and another, less than 6 months old at the time, killed 400 rats in 4 weeks.[118]

Nonrodent Prey Capture

Studies of ingested material in feral cat populations confirm that mice are the cat's primary food. Other prey varies seasonally but includes rats, rabbits, birds, and insects. The availability of commercial food or table scraps does not decrease the consumption of wild prey.[31, 56]

Birds do not make up as much of the cat's diet as is commonly believed. Spring and summer hatches provide most of the supply, and cats that hunt near roads apparently kill more birds than those hunting in fields.[34, 88] Special hunting skills are required to catch flying prey, so not all cats are successful. The best hunters attack as soon as they spot the bird because ambush techniques often send the intended prey hopping or flying. The bird usually is caught with one or both forepaws and instantly brought to the mouth for the nape bite. If the bird is long-necked, the nape bite may be directed close to the head or the shoulder. The latter instinctively is more commonly used because the size disparity is greater between body and neck than between head and neck. The best hunters do not release the catch for a better nape bite because the bird would escape. Except for a few feathers, which may be plucked, the entire animal usually is eaten, beginning with the head.[10, 20]

Once a cat starts hunting birds, it is almost impossible to prevent its continuation. At best, throwing things at the cat causes it to hunt on the sly. To avoid having a bird-catching cat, a kitten whose mother does not hunt birds should be selected, or it should be adopted at about 6 weeks of age. In both cases the kitten should be confined and not allowed exposure to birds until after it is 1 year old.[59]

Rabbits that are caught usually are juveniles, probably because full-grown ones are too powerful.[112] Even then the difficulty of the catch is still greater than for other species.[112]

Another, less common prey for the cat is the fish. Although most cats leave fish alone, a few are noted for pursuit of the family's goldfish. The fishing cat of Malaysia is adept at hooking fish with its forepaws, as are certain individuals that live in coastal regions or near lakes and streams. Fishing in fact is one of the earliest skills for which selection was made in domestication. Like good bird hunters, good fishers do not let the catch go to obtain a better nape bite because that leads to the fish's escape. Cats that have no early fishing experience may run away from a fish flopping along a shore.

FOOD PREFERENCES

Initial gustatory responses appear as early as the 1st day of life and basically involve differentiation of salty milk from regular milk.[30] By 10 days responses also are seen to bitter, sweet, and sour.[30, 113] Maturation involves changes in ingestive behavior, but environment probably is the strongest influence on food preferences. The specific prey introduced by the queen or the food type fed by owners to the juvenile often determines the patterns in the adult, with food preferences usually established before 6 months of age. If the kitten was not exposed to a variety of foods, food preferences can be so limited that the cat may refuse to eat anything except its one or two choices. Cats are extremely particular, and the assumption that a cat eventually will eat a nutritious food when it becomes hungry is not correct. Cats may literally starve to death rather than eat an unacceptable meal. Queens have been known to eat their young while in this state, never touching the available food.[11] Foods should be changed gradually by mixing well 20 per cent to 25 per cent of the new food with the old. The first mixture should be offered until it is readily accepted, which usually takes up to 14 days. Then the mixture may be further changed by introducing another 20 per cent to 25 per cent of the new food. These steps should be repeated until the new diet is being fed exclusively.

Initial selection of a free-choice food depends on odor, which can provide the sole basis for dietary selection.[20, 92] If the smell is acceptable, the front of the tongue brings in the next information. Undesirable odors, tastes, or textures can overrule the metabolic need for nutrition and are more important as negative factors than as positive ones.[29] This explains why some cats will eat a novel diet if it is aesthetically acceptable.[60] It is related to the relatively rapid acceptance of most new foods. Rejection can recur after a period without a particular type of food.[21] Meat is the food of choice, and older cats prefer kidney.[20, 113] They also choose fish and commercial cat food over rats.[66] Cold, dead rats are slightly more palatable than the fresh kill.[66] Ranked in decreasing order of general feline preference is flesh from sheep, cattle, horses, pigs, chicken, and fish. Whether a meat is raw or cooked is relatively unimportant; foods at body temperature are preferable to those at higher or lower temperatures.[20, 92, 113] Moisture, which may help to release odors, enhances palatability; spicy foods usually are disliked.[20, 113] Sucrose does not increase palatability in cats like it does in other species.[67] One cat raised by a Jewish rabbi observed Jewish laws by not drinking milk when eating meat, even though both were available, illustrating that variations do occur based on individual factors and environmental influences.[77]

Prey preference can exist not only in hunting but also in consumption. Mousers catch all kinds of mice but refuse to eat certain types of mice, birds, moles, and shrews. Snakes, frogs, and toads seldom are eaten, although they may be hunted and caught.[10]

The immediate ancestors of the cat ate small prey, consuming frequent small meals rather than following the "feast or famine" principle. If allowed to set their own schedule, cats will eat up to 13 small, evenly sized meals a day.[60, 62, 109, 112] When fed periodically, cats tend to be more aggressive and less cooperative than if fed free-choice.[42] A great deal of time may be spent hunting. Females spend 26 per cent to 46 per cent of the day hunting, compared with 5 per cent to 34 per cent spent by males, during bouts averaging 30 minutes (range of 5 to 133 minutes).[112] As little as 1 per cent of the waking time may be spent eating.[60] Males eat more, but females show more variation in body weight, primarily because of changes in eating and activity patterns related to estrous cycles. Based on high-protein body needs, a cat consumes about 75 g of dry food or 250 g of canned food each day (each about 250 calories), or about 30 kg of dry or 90 kg of canned food per year.[28, 93] Caloric intake fluctuates somewhat on a 4-month cycle, along with cyclic changes in body weight, food intake, and thyroid activity.[67, 98]

Regulation of ingestive behavior is not completely understood. Several theories have been advanced, but each has exceptions, so that feeding may really be regulated by multiple factors. Theories include palatability of food, blood levels of amino acids, and hepatic glucoreceptors.[67, 105]

Food preferences are not restricted to meat, and that may again reflect the wild heritage. Grass and other vegetable matter can be found in the feces or the stomachs of about a third of feral cats. Animals that serve as normal prey for F. catus are primarily vegetarians, so that when the prey is eaten, vegetable matter becomes part of the cat's diet. Therefore, most of the vegetative matter consumed has already been partially processed by the prey's intestinal tract. Although cats can digest a small amount of fresh vegetable starch, large amounts of uncooked carbohydrate may cause vomition or diarrhea. Because cats lack the ability to break down the beta bonds of cellulose to glucose, fresh grass remains unchanged within the gastrointestinal system and may become irritative.[12] Because the indoor cat is most apt to consume large quantities infrequently, grass commonly has been assigned the role of a purgative for such things as hair balls. If the cat is introduced to small portions of vegetable matter early in life, it can be fairly omnivorous. Garbage also is commonly eaten, representing an opportunistic adaptation.[43]

Protocol when more than one cat approaches a food bowl is not governed by social status, as in other species. Instead, cats usually adhere to the first come, first served principle. Because cats do not know how to behave toward one another when eating together, the individual arriving later may choose to wait. Who eats first or how many eat at the same time depends on individuals rather than on age, sex, or other dominance factors. (See Fig. 4–4.) Seldom will one cat take prey from another.[10]

WATER CONSUMPTION

Around the 5th week of life a young kitten begins drinking from dishes. By adulthood the average cat requires about 200 mL of water per day. Water is available to an animal from three sources: drinking water, water in food, and water from nutrient metabolism of fat and energy.[106] A canned food diet is 74 per cent water, making 185 mL available directly, with about 15 mL more from fat metabolism. The cat does not need to drink. Dry food has only 10 per cent water, thus supplying 7.5 mL, with another 7.5 mL available from fat metabolism.[28] In this case, 185 mL of water must be ingested directly.

A kitten learns to drink by first lowering its head until the mouth touches the water. The head is then raised, and water is licked from around the mouth. The adult cat usually crouches over the water source and uses its tongue to bring water into its mouth (Fig. 7–3). For this, the tip of the tongue is curled caudally, forming a ladle to lift the liquid into the mouth, and the cat usually laps four or five times before swallowing.[10] Some house cats prefer to drink from the toilet bowl or a dripping faucet. One of two postures is used. If possible, the cat prefers to keep both hind feet on the floor, leaning or stretching as necessary to lap the water. If this is impossible, the cat straddles the toilet or sink, bracing itself while it drinks. More than one cat has lost its balance, and some no longer use that water source.

A few cats, in addition to using the regular form of drinking, have

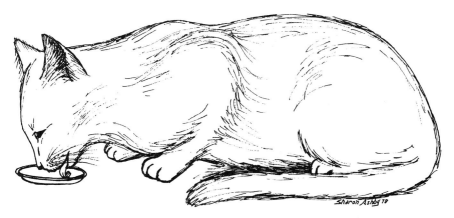

FIGURE 7-3. The most common drinking posture, with ladled tongue.

been observed to drink by dipping a paw into the water and then sucking moisture from it (Fig. 7-4). If this occurs when fresh water is being added, it may represent a play behavior. However, this behavior has been seen when fresh water was not a factor. In one colony a female cat displayed the behavior and later so did a female kitten, a daughter of one of the first cat's littermates. Paw-dipping may, therefore, be a genetic trait because the kitten's mother was not a dipper and observational learning could not have occurred.

FIGURE 7-4. A cat drinking water by dipping its paw and sucking from it.

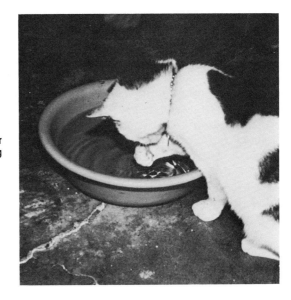

NEURAL AND HORMONAL REGULATION

Food Consumption

The Hypothalamus. The hypothalamus is well known for its control over appetite and ingestive behavior, and specific areas control specific functions. The lateral hypothalamus is considered the feeding center. Electrical and adrenergic stimulation of that area result in greatly increased food intake even in satiated cats. The intake increase, which occurs over a period of time, indicating a humoral mechanism, can be as much as 1000 per cent greater than normal.[32] In addition, stimulation results in increased activity, which simultaneously increases the likelihood of encountering food.[5] Destruction of the lateral hypothalamus results in aphagia. Conversely, the ventromedial hypothalamus controls satiety. Stimulation of this area causes anorexia, whereas its destruction results in hyperphagia, which leads to obesity. Experimentally, alterations of the lateral hypothalamus take precedence over those of the ventromedial hypothalamus, which indicates that although the lateral hypothalamus normally may control feline ingestive behavior, the ventromedial portion may exhibit inhibitory control over it.[6]

Aggression plays a significant role in food consumption because it is necessary for food capture in the wild. Specific areas of neurologic control have in the past been hard to identify because studies of affective aggression often included predatory aggression. Most forms of aggression are controlled by the hypothalamus, but not by the same portion that controls predation. Stimulation of the lateral hypothalamus results in normal rat-hunting behaviors, from stalking through the nape bite, even in cats that have never exhibited this behavior before the experiment. These stimulated attacks are not indiscriminate, as frequently is the case with the forms of aggression controlled by nearby portions of the hypothalamus; rather, specific prey is selected.[79, 110] Postural displays are another distinguishing characteristic of predatory aggression and do not follow the pattern of affective aggression. Even the active neurotransmitters differ in the two situations.[4, 15, 99]

Stimulation of the lateral hypothalamus has another neurologic effect related to predatory behavior. Two sensory areas around the cat's mouth become more sensitive, based primarily on the intensity of the stimulation to the brain. The perioral region becomes increasingly sensitive to touch and causes a reflex movement of the head, bringing the mouth closer to the tactile stimulus.[85] In addition, a touch reflex at the edge of the lips results in the mouth being opened.[85]

Hunger has been associated with increased excitatory changes in the hypothalamus; when the cat is satiated neural activity throughout the brain decreases.[3] In this way relative hunger may neurologically regulate stimulation of predatory behavior.[16]

Other Brain Areas. In cats of any age other parts of the brain also affect ingestive behavior but to a lesser degree than the hypothalamus.[8] In fact, all parts of the brain except the cerebellum and primary sensorimotor cortical areas modify this behavior.[53] Destructive lesions of lateral positions of the amygdala may result in hyperphagia or at least increased licking and mouthing.[51, 53, 71] Conversely, aphagia can result from lesions of the amygdala, whereas hyperphagia follows amygdala stimulation.[53, 89] A more specific relation between the hypothalamus and ingestive behavior probably is related to suppressing and facilitating certain regions of the amygdala. Although ingestion is elicited by stimulation of the hypothalamus, it can be modulated by means of the amygdala. Physiologic differences exist in the limbic systems of predatory and nonpredatory cats. Rat-killers show a significantly higher threshold for elicitation of after-discharge (ADT) from the amygdala than do nonpredatory cats, and cats with the lowest ADTs have the weakest attack tendencies.[2] This indicates neurologic differences between the two groups.

Destructive cortical lesions of the frontal and temporal lobes may increase food intake, although those of the frontal lobe have been reported to have the opposite effect.[7, 53, 78, 89] Removal of the frontal lobes has led to the reappearance of certain portions of kittenlike sucking behavior, including the milk tread movements of the forepaws and the clumsy motions.[78] Again, these areas probably modify hypothalamic cues.[7] Complete removal of the cerebral cortex results in complete anorexia.[119]

Electrical stimulation of the neural septum and tegmentum can override the aphagia of hypothalamic destruction.[27, 53] In the normal animal these areas probably serve as modifiers of appetite control.[89]

Electroencephalographic studies of patterns associated with ingestive behavior demonstrate different tracings for different activities. The sensorimotor rhythm is the slow-wave pattern associated with the motionless stances of hunting behavior. In contrast, ingestive reinforcement synchronization is a different type of slow-wave rhythm, which appears during food consumption. Interestingly, the latter pattern is identical to that seen during drowsiness, indicating the same neural status for both satiety and drowsiness.[111] Kittens also show slow-wave patterns with food searching and with satiation.[8]

Water Consumption

Water consumption is governed by an area of the lateral hypothalamus near the location that controls eating.[5, 52] Onset of water consumption caused by electrical or cholinergic stimulation of this area is delayed somewhat longer than that of food intake. However, the drinking behavior has a longer duration. This indicates that a separate humoral mechanism is related to water consumption. As expected, destruction of the lateral hypothalamus results in adipsia. Stimulation of the amygdala electrically or cholinergically also can increase water consumption; stimulation of other neural areas, such as the septum, has varying effects on this behavior. Discrete areas in the dorsal, rostral pons are responsive to hypovolemia, and their destruction greatly increases basal water intake.[114] Cats with midbrain lesions occasionally dip their paws into water and move them about.[76]

Hormonal Control

In attempting to study feline affective aggression by observing cats attacking mice, researchers in the past studied predatory aggression and looked at the behavioral effects of a number of hormones, drugs, and neurohormones. The findings of those studies are valid for predatory aggression only. Hormonal influences on predatory behavior are sex-dependent, probably a result of the early neonatal sex differentiation in the brain. In general, the male cat has a lower threshold for elicitation of hunting behaviors than does his female counterpart.[68] Castration tends to increase attack latency, whereas ovariectomy tends to have the opposite effect.[60, 68] These characteristics vary with the individual, however, so the results of neutering are not always predictable.

INGESTIVE BEHAVIOR PROBLEMS

Abnormal Nursing Behavior

Very young kittens have an innate need to suck. Nutritional sucking normally continues until weaning; nonnutritional sucking decreases during this period. Many kittens that are undernourished because of an inadequate milk supply from the mother, early weaning, or orphaning and that must be fed by bottle or stomach tube develop maladaptive reactions to stress and nonnutritional sucking vices. To satisfy their natural nursing drive, these kittens suck the bodies of littermates or themselves if no littermates are available. This sucking can become a severe habit, to the point of seriously traumatizing the skin. Pendulous portions of the body, such as ears, tails, folds of the flank, vulvas, and scrotums, are most frequently sucked. Some of these deprived kittens attempt to nurse human skin, the family dog, a stuffed toy, or, occasionally, objects such as buttons or clothing. This behavior, called prolonged sucking, represents an extension of normal, as does maternal nursing by a kitten over a year of age, and thus both atypical behaviors may be related to variations of normal weaning.[13] In prolonged cases of inappropriate sucking, which can last as long as 2 years, the kitten usually sucks during periods of relaxation, often kneading and purring at the same time.[11] The sucking eventually stops while the kneading and purring continue. With time these disappear as well.

Because this excessive sucking can be upsetting to owners, as well as traumatic to the skin, measures can be taken to speed up the "weaning" process. Under natural conditions the queen shows increasing avoidance of kittens being weaned and even displays mild aggression by batting their noses with her paw. Humans can separate littermates when they are sucking each other or thump the kitten on its nose and say "no" if it tries to nurse human skin. Another technique is to pick up the kitten by the nape of the neck, say "no," and put the kitten down, away from the sucked object.

Some of these kittens become stealthy in their approaches, suddenly grabbing and sucking the skin that is being kept from them. In these situations aversive conditioning techniques may be useful. For taste aversion, the cat is allowed to smell a foul-tasting substance, such as a mixture of Tabasco and pepper sauce or a commercial product used to stop chewing. At the same time, a substantial dose is introduced into its mouth so that the cat will associate the bad taste with a particular odor. From that point, the smell of the substance, whether alone or mixed with household shortening for smearability, initiates an avoidance reaction. Thus the nursed region or object can be spread with hot sauce, and the nursing habit can be broken. Another form of aversive conditioning, smell aversion, involves the use of a spray can. The owner shows the can to the cat and, aiming the spray 90 degrees from the cat's face, releases it while rapidly advancing the can toward the cat. The purpose is to threaten the cat with the advancing, hissing can so that the cat associates the smell emitted with the threat. Then, with the cat absent, the owner sprays the sucked objects and allows the mist to settle before readmitting the cat to the room. This technique varies in success because the amount of threat perceived by each cat and the offensiveness of the odor chosen may differ widely.

Medroxyprogesterone acetate (Depo-Provera) (50 mg I.M. for spayed females; 100 mg I.M. for males) and megestrol acetate (Ovaban) (1 mg/lb/day P.O. for 7 days, 0.5 mg/lb/day P.O. for 7 days, and then 0.5 mg/lb/wk P.O. for maintenance) have been successful in stopping self-sucking.[17]

A second type of abnormal nursing behavior, called wool-sucking, is almost exclusively seen in Siamese or part-Siamese cats, suggesting the possibility of genetic transfer of the trait. Burmese also have recently been implicated.[18, 65] Many of these cats do not develop the abnormal sucking behavior until they approach puberty.[57, 58] The usual owner complaint is that the cat has orally destroyed a woolen article or other piece of clothing by sucking or chewing it, or that the cat constantly tries to suck the armpit region of a family member. The cat may be seeking the odor of lanolin or that associated with the human sweat glands, whether from the human axilla itself or from the portion of a shirt soiled by the axilla.[38, 46, 47] These cats sleep with, lick, suck, chew, knead, and, on occasion, ingest pieces of the object. Most stop the behavior by 2 years of age, but others never do.[57, 58]

Several techniques have been used to stop wool-sucking, and often euthanasia was the last resort. Access to woolen objects can be limited to one item by putting away other potential targets.[13] The cat's carnassial teeth have been removed to prevent the objectionable damage without altering the behavior.[36] A lanolin-containing product may be fed to the cat in an attempt to satiate the desire for lanolin. Thyroid hormone (0.5 g/day P.O.) works well for some cats, as has aversive conditioning using the hot sauce mixture, the spray can (such as a deodorant), or both.[19] In early stages the thump on the nose and "no" may work. Some Siamese cat breeders delay weaning until at least 12 weeks, hoping to decrease the incidence of the problem.[58]

Hunting Behavior Problems

Atypical or Abnormal Variations. Some cats, primarily females, bring dead prey home and either leave it outside or present it to their owners. This may represent the cat's natural tendency to carry dead prey home or to a quiet spot before eating, or it may represent a maternal behavior— bringing prey home for phantom kittens.[10, 46] The same behaviors can be represented when a cat places a toy mouse in the food bowl. Taste preference tests show that a cat will leave a killed rat to eat commercial food, giving rats the lowest of food preferences.[66] This unpalatability is another reason a cat may bring prey home and not eat it. Presentation of live prey may again represent a much lowered maternal threshold of bringing live prey so that phantom kittens can practice their hunting skills. The presentation also may indicate that there was enough psychological excitement for the cat to catch prey but not enough to kill it, whether because of too many recent catches or lack of training as a kitten. Conversely, when too much excitement has been generated, the cat may have to dissipate some of it by repeatedly ambushing the corpse and tossing it into the air.[39] As the energy of excitement wears off, the prey is eaten.

Cats that attack the ankles of people walking across a room are exhibiting another form of abnormal prey-killing. This behavior usually is displayed by house cats that are not allowed outside and is most common between puberty and 2 years of age, during a time of "psychological adolescence."[23] For these animals, predatory aggression has been significantly repressed and the threshold to stalk prey is greatly lowered, so that anything moving initiates prey chase and attack. The threshold can be lowered to the point that the ambush activities appear as true vacuum (spontaneous) activities.[39, 118] To prevent this behavior, one must provide other methods for releasing this energy. For young kittens, another kitten playmate is successful; for both older and younger cats, toys that move, such as a ball, or playmates, such as other pets, work well.[91] Owners also should encourage the cat to play with these objects by occasionally initiating the movement. Progestin therapy has been suggested for animals that show extremely abnormal hunting behavior.[87]

Undesirable Prey. Cannibalism is considered one of the least desirable of the atypical behaviors, although it seldom is truly abnormal in the cat except in stressful situations. The subject is considered in more detail in Chapter 6.

Eating birds or other prey and stealing food from counters may be considered undesirable by owners, but these behaviors are difficult to control. Aversive conditioning may deter the cat when the owner is present, but without the human's presence, cats ignore their lessons. Bird corpses and partially eaten chicken legs have been tied around a cat's neck in an effort to stop the cat from eating these things.[45] A combination of smell aversion and remote punishment probably is more successful.[62] Some foods become undesirable if the food causes an unpleasant experience for the cat, such as vomition, nausea, or foul taste. Objects and verbiage have been hurled at cats, but these usually only create animosity between the animal and its owner.

Burying Food

Cats occasionally cover food, although this is not a common behavior in the wild. In the home, covering usually is elicited by presentation of a different food. Or a cat may partially consume a food and then cover it as though it were fecal matter. Odors associated with defecation stimulate neural centers to induce covering, and therefore the odor of the food or prey, rather than a desire for its preservation, probably initiates the covering.[70]

Excessive Food Intake

Cats, especially those that are nervous or have not eaten for some time, have been known to bolt food, even to the point of inducing regurgition. Most cats reingest the food, although some are not especially interested in it. In either case, small meals fed frequently are recommended to reduce or prevent the behavior.

Obesity does occur in the cat, although the rate of obesity is about 10 per cent and often is related to overeating as the result of certain psychological stresses and an overabundant, highly palatable, calorie-dense food supply.[64, 66, 67] Invasion of privacy, overcrowding, changes in routine, and postreaction to malnutrition can be initiating stresses. Physical conditions, such as chronic pancreatitis, also may result in compulsive eating. Changes in metabolism, such as with hypothyroidism, also should be considered.[64]

The amount of adipose tissue normally carried by a cat is regulated by several factors. Genetics is of minor importance in the overeating behavior of *F. catus* except to regulate thinness. Early dietary history, caloric concentration of food, palatability, the amount of neural activation, whether from stress or exercise, and the cat's hormonal state must be considered.[55, 81] A direct correlation between lack of estrogen from an ovariohysterectomy and obesity has not been made in the cat.[62] There is, however, evidence in other species. Under extreme conditions cats can become as much as 74 per cent fat.[22] Joseph, the heaviest cat on record, weighed 48 lbs, and other cats of 40 to 46 lbs have been reported.[9, 44, 118] Synthetic progestins (including megestrol acetate and medroxyprogesterone acetate), diazepam, corticosteroids, and metabolic steroids are well known for producing marked increases in appetitive behavior.

Few treatments other than the reduction of caloric intake have been highly successful in controlling obesity. Food palatability can be decreased, bulk increased, and access regulated. Reduced food intake may increase irritability in the cat, but this method can be successful if the owner can be adequately motivated to carry out the program.

Anorexia

Anorexia nervosa is one of the more serious problem behaviors encountered in cats, particularly in nervous cats such as the Siamese. This condition commonly is produced by emotional or physical stress, such as hospitalization, overcrowding, introduction of new people or animals, loss of a close companion, and excessive handling. Diseases that impair the sense of smell can cause some degree of anorexia, as can about 95 per cent of all cat diseases.[14] In addition to pylorospasm, vomition, halitosis, ulcers, systemic pain, polydipsia, and adipsia, sympathetic physical signs may accompany this condition. Anorexia nervosa lasts from a few days to a week, although extended bouts are not uncommon. One cat survived without food or water when accidentally isolated for 52 days, although that is certainly extreme.[118]

Sick and convalescing cats need full nutrition, so food intake should be strongly encouraged. Even an otherwise healthy cat deprived of food cannot exist long without starting to deplete its body's reserve. A dark, quiet place near food and water may provide enough security for the troubled cat. Mild tranquilization, especially with drugs of the benzodiazepine group noted for antianxiety action, usually is successful. Diazepam (0.05 to 0.4 mg/kg I.V.) can be useful in the anorexic cat if food is presented immediately.[86] These results may be related in part to the antianxiety tranquilizing effects; diazepam also has been shown to escalate predation, probably at the lateral hypothalamus.[96] Oxazepam (3 mg/kg P.O.) is particularly good in this situation.[48] In extreme cases light anesthetization can be used, allowing the cat to recover with food nearby. Force-feeding with minimal handling, a pharyngotomy tube, progestins, and anabolic steroids can be used when appropriate.

House Plant Ingestion

Eating house plants is a common variation of ingestive behavior in cats that do not get vegetable matter in their diet. By providing a small flower pot with grass or catnip, an owner often can eliminate the problem. For the cat that has developed a habit or preference, putting the plant where the cat cannot get to it or using aversive taste-smell conditioning with pepper sauce or vinegar usually works. An additional aversive technique is useful in these situations: By aiming a fine-mist water sprayer at the plant usually chewed and rigging a string to trigger the device from a distance, the owner can hide and remotely spray the cat when it disturbs the plant.[61, 69] Appropriately placed mousetraps or other scare tactics that are set off by the cat's presence also have been used.

Excessive Salivation

Excessive salivation or minimization of swallowing, or both, is common in the extremely relaxed cat, most frequently during petting. It probably represents parasympathetic stimulation.

Food Allergies

Food allergies are difficult to substantiate but do occur in the cat.[90] The full ramification of their effects are unknown but include aggression, irritableness, and seizures. The incidence of these behaviors can be related to the introduction or deletion of certain foods in the cat's diet.

Food Aversion

Cats can develop an aversion to a certain food as the result of an allergy or because of an associated experience. The nausea and vomiting caused by lithium chloride are related to the food eaten at the same time.[62] Being traumatized while eating a certain food results in the same type of aversion.

Oral Medications

There are several techniques for giving oral medications, but speed and dexterity often are necessary. Up to 10 mL of a liquid can be introduced at one time between the teeth and the buccal wall with an eyedropper or a syringe.[24] Small amounts of liquid, gel, or paste will be ingested by a cat that is grooming if the material is placed on the hair or nose. To give medication in the food, a small amount of medicine is first placed on the cat's nose to satiate its olfactory system. The cat will lick it off and satiate its gustatory system so that the rest of the medication in the food will be eaten undetected.

To give tablets, minimal restraint is best, and the tablet must get into the laryngopharynx quickly so that it neither dissolves nor is tasted or smelled. While holding the head back, one uses the thumb and third finger to push the sides of the cat's mandible and hold it open, after the index finger of the opposite hand has opened the mouth by pushing down on the lower incisors (Fig. 7–5). The cat usually tries to back away. After putting the tablet in place, one holds the mouth closed until the cat licks its nose or otherwise indicates that it has swallowed. If the animal still does not swallow, a sudden puff of air on the nose may startle it into doing so.

Another technique to administer tablets requires that the cat face the person. Using the restraining arm, one places the hand on the cat's head so that the thumb grasps one ear, the palm is near its other ear, and the fingers are at its throat. The cat's skull is rotated, without raising its

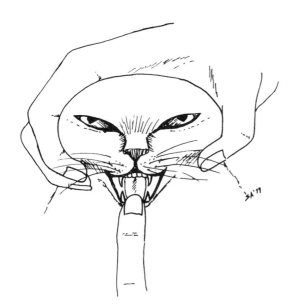

FIGURE 7–5. A technique used to open the cat's mouth.

head, until its nose points toward the ceiling. About 90 per cent of cats in this position will relax the muscles of mastication so that the mouth can easily be opened.[63] Again, the head is held until the cat has swallowed.

CASE PRESENTATIONS

CASE 7–1. Four-month-old Siamese female. The kitten was obtained at 8 weeks of age and had sucked the owner's skin periodically ever since. When skin was not available, it would suck on an article of clothing.

Diagnosis. Prolonged sucking (persistent nursing behavior).

Treatment. Behavior modification was achieved with the spray can technique, using spray deodorant. The kitten was picked up by the back of the neck, reprimanded with "no," and moved away from the item being sucked whenever it was caught at the behavior.

CASE 7–2. Two-year-old Burmese neutered male. The cat chewed house plants, ruining the owner's prized collection. The animal was not allowed outside and normally was fed canned cat food.

Diagnosis. Destructive chewing that is normal plant ingestion owing to lack of access to other vegetable matter.

Treatment. Behavior modification was achieved by coupling the odor and taste of vinegar with the plants. The owner also grew two flowerpots of grass in an area separate from her other plants so that the cat would have access to some vegetable matter.

CASE 7–3. Two 2½-year-old Siamese neutered female littermates. Both cats were obtained at 13 weeks of age from a breeder, and at 4 months the owner noticed that both cats were sucking a woolen scarf. They gradually began to suck other woolen objects, with increasing amounts of damage.

Diagnosis. Wool-sucking.

Treatment. Behavior modification was not successful using the spray can technique but was achieved by coupling the odor and taste of a pepper sauce with the cats' favorite woolen objects. At first other woolen items were kept away from the cats, but after 30 days during which there was no wool-sucking, other woolen items gradually were reintroduced. Wool-sucking did not resume in either cat.

CASE 7–4. Two-year-old domestic shorthair female. The cat was part of a small, private research colony that at the time of the problem was testing flavorings for cat food. The cat had been raised on a dry-nugget diet, but during the experiment it was put on a beef-flavored, gelatin-textured, cubed ration. Because the investigator did not understand, the cat's diet was not changed when it would not eat and it eventually died.

Diagnosis. Death by starvation probably because of the unacceptable texture or flavor of the experimental diet.

CASE 7–5. Five-year-old domestic longhair neutered male. This cat was one of seven cats in a home, and all had been doing well until the owners got a new piano. This cat started fighting with the others and was given to a new home. The new owners really liked the cat and brought it to the veterinarian after 1 week of its not eating.

Diagnosis. Psychogenic anorexia related to the environmental stress of a change and a move.

Treatment. The cat was given a 3-week treatment of megestrol acetate (reducing dose starting at 5 mg P.O. s.i.d.) and presented food for 20-minute periods four times a day. The cat's appetite gradually picked up, and it was a well-adjusted animal within 4 months.

CASE 7–6. Fourteen-week-old domestic shorthair male. The kitten was probably 4 weeks old when the owners obtained it from a pet store. It had always sucked its foot and had recently started to suck a few items of clothing.

Diagnosis. Prolonged sucking caused by early weaning.

Treatment. The owners were able to keep most clothing away from the kitten so that it only sucked its foot. Because no physical injury was occurring, the owners did not mind the behavior. It is expected to decrease as the kitten grows older.

CASE 7–7. Two-and-one-half-year-old domestic shorthair neutered female. The cat has a history of anorexia when stressed, and at one time had a feeding tube placed during a 26-day fast. Three days before presentation the cat had stopped eating again.

Diagnosis. Anorexia nervosa.

Treatment. After careful investigations it was determined that there had been a recent change in the formulation of the brand of cat food this cat ate. The cat gradually resumed eating after 2 weeks of almost nothing, and on the evening before another feeding tube was to be installed.

CASE 7–8. Four-year-old domestic shorthair neutered female. The initiating complaint was a 3-month duration of eating strange objects, such as stamps, envelopes, photographs, and soap. The cat had been put on a reducing diet about 3 months before the development of the behavior problem.

Medical Workup. No abnormalities were noted except that the cat weighed 12.4 lbs and should have weighed 8 lbs.

Diagnosis. Pica.

Treatment. Many of the products this cat sought may have had rendered animal parts, so it was decided to try to prevent access to those items. In addition, the cat was given low-calorie, high-fiber treats, such as popcorn, which it really liked.

CASE 7–9. One-year-old Siamese-cross neutered female. About 4 weeks before presentation the cat had started to chew on fabric, particularly cotton and synthetic materials. The only items selected were ones the owners had recently worn.

Diagnosis. Wool-sucking of objects with owner smell.

Treatment. The owners were careful to put away clothing they had worn. They selected a sweater that had been ruined and used taste aversion with it to decrease the tendency of the cat to ruin other items that accidentally might be left out.

CASE 7–10. One-year-old Siamese-cross neutered female. Around the time this animal was neutered, it began to nurse and eat cloth items. It started with the lady owner's clothes and progressed to dirty clothes in the laundry, T-shirts, cotton socks, a blanket, napkins, a woolen afghan, and cotton underwear.

Diagnosis. A variation of wool-sucking.

Treatment. Preventing access to possible targets and taste aversion to selected material were not successful. Because of the degree of the problem, the cat eventually became an outdoor pet.

CASE 7–11. Five-month-old domestic shorthair male. The owners got this kitten when it was 4 weeks old, and since then it had nursed on everything. The owners thought that the problem was getting worse because the cat then nursed on the owner's hair and ears, its paw, towels, and blankets. The cat also would knead with its front paws.

Diagnosis. Prolonged sucking.

Treatment. Access was limited to the cat's own paw, but it continued to try to suck on the owner. The cat was given to an animal shelter because the owner could not cope with the problem, and living in an apartment prevented the owner from making the cat an outdoor animal.

CASE 7–12. Four-month-old domestic shorthair male. The kitten was presented for the problem of self-sucking. Originally it would suck on its sister, until they were separated. Then it started sucking on its own penis and prepuce.

Diagnosis. Prolonged sucking.

Treatment. Access to its own body parts were limited by an Elizabethan collar. Because the behavior would recur if the collar was removed, the owner intended to keep the collar on for several months.

Also see case 2–2.

REFERENCES

1. Adamec, R.: The behavioral bases of prolonged suppression of predatory attack in cats. Aggr. Behav. 1:297, 1975.
2. Adamec, R. E.: The neural basis of prolonged suppression of predatory attack. I. Naturally occurring physiological differences in the limbic systems of killer and non-killer cats. Aggr. Behav. 1:315, 1975.
3. Adamec, R. E.: Hypothalamic and extrahypothalamic substrates of predatory attack: Suppression and the influence of hunger. Brain Res. 106:57, Apr. 16, 1976.
4. Allikmets, L. H.: Cholinergic mechanisms in aggressive behaviour. Med. Biol. 52:19, Feb. 1974.
5. Anand, B. K.: Nervous regulation of food intake. Physiol. Rev. 41:677, 1961.
6. Anand, B. K., and Brobeck, J. R.: Hypothalamic control of food intake in rats and cats. Yale J. Biol. Med. 24:123, 1951.
7. Anand, B. K., Dua, S., and Chhina, G. S.: Higher nervous control over food intake. Indian J. Med. Res. 46:277, 1958.
8. Anokhin, P. K., and Shuleikina, K. V.: System organization of alimentary behavior in the newborn and the developing cat. Dev. Psychobiol. 10:385, 1977.
9. Austin American-Statesman, Feb. 16, 1978.
10. Beadle, M.: The Cat: History, Biology, and Behavior. New York: Simon & Schuster, 1977.
11. Beaver, B. V.: Feline behavioral problems. Vet. Clin. North Am. 6:333, 1976.
12. Beaver, B. V.: Grass eating by carnivores. Vet. Med. Small Anim. Clin. 76:968, 1981.
13. Beaver, B. V.: Disorders of behavior. In Sherding, R. G., ed.: The Cat: Diseases and Clinical Management. New York: Churchill Livingstone, 1989.
14. Berkson, G.: Maturation defects in kittens. Am. J. Ment. Defic. 72:757, 1959.
15. Berntson, G. G., and Leibowitz, S. F.: Biting attack in cats: Evidence for central muscarinic mediation. Brain Res. 51:366, 1973.
16. Biben, M.: Predation and predatory play behaviour of domestic cats. Anim. Behav. 27:81, 1979.
17. Bigbee, H. G.: Personal communication.
18. Blackshaw, J. K.: Abnormal behaviour in cats. Aust. Vet. J. 65:395, 1988.
19. Bloxham, J. C.: Replies to dialog. Fel. Pract. 3:6, Mar.-Apr. 1973.
20. Boudreau, J. C., and Tsuchitani, C.: Sensory Neurophysiology. New York: Van Nostrand Reinhold Co., 1973.
21. Bradshaw, J. W. S.: Mere exposure reduces cat's neophobia to unfamiliar food. Anim. Behav. 34:613, 1986.
22. Brobeck, J. R.: Mechanism of the development of obesity in animals with hypothalamic lesions. Physiol. Rev. 26:541, 1946.
23. Brunner, F.: The application of behavior studies in small animal practice. In Fox, M. W., ed.: Abnormal Behavior in Animals. Philadelphia: W. B. Saunders Co., 1968.
24. Bryant, D.: The Care and Handling of Cats. New York: Ives Washburn, 1944.
25. Caro, T. M.: The effects of experience on the predatory patterns of cats. Behav. Neural Biol. 29:1, May 1980.
26. Caro, T. M.: Effects of the mother, object play, and adult experience on predation in cats. Behav. Neural Biol. 29:29, May 1980.
27. Chase, M. H., and Wyrwicka, W.: Facilitation of feeding in aphagic cats by rewarding brain stimulation. In Novin, D., Wyrwicka, W., and Bray, G. A., eds.: Hunger: Basic Mechanisms and Clinical Implications. New York: Raven Press, 1976.
28. Collins, D. R.: Drinking water requirements of cats. Mod. Vet. Pract. 51:27, Oct. 1970.

29. Collins, D. R.: Feline anorexia: The veterinarian's enigma. Fel. Pract. 2:17, Jan.-Feb. 1972.
30. Cruickshank, R. M.: Animal infancy. In Carmichael, L., ed.: Manual of Child Psychology. New York: John Wiley & Sons, 1946.
31. Davis, D. E.: The use of food as a buffer in a predator-prey system. J. Mammal. 38:466, 1957.
32. Delgado, J. M. R., and Anand, B. K.: Increase of food intake induced by electrical stimulation of the lateral hypothalamus. Am. J. Physiol. 172:162, 1953.
33. Eaton, R. L.: The evolution of sociality in the Felidae. In Eaton, R. L., ed.: The World's Cats. 3rd ed. Seattle: Carnivore Research Institute, 1976.
34. Eberhard, T.: Food habits of Pennsylvania house cats. J. Wildl. Mgt. 18:284, 1954.
35. Elton, C. S.: The use of cats in farm rat control. Br. J. Anim. Behav. 1:151, 1953.
36. Eschenroeder, H. C., Coughlin, B. E., and Clarke, A. P.: Wool-eating cats. Fel. Pract. 6:5, Nov. 1976.
37. Ewer, R. F.: Sucking behaviour in kittens. Behaviour 15:146, 1959.
38. Ewer, R. F.: Further observations on suckling behaviour in kittens, together with some general considerations of the interrelations of innate and acquired responses. Behaviour 17:247, 1961.
39. Ewer, R. F.: Ethology of Mammals. London: Paul Elek, Ltd., 1968.
40. Ewer, R. F.: The Carnivores. Ithaca, NY: Cornell University Press, 1973.
41. Ewer, R. F.: Viverrid behavior and the evolution of reproductive behavior in the Felidae. In Eaton, R. L., ed.: The World's Cats. Seattle: Feline Research Group, 1974.
42. Finco, D. R., Adams, D. D., Crowell, W. A., et al.: Food and water intake and urine composition in cats: Influence of continuous versus periodic feeding. Am. J. Vet. Res. 47:1638, 1986.
43. Fitzgerald, B. M.: Diet of domestic cats and their impact on prey populations. In Turner, D. C., and Bateson, P., eds.: The Domestic Cat: The Biology of Its Behaviour. New York: Cambridge University Press, 1988.
44. Fireman, J.: Cat Catalog. New York: Workman Publishing Co., 1976.
45. Forbush, E. H.: The Domestic Cat: Bird Killer, Mouser, and Destroyer of Wild Life, Means of Utilizing and Controlling It. Boston: Wright & Potter Printing Co., 1916.
46. Fox, M. W.: Understanding Your Cat. New York: Coward, McCann & Geoghegan, 1974.
47. Fox, M. W.: The behaviour of cats. In Hafez, E. S. E., ed.: The Behaviour of Domestic Animals. 3rd ed. Baltimore: Williams & Wilkins Co., 1975.
48. Fratta, W., Mereu, G., Chess, P., et al.: Benzodiazepine-induced voraciousness in cats and inhibition of amphetamine-anorexia. Life Sci. 18:1157, 1976.
49. Galambos, R.: Processing of auditory information. In Brazier, M. A. B., ed.: Brain and Behavior. Vol. 1. Washington, DC: American Institute of Biological Sciences, 1961.
50. Glasofer, S.: Practice pointers. Vet. Med. Small Anim. Clin. 67:718, 1972.
51. Green, J. D., Clemente, C. D., and DeGroot, J.: Rhinencephalic lesions and behavior in cats. J. Comp. Neurol. 108:505, 1957.
52. Grossman, S. P.: Eating or drinking elicited by direct adrenergic or cholinergic stimulation of hypothalamus. Science 132:301, 1960.
53. Grossman, S. P.: Neurophysiologic aspects: Extrahypothalamic factors in the regulation of food intake. Adv. Psychosom. Med. 7:49, 1972.
54. Hart, B. L.: Maternal behavior. II. The nursing-suckling relationship and the effects of maternal deprivation. Fel. Pract. 2:6, Nov.-Dec. 1972.
55. Hart, B. L.: Feeding behavior. Fel. Pract. 4:8, Jan.-Feb. 1974.
56. Hart, B. L.: Predatory behavior. Fel. Pract. 4:8, Mar.-Apr. 1974.
57. Hart, B. L.: Quiz on feline behavior. Fel. Pract. 6:10, May 1976.
58. Hart, B. L.: Behavioral aspects of selecting a new cat. Fel. Pract. 6:8, Sept. 1976.
59. Hart, B. L.: Behavioral aspects of raising kittens. Fel. Pract. 6:8, Nov. 1976.
60. Hart, B. L.: Appetite and feeding: Problems with too much or too little. Fel. Pract. 8:10, Sept. 1978.
61. Hart, B. L.: Water sprayer therapy. Fel. Pract. 8:13, Nov. 1978.
62. Hart, B. L., and Hart, L. A.: Canine and Feline Behavioral Therapy. Philadelphia: Lea & Febiger, 1985.

63. Hilton, F. E.: Medicating a cat: "The Hilton modification." Fel. Pract. 6:44, Nov. 1976.
64. Houpt, K.: Ingestive behavior problems of dogs and cats. Vet. Clin. North Am. [Small Anim. Pract.] 12:683, 1982.
65. Houpt, K. A.: Feeding and drinking behavior problems. Vet. Clin. North Am. [Small Anim. Pract.] 21:281, 1991.
66. Houpt, K. A., and Smith, S. L.: Taste preferences and their relation to obesity in dogs and cats. Can. Vet. J. 22:77, Apr. 1981.
67. Houpt, K. A., and Wolski, T. R.: Domestic Animal Behavior for Veterinarians and Animal Scientists. Ames: Iowa State University Press, 1982.
68. Inselman-Temkin, B. R., and Flynn, J. P.: Sex-dependent effects of gonadal and gonadotropic hormones on centrally-elicited attack in cats. Brain Res. 60:393, 1973.
69. Jacobs, D. L.: Behavior modification technique. Fel. Pract. 8:6, Mar. 1978.
70. Kleiman, D. G., and Eisenberg, J. F.: Comparisons of canid and felid social systems from an evolutionary perspective. Anim. Behav. 21:637, 1973.
71. Kling, A., Kovach, J. K., and Tucker, T. J.: The behaviour of cats. In Hafez, E. S. E., ed.: The Behaviour of Domestic Animals. 2nd ed. Baltimore: Williams & Wilkins Co., 1969.
72. Koepke, J. E., and Pribram, K. H.: Effect of milk on the maintenance of sucking behavior in kittens from birth to six months. J. Comp. Physiol. Psychol. 75:363, 1971.
73. Kovach, J. K., and Kling, A.: Mechanisms of neonate sucking behavior in the kitten. Anim. Behav. 15:91, 1967.
74. Kuo, Z. Y.: The genesis of the cat behavior toward the rat. J. Comp. Psychol. 11:1, 1930.
75. Kuo, Z. Y.: Further study on the behavior of the cat toward the rat. J. Comp. Psychol. 25:1, 1938.
76. Lakso, V., and Randall, W.: Fishing behavior after lateral midbrain lesions in cats. J. Comp. Physiol. Psychol. 68:467, 1969.
77. Landers, A.: Cat, dog follow kosher household rules. The Bryan Eagle 102:6A, 1978.
78. Langworthy, O. R.: Behavioral disturbances related to the decomposition of reflex activity caused by cerebral injury: An experimental study of the cat. J. Neuropathol. Exp. Neurol. 3:87, 1944.
79. Levinson, P. K., and Flynn, J. P.: The objects attacked by cats during stimulation of the hypothalamus. Anim. Behav. 13:217, 1965.
80. Leyhausen, P.: Cat Behavior: The Predatory and Social Behavior of Domestic and Wild Cats. New York: Garland STPM Press, 1978.
81. Levitsky, D. A.: Obesity and the behavior of eating. Gaines Dog Res. Prog., p. 4, 1972.
82. Liberg, O.: Predation and social behaviour in a population of domestic cat. An evolutionary perspective. Ph.D. diss., Department of Animal Ecology, University of Lund, Sweden, 1981.
83. Lorenz, K., and Leyhausen, P.: Motivation of Human and Animal Behavior. New York: Van Nostrand Reinhold Co., 1973.
84. Macdonald, D. W., Apps, P. J., Carr, G. M., and Kerby, G.: Social Dynamics, Nursing Coalitions, and Infanticide Among Farm Cats, Felis catus. Berlin: Paul Parey Scientific Publ., 1987.
85. MacDonnell, M. F., and Flynn, J. P.: Control of sensory fields by stimulation of hypothalamus. Science 152:1406, 1966.
86. Macy, D. W., and Gasper, P. W.: Diazepam-induced eating in anorexic cats. J. Am. Anim. Hosp. Assoc. 21:17, 1985.
87. McFarland, C. A., and Hart, B. L.: Aggressive behavior. Fel. Pract. 8:13, July 1978.
88. McMurry, F. B., and Sperry, C. C.: Food of feral house cats in Oklahoma, a progress report. J. Mammal. 22:185, 1941.
89. Morgenson, G. J., and Huang, Y. H.: The neurobiology of motivated behavior. Prog. Neurobiol. 1:55, 1973.
90. Morris, M. L., and Teeter, S. M.: Allergy: A Commentary on Nutritional Management of Small Animals. Topeka, KS: Mark Morris Assoc., 1977.
91. Mosier, J. E.: Common medical and behavioral problems in cats. Mod. Vet. Pract. 56:699, 1975.

92. Mugford, R. A.: Comparative and developmental studies of feeding behaviour in dogs and cats. Br. Vet. J. 133:98, 1977.
93. Papurt, M. L.: Exaggerated cost of feeding a Great Dane. Vet. Med. Small Anim. Clin. 2:513, 1977.
94. Pearson, O. P.: Carnivore-mouse predation: An example of its intensity and bioenergetics. J. Mammal. 45:177, 1964.
95. Pearson, O. P.: The prey of carnivores during one cycle of mouse abundance. J. Anim. Ecol. 35:217, 1966.
96. Pellis, S. M., O'Brien, D. P., Pellis, V. C., et al.: Escalation of feline predation along a gradient from avoidance through "play" to killing. Behav. Neurosc. 102:760, 1988.
97. Pfaffmann, C.: Differential responses of the new-born cat to gustatory stimuli. J. Genet. Psychol. 49:61, 1936.
98. Randall, W. L., and Parsons, V. L.: The concomitancy in the rhythms of caloric intake and behavior in cats: A replication. Psychon. Sci. 15:35, 1969.
99. Reis, D. J.: Central neurotransmitters in aggression. Res. Publ. Assoc. Res. Nerv. Ment. Dis. 52:119, 1974.
100. Rogers, W. W.: Controlled observations on the behavior of kittens toward rats from birth to five months of age. J. Comp. Psychol. 13:107, 1932.
101. Rosenblatt, J. S.: Suckling and home orientation in the kitten: A comparative developmental study. In Tobach, E., Aronson, L. R., and Shaw, E., eds.: The Biopsychology of Development. New York: Academic Press, 1971.
102. Rosenblatt, J. S.: Learning in newborn kittens. Sci. Am. 227:18, 1972.
103. Rosenblatt, J. S., Turkewitz, G., and Schneirla, T. C.: Early socialization in the domestic cat as based on feeding and other relationships between female and young. In Foss, B. M., ed.: Determinants of Infant Behaviour. New York: John Wiley & Sons, 1961.
104. Rosenblatt, J. S., Turkewitz, G., and Schneirla, T. C.: Development of suckling and related behavior in neonate kittens. In Bliss, E. L., ed.: Roots of Behavior. New York: Harper & Row, 1962.
105. Russek, M.: Hepatic receptors and the neurophysiological mechanisms controlling feeding behavior. Neurosci. Res. 4:213, 1971.
106. Sauer, L. S., Hamar, D., and Lewis, L. D.: Effect of diet composition on water intake and excretion by the cat. Fel. Pract. 15:16, July-Aug. 1985.
107. Schneirla, T. C., and Rosenblatt, J. S.: Behavioral organization and genesis of the social bond in insects and animals. Am. J. Orthopsychiatry 31:223, 1961.
108. Schneirla, T. C., Rosenblatt, J. S., and Tobach, E.: Maternal behavior in the cat. In Rheingold, H. L., ed.: Maternal Behavior in Mammals. New York: John Wiley & Sons, 1963.
109. Scott, P. P.: Diet and other factors affecting the development of young felids. In Eaton, R. L., ed.: The World's Cats. 3rd ed. Seattle: Carnivore Research Institute, 1976.
110. Siegel, A., and Edinger, H.: Neural control of aggression and rage behavior. In Morgane, P. J., and Panksepp, J., eds.: Behavioral Studies of the Hypothalamus. Vol. 3, Pt. B. New York: Marcel Dekker, 1981.
111. Sterman, M. B., Wyrwicka, W., and Roth, S.: Electrophysiological correlates and neural substrates of alimentary behavior in the cat. Ann. N.Y. Acad. Sci. 157:723, 1969.
112. Turner, D. C., and Meister, O.: Hunting behaviour of the domestic cat. In Turner, D. C., and Bateson, P., eds.: The Domestic Cat: The Biology of Its Behaviour. New York: Cambridge University Press, 1988.
113. Walker, A. D.: Taste preferences in the domestic dog and cat. Gaines Dog Res. Prog., p. 1, Summer 1975.
114. Ward, D. G., and Ward, J. H.: Control of water intake: Evidence for the role of a hemodynamic pontine pathway. Brain Res. 262:314, 1983.
115. Weigel, I.: Small cats and clouded leopards. In Grzimek, H. C. B., ed.: Grzimek's Animal Life Encyclopedia. Vol. 12. New York: Van Nostrand Reinhold Co., 1975.
116. West, M.: Social play in the domestic cat. Am. Zool. 14:427, 1974.
117. Widdowson, E. M.: Food, growth, and development in the suckling period. In Graham-

Jones, O., ed.: Canine and Feline Nutritional Requirements. New York: Pergamon Press, 1965.
118. Wood, G. L.: Animal Facts and Feats. Garden City, NY: Doubleday & Co., 1972.
119. Worden, A. N.: Abnormal behaviour in the dog and cat. Vet. Rec. 71:966, 1959.

ADDITIONAL READINGS

Adamec, R. Behavioral and epileptic determinants of predatory attack behavior in the cat. Can. J. Neurol. Sci. 2:457, 1975.

Adamec, R. E. The interaction of hunger and preying in the domestic cat (Felis catus); an adaptive hierarchy? Behav. Biol. 18:263, 1976.

Anand, B. K., and Dua, S. Feeding responses induced by electrical stimulation of the hypothalamus in cat. Indian J. Med. Res. 43:113, 1955.

Anand, B. K., Dua, S., and Shoenberg, K. Hypothalamic control of food intake in cats and monkeys. J. Physiol. (Lond.) 127:143, 1955.

Bandler, R., and Flynn, J. P. Visual patterned reflex present during hypothalamically elicited attack. Science 171:817, 1971.

Beaver, B. V. Reflex development in the kitten. Appl. Anim. Ethol. 4:93, 1978.

Berntson, G. G., Hughes, H. C., and Beattie, M. S. A comparison of hypothalamically induced biting attack with natural predatory behavior in the cat. J. Comp. Physiol. Psychol. 90:167, 1976.

Berry, C. S. An experimental study of imitation in cats. J. Comp. Neurol. Psychol. 18:1, 1908.

Brown, J. L., and Hunsperger, R. W. Neuroethology and motivation of agonistic behaviour. Anim. Behav. 11:439, 1963.

Chertok, L., and Fontaine, M. Psychosomatics in veterinary medicine. J. Psychosom. Res. 7:229, 1963.

Chi, C. C., and Flynn, J. P. Neural pathways associated with hypothalamically elicited attack behavior in cats. Science 171:703, 1971.

Cooper, J. B. A description of parturition in the domestic cat. J. Comp. Psychol. 37:71, 1944.

Courthial, A. S. The persistence of infantile behavior in a cat. J. Genet. Psychol. 36:349, 1929.

Egger, M. D., and Flynn, J. P. Effects of electrical stimulation of the amygdala on hypothalamically elicited attack behavior in cats. J. Neurophysiol. 26:705, 1963.

Eleftheriou, B. E., and Scott, J. P. The Physiology of Aggression and Defeat. New York: Plenum Publishing Corp., 1971.

Errington, P. L. Notes on food habits of the southern Wisconsin house cat. J. Mammal. 17:64, 1936.

Everett, G. M. The pharmacology of aggressive behavior in animals and man. Psychopharmacol. Bull. 13:15, 1977.

Ewert, J. P. Neuroethology. New York: Springer-Verlag, 1980.

Fitzgerald, B. M., and Karl, B. J. Food of feral house cats (Felis catus L.) in forest of the Orongorongo Valley, Wellington. N.Z.J. Zool. 6:107, 1979.

Fox, M. W. New information on feline behavior. Mod. Vet. Pract. 56:50, Apr. 1965.

Fox, M. W. Psychomotor disturbances. In Fox, M. W., ed.: Abnormal Behavior in Animals. Philadelphia: W. B. Saunders Co., 1968.

Fox, M. W. Psychopathology in man and lower animals. J. Am. Vet. Med. Assoc. 159:66, 1971.

Fraser, A. F. Behavior disorders in domestic animals. In Fox, M. W., ed. Abnormal Behavior in Animals. Philadelphia: W. B. Saunders Co., 1968.

Gonyea, W., and Ashworth, R. The form and function of retractile claws in the Felidae and other representative carnivorans. J. Morphol. 145:229, 1975.

Hart, B. L. The brain and behavior. Fel. Pract. 3:4, Sept.-Oct. 1973.

Hart, B. L. Disease processes and behavior. Fel. Pract. 3:6, Nov.-Dec. 1973.

Hart, B. L. Behavior of the litter runt. Fel. Pract. 4:14, Sept.-Oct. 1974.

Hart, B. L. A quiz on feline behavior. Fel. Pract. 5:12, May-June 1975.

Hart, B. L. Psychosomatic aspects of feline medicine. Fel. Pract. 8:8, July-Aug. 1978.

Hirsch, E., Dubose, C., and Jacobs, H. L. Dietary control of food intake in cats. Physiol. Behav. 20:287, 1978.

Houdeshell, J. W., and Hennessey, P. W. Megestrol acetate for control of estrus in the cat. Vet. Med. Small Anim. Clin. 72:1013, 1977.

Houpt, K. A. Animal behavior as a subject for veterinary students. Cornell Vet. 66:73, 1976.

Hubbs, E. L. Food habits of feral house cats in the Sacramento Valley. California Fish and Game 37:177, 1951.

Huidekopper, R. S. The Cat. New York: D. Appleton & Co., 1895.

Hutchinson, R. R., and Renfrew, J. W. Stalking attack and eating behaviors elicited from the same sites in the hypothalamus. J. Comp. Physiol. Psychol. 61:360, 1966.

Jackson, W. B. Food habits of Baltimore, Maryland, cats in relation to rat populations. J. Mammal. 32:458, 1951.

Jenkins, T. W. Functional Mammalian Neuroanatomy. Philadelphia: Lea & Febiger, 1972.

Joshua, J. O. Abnormal behavior in cats. In Fox, M. W., ed.: Abnormal Behavior in Animals. Philadelphia: W. B. Saunders Co., 1968.

Kalber, L. A. Dog and cat food trends. J. Am. Vet. Med. Assoc. 161:1678, 1972.

Katz, R. J., and Thomas, E. Effects of scopolamine and α-methylparatyrosine upon predatory attack in cats. Psychopharmacologia 42:153, 1975.

Katz, R. J., and Thomas, E. Effects of a novel anti-aggressive agent upon two types of brain stimulated emotional behavior. Psychopharmacology (Berlin) 48:79, 1976.

Kuo, Z. Y. Studies on the basic factors in animal fighting. VII. Interspecies coexistence in mammals. J. Genet. Psychol. 97:211, 1960.

Kuo, Z. Y. The Dynamics of Behavior Development. New York: Plenum Publishing Corp., 1976.

Levinson, B. M. Man and his feline pet. Mod. Vet. Pract. 53:35, Nov. 1972.

Leyhausen, P. The communal organization of solitary mammals. Symp. Zool. Soc. Lond. 14:249, 1965.

Lubar, J. F., and Numan, R. Behavioral and physiological studies of septal function and related medial cortical structures. Behav. Biol. 8:1, 1973.

MacDonnell, M. F. Some effects of ethanol, amphetamine, disulfiram and p-CPA on seizing of prey in feline predatory attack and on associated motor pathways. Q.J. Stud. Alcohol 33:437, 1972.

MacDonnell, M. F., Fessock, L., and Brown, S. H. Ethanol and the neural substrate for affective defense in the cat. Q.J. Stud. Alcohol 32:406, 1971.

MacDonnell, M. F., Fessock, L., and Brown, S. H. Aggression and associated neural events in cats. Effects of p-chlorophenylalanine compared with alcohol. Q.J. Stud. Alcohol 32:748, 1971.

McDougall, W., and McDougall, K. D.: Notes on instinct and intelligence in rats and cats. J. Comp. Psychol. 7:145, 1927.

McMurry, F. B. Three shrews, Cryptotis parva, eaten by a feral housecat. J. Mammal. 26:94, 1945.

Mereu, G. P., Fratta, W., Chessa, P., and Gessa, G. L. Voraciousness induced in cats by benzodiazephines. Psychopharmacologia 47:101, 1976.

Morgane, P. J., and Kosman, A. J. Alterations in feline behaviour following bilateral amygdalectomy. Nature 180:598, 1957.

Polsky, R. H. Developmental factors in mammalian predation. Behav. Biol. 15:353, 1975.

Roberts, W. W., and Bergquist, E. H. Attack elicited by hypothalamic stimulation in cats raised in social isolation. J. Comp. Physiol. Psychol. 66:590, 1968.

Roberts, W. W., and Keiss, H. O. Motivational properties of hypothalamic aggression in cats. J. Comp. Physiol. Psychol. 58:187, 1964.

Schmidt, J. P. Psychosomatics in veterinary medicine. In Fox, M. W., ed. Abnormal Behavior in Animals. Philadelphia: W. B. Saunders Co., 1968.

Sharp, J. C., Nielson, H. C., and Porter, P. B. The effect of amphetamines upon cats with lesions in the ventromedial hypothalamus. J. Comp. Physiol. Psychol. 55:198, 1962.

Sheard, M. H. Behavioral effects of p-chlorophenylalanine: Inhibition by lithium. Commun. Behav. Biol 5(pt. A):71, 1970.

Starer, E. Effects of frustration of the nursing process on kittens. J. Genet. Psychol. 105:113, 1964.

Toner, G. C. House cat predation on small animals. J. Mammal. 37:119, 1956.

Voith, V. L., and Marder, A. R. Feline behavioral disorders. In Morgan, R. V., ed. Handbook of Small Animal Practice. New York: Churchill Livingstone, 1988.

Wemmer, C., and Scow, K. Communication in the Felidae with emphasis on scent marking and contact patterns. In Sebeok, T. A., ed. How Animals Communicate. Bloomington: Indiana University Press, 1977.

Wyrwicka, W. Lateral hypothalamic "feeding" sites and gastric acid secretion. Experientia 32:1287, 1976.

Wyrwicka, W. The problem of motivation in feeding behavior. In Novin, D., Wyrwicka, W., and Bray, G. A., eds. Hunger: Basic Mechanisms and Clinical Implications. New York: Raven Press, 1976.

8

Feline Eliminative Behavior

ELIMINATIVE BEHAVIOR DEVELOPMENT

Infantile Patterns

The neonate cannot voluntarily urinate and defecate. Instead, eliminative behaviors are controlled for several weeks by the urogenital reflex. Stroking of the kitten's perineal region or caudal abdomen results in urination and defecation. When the young are not mobile enough to leave the nest, it is critical to their survival in the wild that the nest be reasonably undetectable, which requires that it have relatively little odor. Because the kittens can eliminate only when the queen is present to tactilely stimulate them, the urogenital reflex assures that she can consume their wastes and prevent their soiling the nest. Even after this period of relative kitten immobility, the queen continues to stimulate this reflex because the home nest remains the center of activity until the kittens are about 6 weeks of age, when it begins to share significance with other sites specific for feeding, playing, and eliminating.[48] The anogenital reflex disappears between 23 and 39 days of age, although kittens can voluntarily eliminate by 3 weeks of age.

Most of the queen's grooming and ingestion of waste initially occur during nursing or shortly thereafter; as the kittens grow older the queen may directly approach certain individuals. The kitten commonly assumes dorsal recumbency with the limbs abducted. Younger kittens are passive until the grooming-toilet session is completed, whereas older ones tend to squirm more.

Kittens have a natural tendency to "earth-rake" loose sand and dirt as a prelude to the use of this behavior in elimination. Around 30 days of age a kitten begins to spend time in a litter box or in soft dirt, moving the particles from one side to another. Ingestion of litter or dirt as a form of oral exploration also is common at this time. This oral behavior usually is followed within a few days by the species' behaviors of eliminating in a certain area and covering the elimination.

The neural mechanism for eliminative behavior can be demonstrated to be functional by electrical stimulation of the hypothalamus at 2 weeks of age. Thus neurologic maturation of these pathways has occurred as long as 2 weeks before the actual onset of the behavior.[18, 38] The kittens learn the specific toilet area by observing the queen as well as by olfactory cues.

Litter Training

Because kittens naturally complement innate behaviors, such as burying wastes, with learned patterns, such as where to eliminate, a newly acquired kitten normally does not have to be litter trained. Some individuals, such as orphans and outdoor cats, do not have the opportunity to learn, and the owner must educate them. Young cats also learn surface and location preferences.[10]

It is initially important that any cat be confined to a small area to take advantage of the fastidious feline nature. It is not realistic to expect a kitten that spends most of its time in the living room to reliably use a litter box kept in a back bedroom on the second floor.[4] The owner should place the untrained kitten in the litter pan shortly after each meal and manipulate its forepaws to make digging motions. The kitten should then be allowed to jump out so that this process can be repeated one or two times.[36] For the older outdoor cat, the same procedures can be used, but it often is desirable to use dirt or sand initially and gradually change to litter. With these older individuals, particular care must be taken to keep potted plants out of the area so that the cat does not use the dirt in the pot for its toilet area. The plant also can be protected by putting decorative stones, pine bark chips, moth balls, or aluminum foil on the surface.[4]

Litter training at first may require leaving small traces of excretions in the box so that the smell can be used as a cue. If the kitten uses the area of the litter box but not the box specifically, the owner can place the droppings in the tray to give it the appropriate odor and show the cat where the preferred area is. For the really difficult animal, the entire floor area of the small room, except where the cat's food, bed, and litter pan are, can be covered with a thin layer of litter. This arrangement will necessitate the cat's urinating and defecating on the litter because it will not do so in its bed or food. After 2 to 5 days the owner can reduce the litter-covered area by a fourth, and after another 2 to 5 days, by another fourth. This sequence is repeated until only the area with the litter pan is covered. If necessary, the owner gradually can move the litter pan over a period of several days, using successive approximation to put it in a more desirable location. Cats normally visit the litter box three times a day for two short visits to urinate and one longer visit for defecation. There is a 73 per cent frequency of these trips occurring in the morning.[35]

Certain individuals, especially of popular breeds such as the Persian, may be exceptionally difficult for either the queen or the owner to litter train.[11] This may indicate a genetic problem owing to the popularity of the breed and consequent indiscriminate breeding. Perhaps house trainability was not considered in selection, or cat domestication in general has created the difficulty.

ADULT URINATION

Eliminative Urination

Urinary postures and associated behaviors ordinarily are similar between the sexes. The cat usually digs a small hole in soft dirt or litter with its forepaws and then positions itself so that the urine is expressed into this area. The cat assumes a posture almost like that of sitting, except that the pelvic limbs are slightly abducted and the tail is held more rigidly, usually pointed caudally (Fig. 8–1). Urine is forcefully ejected in a stream, probably because of abdominal press and urinary bladder contraction. When finished, the cat stands and moves dirt or litter over

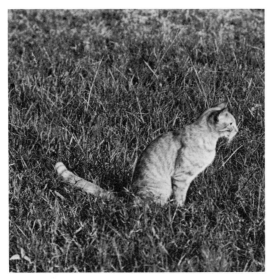

FIGURE 8–1. The urination posture of a cat.

the urine with its forepaws (Fig. 8–2). Covering of feces is limited to core areas in many outdoor cats. Thus, away from a home location, cats often do not attempt to bury feces. Kuiat cats are unique because, if at all possible, they will stand on the four corners of the litter box when eliminating.

Although the cat instinctively eliminates in loose dirt, it can learn to use other locations either by itself or by special learning techniques. Litter box substance is relatively easily changed from dirt or clay to loose material such as wood shavings or shredded newspaper. Unshredded newspapers may even be acceptable to the cat. In fact, cats frequently choose to use whole newspaper lying around the home instead of a litter box.

Some cats learn on their own to urinate in a sink, a bathtub, or a toilet. If this practice is undesirable, the owner can fill the tub with a few inches of water for several days and place a litter box next to the tub. The water technique will not work if the cat straddles the sink when it urinates. In this case, an object like a cactus can be placed in the sink, with the litter box nearby. For the cat that continues this behavior or that urinates in the toilet, the sink or toilet seat is lined with aluminum foil or plastic wrap and then filled with litter. Once the cat learns to use the litter, the owner moves the litter to a box beside the sink or toilet.[9, 32] As the box is used, the owner gradually can move it short distances at a time until it is located in the preferred spot. The reverse technique can be used to train a cat to urinate in the toilet (Fig. 8–3). The owner gradually brings the litter box next to the toilet and then fastens plastic wrap securely enough to the toilet seat to hold quite a bit of litter,

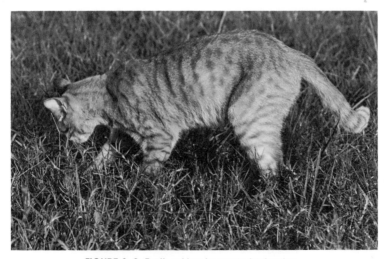

FIGURE 8–2. Earth-raking to cover fresh urine.

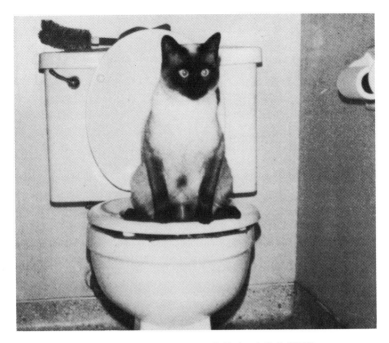

FIGURE 8–3. A toilet-trained cat. (From Fel. Pract. 5:12, Sept.-Oct. 1975.)

creating a litter box. After a few days the cat will accept a decrease in the amount of litter. As the plastic becomes visible, the owner puts some holes in it to drain the urine. The last stage is the removal of the plastic and litter. Because this posture is somewhat awkward for the cat, sometimes the animal may slip off the toilet seat, and repetition of some of the procedures may be necessary to retrain it.[23, 32]

Marking Urination

Spraying urination is used by cats, especially intact males, to mark territorial boundaries. To spray urine, the cat stands with its tail erect and quivering, although a few flex their elbows to lower the forequarters[56] (see Fig. 3–16). Urine is ejected onto a vertical object in spurts that cover a relatively larger surface than does normal urination, at a level 1 to 2 ft high. A tomcat uses spraying most frequently along the edges of his territory to attract estrous females, reassure himself, and signal other males of his presence, thus minimizing the frequency and severity of encounters with intruders.[20] Because this marking behavior is sexually dimorphic, it occasionally is used by females and castrated males when environmental situations become excessively frustrating.

Emotional states affect renal circulation and thus urine formation.

Excitatory states result in vasoconstriction, as in the intestinal vessels, because of neurogenic factors and a humoral component. During natural sleep there is renal vasodilation, probably as a result of vascular autoregulation.[39] These physiologic factors result in decreased urine output during excitement and increased output during sleep.

ADULT DEFECATION

Behaviors associated with defecation resemble those used for normal urination—posturing is similar, as is the digging and covering procedure. Only near the edges of a territory might a cat leave feces uncovered, although the general consensus is that cats do not mark with feces.[6, 18, 19, 21] The earth-raking associated with burying feces is initiated by the odor of fecal matter, and thus may be performed on the floor by cats that miss the litter box, although they move only air.[37] Odors from other sources, including some foods, also can stimulate this behavior. The artificial selections of domestication have changed some of the genetic factors of this behavior, and consequently some cats do not bury their feces. Conversely, some cats are so fastidious that they cover not only their feces, but also any other cat's exposed feces.

There is no one toilet area for the free-roaming cat, so feces are widely spread. This dispersal, along with the covering behavior, serves as a form of parasite control. Because the concentrated odor of fecal matter may inhibit the use of a certain area, litter pans must be frequently cleaned.

ELIMINATIVE BEHAVIOR PROBLEMS

Housesoiling is the most common problem in cats.[3] An estimated 10 per cent of pet cats show an elimination problem at some time in their lives.[10] To work effectively with these cats, history taking is the most important part of the workup. There are a number of methods that can be used, including a taxonomy.[2] Regardless of the specific approach, it is important to determine which cat is soiling, what specific type of elimination is occurring, where the cat is eliminating, and how long the behavior has been occurring. The history of litter box use by the cat and box maintenance by the owner also is necessary. In multicat households an owner may assume that a particular cat has been housesoiling because it "looks guilty" or because he or she does not particularly like the animal. Because treatment of the wrong cat is not successful, the true problem animal must be found. Isolation of individuals may indicate which cat is soiling. Another option is to give fluorescein orally or subcutaneously to a single cat and check fresh urine spots with an ultraviolet light.[29, 32, 33]

The specific type of eliminative problem needs to be determined. Differentiate feces from urine and spraying from urination. If the owner has not seen the cat avoid the litter box, determine if the spots are on vertical surfaces, such as a wall or drape, or if a specific item is targeted, such as the owner's pillow, dirty clothes, or favorite chair. Yes answers indicate that spraying (or urine-marking) is the problem.

Where the housesoiling occurs may indicate why or suggest an appropriate course of action. Owners may indicate that the cat is soiling all over the house when the actual problem may be confined to one or two rooms or even spots. Areas near windows and doors or where cats can see outside are favorite targets for spraying when strange cats roam, especially during the mating season. When items belonging to a certain person are urinated on, there is a disturbance with that individual that bothers the cat. If the problem is confined to a single room, it can be closed off and the problem easily stopped.

Another important piece of information needed is how long the housesoiling behavior has been occurring. A single episode of missing the litter box seldom requires intervention, whereas a 5-year history of not using the box is difficult to change. If the cat never learned to use a litter box, it is not reasonable to expect that it will begin just because it moves to a new home or the owners get a new carpet.

The nonuse of a litter box can be classified in several ways. One way, the method used here, is to determine the type of housesoiling—defecation, urination, or spraying (urine marking). Another is to look at cause, such as litter aversion, surface preference, location preference, or location aversions.[9, 10, 16, 17, 41, 54, 55]

Urine-spraying

Spraying is a common behavior problem, constituting up to 44 per cent of the housesoiling complaints.[3, 5, 8, 13, 45] Although it is normal for the cat, it may not be acceptable to the owner. Because it usually is related to sexual behavior, spraying is most commonly described as a problem of tomcats during the mating season. The resident cat may spray to scent-mark whenever it becomes uncomfortable with its surroundings, such as when there is decreased attention, punishment, change in routine, overcrowding, or introduction of a new cat. The incidence of spraying increases from 25 per cent in single-cat households to 100 per cent when there are more than 10 cats.[9] Females and neutered males also may mark, but the behavior for them usually requires a higher threshold than for tomcats. An estrous female may spontaneously mark. The remedy basically consists of altering either the cat's normal response or the stimulus.

Either of these may be accomplished by eliminating the environmental source of the problem, isolating the resident cat from the offending environment, or minimizing the hormonal influence of the situation.

Certain episodes of housesoiling seem to involve vindictiveness on the cat's part, almost as though the cat were punishing its owner for some slight. Spiteful eliminations probably do occur, such as when the cat urinates on the owner's bed or clothes immediately after a scolding or after a new cat is introduced, but establishing definite proof of spitefulness is extremely difficult. When the resident cat deposits urine on specific objects, it indicates that the cat has singled out that relationship as less than desirable. The person often is found not to like cats, and the cat's behavior does not help. The simplest solution involves having the targeted person feed the cat. It is best if the cat can be given one or two small meals of canned food so that it has a strong desire to approach. Other people in the household should minimize their interaction with the cat during this time.

Castration eliminates spraying behavior in 87 per cent of tomcats. Of these, 78 per cent exhibit a rapid postsurgical change and the remaining 9 per cent change gradually over a few months.[30] About 10 per cent of prepubertally gonadectomized cats start spraying later in life, indicating that learning is not a factor.[31, 32] Males are more apt to spray if there are female cats in the household.[31, 32] Drug therapy is generally satisfactory for the 13 per cent of older males in which castration is not successful, the tomcats in which castration is undersirable, males already castrated, and ovariohysterectomized females. The progestins are most effective, and if one type does not produce satisfactory results, its use may be repeated or another type tried. Medroxyprogesterone acetate (Depo-Provera; 50 mg I.M. for ovariohysterectomized females; 100 mg I.M. for males) and megestrol acetate (Ovaban, Megace; 5 to 10 mg/day P.O. for 7 days and then weekly for 4 to 6 weeks) are the most commonly used forms. These products are effective in about one-third of cases, working better in males and in single-cat households.[26, 29] The progestins depress spermatogenesis and stimulate the appetite, in addition to having some serious side effects if used long term.[46, 47] A single injection of medroxyprogesterone acetate eliminates spraying for up to a month before retreatment is necessary, although it lasts even longer in about one-fourth of the cats.[49] Other hormones, such as repository stilbestrol (0.5 mL per large cat I.M.), ethylestranol (50 to 75 mg S.C. followed by 5 mg/day P.O. until the spraying stops), and progesterone (2.2 mg/kg), have been used to control spraying, but their side effects also can be serious.[6, 44, 49] The antianxiety tranquilizers, particularly diazepam (Valium; 1 to 5 mg/day P.O.), are the drugs of choice if stress is the precipitating factor in housesoiling.[4] They are more helpful than hormonal therapy when the problem involves females and/or multicat households.[40, 42] In all cases, best results can be expected if the initiating factors are removed at the time treatment begins and the drugs are used only initially to decrease stress levels.

In addition to drug therapy, behavior modification has been used to eliminate spraying. If the cat can be constantly observed, a form of aversive conditioning or punishment might be successful. Timing is critical and should start as the behavior starts.[53] A water pistol, a remotely controlled plant sprayer, a noise, a light flash, or a thrown object can deter spraying if used consistently at the moment the cat begins to spray. In another type of aversive conditioning, strips of aluminum foil are hung on the object usually sprayed so that the noise, the reflected spray, or both inhibit the cat.[22, 51, 52] This technique has been successful in a few cases, not because it was aversive, but because the cat was distracted by playing with the foil. Thus the procedure probably should not be considered dependable.[51] Placing food bowls or litter pans near the area that usually is sprayed has met with some success. Isolation in a small room with food, water, and a litter pan may help to alleviate the problem by minimizing some environmental stresses.

New cats should be confined to a single room when first introduced into a home. This allows resident cats to get used to the new smells and noise first, and the new cat can get comfortable in a small territory before spending more time investigating the rest of the house with a gradual introduction. Moving an older cat to a new home also should involve confinement to a small area. This allows the cat to establish a territory, leaving hair and dander as the territorial odor rather than urine. Gradual access to the rest of the house lets the cat explore in a nonthreatening way.

For the chronic, refractory spraying cat, neurosurgical procedures offer some hope. Placing lesions in the medial preoptic area reduced or stopped spraying in six of six male cats; however, side effects made this procedure undesirable as a clinical procedure.[10, 52] Olfactory tractotomy was about 50 per cent successful and was not associated with significant side effects.[10, 27–29, 32] Cutting the ischiocavernosus muscles also has been reported.[42]

Housesoiling

The most frequent complaint related to feline urinary behavior is urination out of the box (50 per cent); defecation is a problem 24 per cent to 29 per cent of the time.[3, 13, 45] Careful questioning of the owner is necessary to determine whether the cat's posture while urinating is in fact typical of spraying or whether it is, as more frequently is the case, typical of normal urination. In taking the history the veterinarian should ascertain whether the cat has ever been litter trained. Only if it has used the litter box correctly at some time should specific causes for house-soiling be sought.

Inappropriate urination or defecation can result from an emotional upset. If that is determined to be the cause, after the stress-initiating factors are minimized, treatment may be necessary with the benzodiaze-pine tranquilizers, progestins for their tranquilizing effect, a deconditioning program, or some combination of these measures.

In many cases the source of the problem of housesoiling is near the litter pan. The fastidious nature of some cats demands that the litter be changed frequently, sometimes more frequently than the owners care to change it, or there may be too few litter pans for the number of cats. The average household does nothing to a litter box except dump it completely every 5 to 7 days. Simply by removing feces once or twice daily, the owner may be able to stop soiling out of the box.[14] This is even more important if several cats use the same box. Ideally, there should be a litter box for each cat and extra if the house is large.[34] Most cats prefer a certain amount of privacy, which an improperly placed litter pan may not provide. Also, sometimes access to the litter pan accidentally is blocked, or the pan is moved. Kittens under 12 weeks of age should not be completely trusted, and any cat brought into a new home should be isolated in a single room until its toilet habits stabilize and anxieties decrease.[12]

Odors associated with certain litters, such as chlorophyll, may prove undesirable to the cat, and the history often connects a litter change with the change in elimination behaviors.[15, 32] Because cats prefer a specific type of litter, changes, if necessary, should be gradual. Odor can serve as a deterrent when excessive amounts of cleaning solutions are used to clean litter pans. Plastic litter boxes should be replaced periodically, since urine reacts with them over time to change their basic odor.

Some cats have come to associate an unpleasant experience with the litter pan and prefer to avoid it. Experiences such as painful defecations or being repeatedly caught at that site and given a pill can adversely condition these cats. Retraining the animal to use the litter pan often is necessary and is best started in a different, isolated location. Once correct habits are reestablished, increased access to the house can be allowed. Using successive approximation, the owner gradually can move the litter pan to a more desirable location.

If the cat attempts to use the litter pan but misses, other measures must be taken. The pan itself should be evaluated. It may be too small or the cat may position itself too near the edge. The solution usually involves supplying a larger litter pan or one with higher sides.

Cats apparently associate pain with location, so any housesoiling cat should be examined medically to be sure there is no medical basis for the problem.[1, 3, 4] When a cat is urinating frequently, not using the litter pan as usual, or both, physical evaluation and a good history are important. Recurrent cystitis, often with small calculi, presents the same signs. Routine diagnostic procedures may not indicate a medical problem even though one exists, since a normal urine pH may not be acceptable for a few individuals, and urine acidifiers may be sufficient to control the problem. A dietary change, ammonium chloride, or even tomato juice on the food has been used successfully.[4, 50] If the animal continues to have a serious problem, the possibility of urinary calculi should be strongly considered. Vinegar has been successful as an oral therapy for atypical urination or spraying, probably because the underlying condition was medical rather than behavioral. Subclinical constipation can result in painful defecations and the cat's choosing to eliminate in a different location. Many of these cats are on special low-residue diets. If the feces can be picked up with a tissue and not cling, the stool probably is too firm. The diet should be changed or a stool softener administered to correct the underlying problem and then an additional litter box should be placed at the chosen defecation spot. After relearning has occurred the box gradually can be moved. Anal sacs also should be checked.

In the very old cat changes in eliminative behavior may be related to age. Certainly there can be loss of sphincter control and associated incontinence, but other painful conditions, such as arthritis, can decrease the animal's desire to move to the litter box, which results in more accidents.[24]

Cats that never used the litter box or have not used it for a long time are not easy to change. Many owners have lost patience too. One suggestion for them is to gradually make the cat an indoor-outdoor cat. Continue to feed it at specific times so that it continues to stay around, and after it learns to eliminate outside it gradually can be allowed back in for longer periods. With the transition being gradual, even declawed cats learn to manage very well. This technique also works well for spraying cats when the owners cannot stand to have the cat indoors any longer. If this is not an option, or if the owners want to keep the cat indoors, it is possible to train a cat to use a litter box. The process is not easy, and owners should be warned about that. The cat is confined to a small room or large carrier and the entire floor is covered with a thin layer of litter. Each week the amount of floor covered by litter is reduced, provided the cat uses the litter area. The litter box eventually is the only litter area. If it is used appropriately for an additional week, gradual access can be given to the rest of the house.[4]

Miscellaneous Behavioral Changes

Emotional states may result in changes other than spraying or breaking house-training. Short-term frustration, fear, or tension can result in nonburial of feces, psychological incontinence, vomition, and diarrhea within 2 to 3 days. If these conditions are prolonged and suppressed, the gastrointestinal tract decreases its activity, which results in constipation and urine retention. Emotional changes can affect the stomach and small intestine as well. In house cats that normally eliminate outside, owners who notice frequent trips in and out may not see the cat actually eliminate.

Cats with upper respiratory tract infections may develop secondary diarrhea or stop using the litter pan. The secondary diarrhea often is associated with mucus ingestion but may be related to emotional stresses of disease and treatment or hospitalization. The anosmia associated with upper respiratory tract disease may be a contributing factor, but experimental destruction of olfactory epithelium usually is not associated with changes in litter pan use.[43]

Once a mild odor of urine or feces becomes associated with an area, that area becomes attractive; therefore, thorough cleaning of soiled spots is a must. Several substances have been used, from carbonated soda water to soapy water with a vinegar-water rinse to commercial products.[7, 24, 36] Other products, such as those mentioned in Chapter 5, help to cover the odor; those that contain ammonia should be avoided because their odor is similar to that of urine.[24] To prevent recurrence, small food bowls or additional litter boxes can be placed where inappropriate urination or defecation occurs.

CASE PRESENTATIONS

CASE 8–1. One-year-old Persian female. The cat was raised in a caged-cattery environment until about 9 months of age, when it went into a home. Although the cat was healthy, it could not seem to adjust to the new life-style, as evidenced by its not using the litter box. When caged, the cat always used the litter box.

Diagnosis. Housesoiling resulting from environmental tensions.

Treatment. The cat was isolated in a small extra bathroom with food, water, and litter until it consistently used the litter box. It was given routine but not excessive attention. When its urinary behavior became consistent, the cat was given access to additional portions of the house until, after 2 months, it had total access.

CASE 8–2. Three-year-old domestic shorthair neutered male. The cat had no previous problems, but the owner noticed a urine spot on the carpet. Since that time she observed that although the cat occasionally used the litter box, area throw rugs, or her husband's clothes, it usually urinated on the single carpet spot. There was no history of household changes. The cat defecated in the litter box.

Diagnosis. Change of preferred urinary location for unknown reasons.

Treatment. Placement of an additional litter box in the cat's selected location after the carpet spot was cleaned resulted in the cat's being retrained to use the litter box.

CASE 8–3. Two-year-old domestic shorthair neutered female. Four months earlier the cat began urinating on the linoleum floor in the kitchen. Treatment for cystitis helped for a short time, but the behavior soon recurred and has persisted.

Medical Workup. Palpation revealed a thickened urinary bladder with a gritty consistency. The urinalysis was normal, but contrast radiography showed foreign matter in the urinary bladder.

Diagnosis. Urinary calculi.

Treatment. Surgical removal of the calculi resulted in an immediate resumption of litter box usage.

CASE 8–4. Eight-month-old domestic shorthair neutered female. The cat was adopted at 12 weeks of age from an animal shelter. The owner complained that the cat urinated but did not defecate in the litter box. Newspaper and several different litters had been tried unsuccessfully. The litter box was kept in a small basement bathroom, and the stools were found in the bathroom but not in the litter box.

Diagnosis. Housesoiling, possibly because the cat did not learn proper behavior as a kitten.

Treatment. The cat was confined to the bathroom with food, water, and a bed area at times when it routinely defecated or when the owner could not watch its activities. Except for the bed area, the entire floor of the bathroom was covered with a thin layer of litter, and the litter box remained in its usual place. Each week the amount of area covered with litter was reduced, and the cat continued to urinate and defecate on litter. By the 5th week the cat was using the litter box only. After an additional week of error-free elimination behavior, the cat was allowed access to the entire house, and there were no further problems.

CASE 8–5. One-year-old domestic shorthair female. The cat came in heat for the first time and started spraying urine near a door and window. This had occurred daily during the previous month.

Diagnosis. Housesoiling by urine-spraying.

Treatment. Because the cat was not to be a breeding animal, the owner chose to control the problem with an ovariohysterectomy.

CASE 8–6. Six-year-old domestic shorthair neutered female. One year before presentation to the referring veterinarian, the cat had started urinating on the hall carpet. The cat was found to have feline urologic syndrome and was placed on a special diet. The problem stopped for a few months but started again with both urine and feces being left on the carpet. No medical problem was found before the referral. The owner put three litter boxes in the garage and cleans them weekly.

Diagnosis. Housesoiling by urination and defecation.

Treatment. A new litter box was added in the hallway, and the cat immediately started using it.

CASE 8–7. Ten-year-old Siamese neutered male. For 4 months the cat occasionally had been urinating on the carpet in the hallway next to the cat room. The owner reported putting up a child gate in the door going into the room with the cat food and litter box to keep out the two dogs. The three resident cats would jump over the gate to get access to the room.

Diagnosis. Housesoiling by urination.

Treatment. Because this cat was a geriatric patient, it was thought that the jumping occasionally would be painful. The owner lifted the child gate so the cat could crawl under and it again used the litter box consistently.

CASE 8–8. One-year-old Persian neutered male. Five months earlier the cat had a protracted bout of problems with feline urologic syndrome, and since that had been cleared up it continued to urinate in about 10 areas in the house. The referring veterinarian had tried megestrol acetate and diazepam, but they were not helpful.

Diagnosis. Housesoiling by urination.

Treatment. The owners were excited about gradually turning this cat into an outdoor animal.

CASE 8–9. Six-year-old domestic shorthair neutered male. The cat had not urinated in the litter box for the past 8 months, and had been eliminating mainly in one corner of one room. There were no known changes in events associated with the litter box.

Diagnosis. Housesoiling by urination.

Treatment. A litter box was added on the normal urination spot, and the cat continued to use that box for urine and the original box for feces.

CASE 8–10. Seven-year-old domestic shorthair neutered male. The cat lived with one other cat, which had been bullying this cat for the past year. For the past month the cat had not been defecating in the litter box.

Diagnosis. Housesoiling by defecation.

Treatment. Another litter box was added in an adjoining room so that the cat could have access to one if the other was being blocked. Feces occasionally was found outside a box, but the major problem stopped.

CASE 8–11. Eight-year-old domestic longhair neutered female. The cat had been on a special dry diet for previous urinary problems and recently started defecating near but out of the litter box. The owner described the stools as being very dry.

Diagnosis. Housesoiling by defecation.

Treatment. The cat was put on a canned diet and a second litter box was added near the first. As the stool softened, the cat started using the added box most of the time.

CASE 8–12. Eight-year-old domestic shorthair neutered male. One of three cats, the cat had been urinating in several places in the house, including on drapes, the piano, the stove, the kitchen countertop, and the wall. It would be especially bad if the owner had been gone a few days. Over the past 3 years the referring veterinarian had tried megestrol acetate and diazepam without success.

Diagnosis. Housesoiling by urine spraying.

Treatment. The owner was not able to identify a specific stressor and was mad at this cat and not willing to put much effort into changing the cat. He decided to make the cat an outdoor cat that could come in occasionally.

CASE 8–13. Nine-year-old domestic shorthair neutered female. Because the cat was an indoor-outdoor cat, the owner did not have a litter box in the house. She had been letting the cat out three times daily to eliminate, but for 4 weeks had been finding urine and feces in a corner of the living room. It was noted that the weather had been particularly bad during that time.

Diagnosis. Housesoiling by urination and defecation probably related to not eliminating when outside because of the nasty weather.

Treatment. Adding a litter box in the corner stopped the problem, and the cat resumed its outside elimination pattern once the weather cleared up.

CASE 8–14. One-and-one-half-year-old domestic shorthair neutered female. The cat had been urinating in the house, even directly in front of the owner, three times a week for a month. The referring veterinarian tried megestrol acetate after finding a normal urinalysis, but there was no change in the behavior. The owner described a recent move and long hours associated with a new job.

Diagnosis. Housesoiling by urine-marking.

Treatment. Attention was given to the cat's schedule, especially as it related to interaction with the owner, and within the next 2 months the behavior gradually improved.

CASE 8–15. Eight-year-old domestic shorthair neutered male. For the past 2 years the cat had not urinated in its litter box, although it did defecate there. After a move 4 months earlier the owner noticed the cat urinating on several spots in the new home.
Diagnosis. Chronic housesoiling by urination.
Treatment. The owner confined the cat for 4 months, and it used the litter box during that time. As soon as it was let out the problem recurred. At that time the owner decided to make the cat an indoor-outdoor animal.

CASE 8–16. Eight-year-old Burmese neutered female. The cat had been urinating on the owner's bed for 8 months and would go on the carpet by the door if it was shut. The litter box was located in the basement utility room.
Medical Workup. The physical examination and urinalysis were within normal limits.
Diagnosis. Housesoiling by urination.
Treatment. The owners were told to keep the bedroom door closed and add another litter box near the door to make it convenient for the cat. This worked reasonably well, except when they occasionally forgot to close the door.

CASE 8–17. One-and-one-half-year-old domestic longhair neutered male. Two weeks before presentation the cat had been found as a stray. Since being introduced into the home it had sprayed at least twice.
Diagnosis. Housesoiling by urine-spraying.
Treatment. Because the history of the animal was not known, the owner decided to return this cat to the outdoors and feed it there.

CASE 8–18. Thirteen-year-old domestic shorthair neutered female. Four days earlier the owners had purchased a new bed and bedspread, and the cat started urinating in the middle of it. The cat was confined to the bedroom because of other cats in the house.
Diagnosis. Housesoiling by urine-marking.
Treatment. The bed was covered with an old blanket that had the owner's smell on it, and the cat stopped the problem. After several weeks the blanket was removed and there was no further problem.

CASE 8–19. Two-year-old Persian neutered male. The owner was the third person who had the cat, and each time it had been given up because it would not use the litter box. It still did not 2 weeks after being introduced into the household.

Diagnosis. Housesoiling by urination and defecation, probably because it had never used a litter box or had forgotten how.

Treatment. Because the owner thought that retraining would take too long, she made the cat an indoor-outdoor animal.

CASE 8–20. Five-year-old domestic shorthair neutered female. This cat and a littermate had been introduced to a kitten 3 months earlier. Since that time the cat would urinate on the owner's clothes.

Diagnosis. Housesoiling by urine-marking.

Treatment. The owner confined the kitten in a separate room so that interactions were minimized. The cat gradually stopped the urination, but it did spend most of its time in areas of the house away from the confinement room.

CASE 8–21. Seven-year-old domestic longhair neutered male. The cat had had bloody urine for 3 weeks. It had become inconsistent in using the litter box and often urinated in the bathroom sink.

Medical Workup. The physical examination did not reveal any abnormalities. The urinalysis had a pH of 8.2, and the red cells were too numerous to count. Culture of the urine was sterile.

Diagnosis. Housesoiling by urination as the result of feline urologic syndrome.

Treatment. The problem cleared up within a week when the cat was placed on a special urine-acidfying diet.

CASE 8–22. Five-year-old domestic shorthair neutered male. For the past year the cat had been defecating near the front entrance of the home. The stool was described as very dry. The diet was a dry special formula food.

Diagnosis. Housesoiling by defecation.

Treatment. The cat was started on a canned food to soften the stools, and a second litter box was put at the problem area.

CASE 8–23. Six-month-old Persian male. The cat had been very sick for the first 3 months in this home. The illness was under control, but it often urinated in two favorite areas.

Diagnosis. Housesoiling by urination, probably as the result of not learning a rigid pattern of litter box use during the illness.

Treatment. Confinement to a spare bathroom for 2 months greatly improved litter box usage. The owner was careful for several more months to confine the cat when she would not be able to supervise its activities.

CASE 8–24. One-year-old domestic shorthair male. The cat stopped defecating in the litter box 4 months earlier, when the owners were on vacation. The family's son was to clean the box, but the frequency of that happening was questioned. The litter box was kept in the bathroom, and feces were found on the opposite side of the room.

Diagnosis. Housesoiling by defecation.

Treatment. An added litter box where the cat chose to defecate reduced the problem to an occasional one.

CASE 8–25. Five-year-old domestic longhair neutered female. The cat had been urinating on the carpet at the top of the stairs and defecating on the carpet at night several times each week for 3 months. The litter box was located in the basement. Historically the cat had broken its leg 1 year ago, and there had been a prolonged recovery period.

Diagnosis. Housesoiling by urination and defecation, probably related to pain experienced when climbing and descending the stairs.

Treatment. A litter box was added on the main floor, and the cat consistently used the box.

Also see cases 3–1, 4–1, 4–7, 5–1, and 10–6.

REFERENCES

1. Beaver, B.: Therapy of behavior problems. In Kirk, R. W., ed.: Current Veterinary Therapy. VIII: Small Animal Practice. Philadelphia: W. B. Saunders Co., 1983.
2. Beaver, B. V.: Taxonomy for Feline Housesoiling. St. Louis: Scientific Proceedings of the American Animal Hospital Association, 1989.
3. Beaver, B. V.: Housesoiling by cats: A retrospective study of 120 cases. J. Am. Anim. Hospital Assoc. 25:631, 1989.
4. Beaver, B. V.: Disorders of behavior. In Sherding, R. G., ed.: The Cat: Diseases and Clinical Management. New York: Churchill Livingstone, 1989.
5. Beaver, B. V.: Psychogenic manifestations of environmental disturbances. In August, J. R., ed.: Consultations in Feline Medicine. Philadelphia: W. B. Saunders Co., 1991.
6. Beaver, B. V. G.: Feline behavioral problems. Vet. Clin. North Am. 6:333, 1976.
7. Beaver, B. V., Terry, M. L., and LaSagna, C. L.: Effectiveness of products in eliminating cat urine odor from carpet. J. Am. Vet. Med. Assoc. 194:1589, 1989.
8. Blackshaw, J. K.: Abnormal behaviour in cats. Aust. Vet. J. 65:395, 1988.
9. Borchelt, P. L., and Voith, V. L.: Diagnosis and treatment of elimination behavior problems in cats. Vet. Clin. North Am. [Small Anim. Pract.] 12:673, 1982.
10. Borchelt, P. L., and Voith, V. L.: Elimination behavior problems in cats. Compendium on Continuing Education 8:197, 1986.
11. Brunner, F.: The application of behavior studies in small animal practice. In Fox, M. W., ed.: Abnormal Behavior in Animals. Philadelphia: W. B. Saunders Co., 1968.
12. Bryant, D.: The Care and Handling of Cats. New York: Ives Washburn, 1944.
13. Chapman, B., and Voith, V. L.: Geriatric behavior problems not always related to age. D.V.M. 18:32, Mar. 1987.
14. Crowell-Davis, S. L.: Elimination behavior problems in cats, pt. I. Vet. Forum, p. 10, November 1986.
15. Crowell-Davis, S. L.: Elimination behavior problems in cats, pt. II. Vet. Forum, p. 14, December 1986.
16. Crowell-Davis, S. L.: Elimination behavior problems in cats, pt. III. Vet. Forum, p. 16, January 1987.

17. Crowell-Davis, S. L.: Elimination behavior problems in cats, pt. IV. Vet. Forum, p. 20, February 1987.
18. Fox, M. W.: The behaviour of cats. In Hafez, E. S. E., ed.: The Behaviour of Domestic Animals. 3rd ed. Baltimore: Williams & Williams Co., 1975.
19. Gorman, M. L., and Trowbridge, B. J.: The role of odor in the social lives of carnivores. In Gittleman, J. L., ed.: Carnivore Behavior, Ecology, and Evolution. Ithaca, NY: Cornell University Press, 1989.
20. Gosling, L. M.: A reassessment of the function of scent marking in territories. Z. Tierpsychol. 60:89, 1982.
21. Hart, B. L.: Normal behavior and behavioral problems associated with sexual function, urination, and defecation. Vet. Clin. North Am. 4:589, 1974.
22. Hart, B. L.: Spraying behavior. Fel. Pract. 5:11, July-Aug. 1975.
23. Hart, B. L.: Learning ability in cats. Fel. Pract. 5:10, Sept.-Oct. 1975.
24. Hart, B. L.: Inappropriate urination and defecation. Fel. Pract. 6:6, Mar. 1976.
25. Hart, B. L.: The client asks you: A quiz on feline behavior. Fel. Pract. 8:10, Mar. 1978.
26. Hart, B. L.: Objectionable urine spraying and urine marking in cats: Evaluation of progestin treatment in gonadectomized males and females. J. Am. Vet. Med. Assoc. 177:529, 1980.
27. Hart, B. L.: Olfactory tractotomy for control of objectionable urine spraying and urine marking in cats. J. Am. Vet. Med. Assoc. 179:231, 1981.
28. Hart, B. L.: Neurosurgery for behavioral problems: A curiosity or the new wave? Vet. Clin. North Am. [Small Anim. Pract.] 12:707, 1982.
29. Hart, B. L.: Urine spraying and marking in cats. In Slatter, D. H., ed.: Textbook of Small Animal Surgery. Philadelphia: W. B. Saunders Co., 1985.
30. Hart, B. L., and Barrett, R. E.: Effects of castration on fighting, roaming, and urine spraying in adult male cats. J. Am. Vet. Med. Assoc. 163:290, 1973.
31. Hart, B. L., and Cooper, L.: Factors relating to urine spraying and fighting in prepubertally gonadectomized cats. J. Am. Vet. Med. Assoc. 184:1255, 1984.
32. Hart, B. L., and Hart, L. A.: Canine and Feline Behavioral Therapy. Philadelphia: Lea & Febiger, 1985.
33. Hart, B. L., and Leedy, M.: Identification of source of urine stains in multi-cat households. J. Am. Vet. Med. Assoc. 180:77, 1982.
34. Houpt, K. A.: Companion animal behavior: A review of dog and cat behavior in the field, the laboratory and the clinic. Cornell Vet. 75:248, 1985.
35. Houpt, K. A.: Personal communication, 1988.
36. Kahn, B.: Out of the frying pan—into the litter pan. Cat Fancy 15:18, Nov.-Dec. 1972.
37. Kleiman, D. G., and Eisenberg, J. F.: Comparisons of canid and felid social systems from an evolutionary perspective. Anim. Behav. 21:637, 1973.
38. Kling, A., Kovach, J. K., and Tucker, T. J.: The behaviour of cats. In Hafez, E. S. E., ed.: The Behaviour of Domestic Animals. 2nd ed. Baltimore: Williams & Wilkins Co., 1969.
39. Mancla, G., Baccelli, G., and Zanchetti, A.: Regulation of renal circulation during behavioral changes in the cat. Am. J. Physiol. 227:536, 1974.
40. Marder, A.: Personal communication, 1987.
41. Marder, A.: Personal communication, 1989.
42. Marder, A.: Personal communication, 1990.
43. McClung, A. W., and Hart, B. L.: Olfactory loss affecting behavior? Fel. Pract. 8:17, May 1978.
44. Mosier, J. E.: Common medical and behavioral problems in cats. Mod. Vet. Pract. 56:699, 1975.
45. Olm, D. D., and Houpt, K. A.: Feline house-soiling problems. Appl. Anim. Behav. Sci. 20:335, 1988.
46. Pemberton, P. L.: Canine and feline behavior control: Progestin therapy. In Kirk, R. W., ed.: Current Veterinary Therapy. VIII: Small Animal Practice. Philadelphia: W. B. Saunders Co., 1983.
47. Romatowski, J.: Use of megestrol acetate in cats. J. Am. Vet. Med. Assoc. 194:700, 1989.
48. Rosenblatt, J. S.: Suckling and home orientation in the kitten: A comparative developmental study. In Tobach, E., Aronson, L. R., and Shaw, E., ed.: The Biopsychology of Development. New York: Academic Press, 1971.
49. Spraying by castrated tomcats. Mod. Vet. Pract. 56:729, 1975.

50. Taton, G. F., Hamar, D. W., and Lewis, L. D.: Evaluation of ammonium chloride as a urinary acidifier in the cat. J. Am. Vet. Med. Assoc. 184:433, 1984.
51. Voith, V. L.: Personal communication, 1978.
52. Voith, V. L.: Therapeutic approaches to feline urinary behavior problems. Mod. Vet. Pract. 61:539, 1980.
53. Voith, V. L.: Treating elimination behavior problems in dogs and cats: The role of punishment. Mod. Vet. Pract. 62:951, 1981.
54. Voith, V. L.: Behavior disorders. In Davis, L. E., ed.: Handbook of Small Animal Therapeutics. New York: Churchill Livingstone, 1985.
55. Voith, V. L., and Marder, A. R.: Feline behavioral disorders. In Morgan, R., ed.: Handbook of Small Animal Practice. New York: Churchill Livingstone, 1988.
56. Whitehead, J. E.: Tomcat spraying. Mod. Vet. Pract. 46:68, 1965.

ADDITIONAL READINGS

Abdel-Rahman, M., Galeano, C., and Elhilali, M. New approach to study of voicing cycle in cat. Preliminary report on pharmacologic studies. Urology XXII:91, 1983.
Beadle, M. The Cat: History, Biology, and Behavior. New York: Simon & Schuster, 1977.
Bernstein, K. S. A physiological reason for defecating outside the litterbox. Vet. Med. Small Anim. Clin. 72:1549, 1977.
Boudreau, J. C., and Tsuchitani, C. Sensory Neurophysiology. New York: Van Nostrand Reinhold Co., 1973.
Campbell, W. E. Correcting house-soiling problems in cats. Mod. Vet. Pract. 66:53, 1985.
Chalifoux, A., and Gosselin, Y. The use of megestrol acetate to stop urine spraying in castrated male cats. Can. Vet. J. 22:211, 1981.
Chertok, L., and Fontaine, M. Psychosomatics in veterinary medicine. J. Psychosom. Res. 7:229, 1963.
Davidson, M. G., and Baty, K. T. Anaphylaxis associated with intravenous sodium fluorescein administration in a cat. Prog. Vet. Comparative Ophth. 1:127, 1991.
Ewer, R. F. The Carnivores. Ithaca, NY: Cornell University Press, 1973.
Fox, M. W. New information on feline behavior. Mod. Vet. Pract. 56:50, Feb. 1965.
Fox, M. W. Aggression: Its adaptive and maladaptive significance in man and animals. In Fox, M. W., ed. Abnormal Behavior in Animals. Philadelphia: W. B. Saunders Co., 1968.
Fox, M. W. Psychomotor disturbances. In Fox, M. W., ed. Abnormal Behavior in Animals. Philadelphia: W. B. Saunders Co., 1968.
Fox, M. W. Psychopathology in man and lower animals. J. Am. Vet. Med. Assoc. 153:66, 1971.
Fox, M. W. Understanding Your Cat. New York: Coward, McCann & Geoghegan, 1974.
Hart, B. L. Behavioral effects of castration. Fel. Pract. 3:10, Mar.-Apr. 1973.
Hart, B. L. Psychopharmacology in feline practice. Fel. Pract. 3:6, May-June 1973.
Hart, B. L. Behavioral effects of long-acting progestins. Fel. Pract. 4:8, Jul.-Aug. 1974.
Hart, B. L. Quiz on feline behavior. Fel. Pract. 6:10, May 1976.
Hart, B. L. Behavioral aspects of raising kittens. Fel. Pract. 6:8, Nov. 1976.
Hart, B. L. Medication for control of spraying. Fel. Pract. 7:16, May 1977.
Joshua, J. O. Abnormal behavior in cats. In Fox, M. W., ed. Abnormal Behavior in Animals. Philadelphia: W. B. Saunders Co., 1968.
Levinson, B. M. Man and his feline pet. Mod. Vet. Pract. 53:35, Nov. 1972.
McCrory, R. G. Urine spraying. Fel. Pract. 3:6, Mar.-Apr. 1973.
Northway, R. B. Manual stimulation of micturition. Med. Vet. Pract. 56:832, 1975.
Riddle, B. L., Deats, P. H., Meyer, H., and Gilbride, A. P. Solution to spraying cats. Fel. Pract. 5:6, Jan.-Feb. 1975.
Schmidt, J. P. Psychosomatics in veterinary medicine. In Fox, M. W., ed. Abnormal Behavior in Animals. Philadelphia: W. B. Saunders Co., 1968.
Vollmer, P. J. Can a cat be retrained to use a litterbox? Vet. Med. Small Anim. Clin. 72:1161, 1977.
Vollmer, P. J. Feline inappropriate elimination, Pt. 1. Vet. Med. Small Anim. Clin. 74:796, 1979.

Vollmer, P. J. Feline inappropriate elimination, Pt. 2. Vet. Med. Small Anim. Clin. 74:928, 1979.

Vollmer, P. J. Feline inappropriate elimination, Pt. 3. Vet. Med. Small Anim. Clin. 74:1101, 1979.

Vollmer, P. J. Feline inappropriate elimination, Pt. 4. Vet. Med. Small Anim. Clin. 74:1241, 1979.

Vollmer, P. J. Feline inappropriate elimination, Pt. 5. Vet. Med. Small Anim. Clin. 74:1419, 1979.

Wemmer, C., and Scow, K. Communication in the Felidae with emphasis on scent marking and contact patterns. In Sebeok, T. A., ed. How Animals Communicate. Bloomington: Indiana University Press, 1977.

Worden, A. N. Abnormal behavior in the dog and cat. Vet. Rec. 71:966, 1959.

9

Feline Locomotive Behavior

A cat's life basically revolves around eating, sleeping, and reproducing. Because of this, the ability to ambulate at various speeds is a necessity. In this regard, the locomotor patterns and their reciprocal sleep patterns have been specialized to allow successful hunting and survival as well as adequate rest. The comparative development of these patterns is shown in Appendix C.

FETAL GROWTH AND MOVEMENTS

The kitten begins in utero the development of movement patterns that will be necessary in the adult. These patterns, as with sensory systems, parallel the development of the nervous system.[49] Neuronal pathways become myelinated in their phylogenetic order of development.[50]

About 25 days after conception, the 15- to 16-mm fetal kitten shows its first spontaneous movement as a unilateral flexion of its head and a passive flexion of its shoulder. After growth of a few more millimeters, spontaneous neck mobility increases and local response to touch develops, along with ventral neck flexion, bilateral flexion of the head and upper neck, and rotation of the head. By the time the embryo is 20 mm from crown to rump, it begins to show flexion of the lumbar and sacral vertebral column and active flexion of the shoulder joint.[90, 91]

During the 26th day after conception (21 to 22 mm), rotation of the trunk first occurs, as does flexion of the elbow. In another 2 days flexion of the hips is seen, probably in passive response to the waves of muscular movements along the body. Motor responses continue to develop, so that by day 30 (27 to 30 mm), flexion of the carpus and slight activation of the masticatory muscles occur. Flexion of the tail can be observed at 33 days (38 mm), as can adduction of the forelimb. During this time of completion of facial and forelimb muscular development, there is flexion of the stifle, extension of the vertebral column and manus, and withdrawal by flexion from a touch sensation. By 36 days (50 mm) the abdominal and intercostal muscles begin to function.[90, 91]

Sometime between 38 and 40 days after conception (60 mm) flexion of the tarsus begins, and tongue muscles begin to function. By 42 days (75 to 80 mm) the pes flexes and the diaphragm starts functioning, although breathing movements are irregular for another 7 days. After an additional 8 days of growth (100 mm) most motor responses have been shown. The pelvic limb is capable of adduction and digital flexion, and the muscles of facial expression and those of the larynx associated with phonation become active.[90]

Spontaneous body-righting capabilities initially are present at about 50 days (100 mm), although they are by no means adultlike and probably are not vestibular in origin.[23, 89, 90] Vestibular righting does not appear until about 4 days (15 mm) later.[89] Several sensory reflexes develop about the same time as the spontaneous body righting, including the scratch, sucking, light blink, and forelimb crossed-extensor reflexes. The ear-scratch reflex develops at this time also, as do ipsilateral flexion and contralateral extension of the forelimb.[20, 90] The coordinated action of the limbs necessary for progressive forward movement occurs near term, indicating that the coordination involved in walking is innate, not learned.[23]

INFANT GROWTH AND MOVEMENTS

Prewalking Movements

At birth the motor skills continue to mature in conjunction with the central nervous system, but additional motor behaviors can be learned. Movements initially involve the whole limb, but with time and maturation, discrete segmental movements are used.[11] Neonatal movements toward the queen are the stiff paddlinglike motion of the forelimbs that matured shortly before birth. These movements are sufficiently coordinated within 8 minutes of birth to pull the suckling for the short distances it must travel. The limbs still lack a great deal of motor coordination and strength because they are unable to bear weight, and the claws are not retractable. The poorly developed motor coordination at this stage functions to prevent the young from wandering. Thermoregulation also is poorly developed until about 2 weeks of age and further serves to keep the kittens close to one another and to the queen. A strong rooting response, the burrowing into warm objects, is present for up to 16 days, giving an indication about the progression of homeostatic mechanisms. (See Fig. 2–8.)

The righting response that occurs when kittens are accidentally pushed over by the queen is continued from the prenatal behaviors; the righting response of cats dropped from a height does not appear until 35 days.[76] Vestibular function develops slowly during the first few days of life. Nystagmus associated with rotatory stimulation appears experimentally at the end of the 1st week, although it has been associated with deviation of the eyes and oscillating eye movements during this early appearance. Vestibular nystagmus becomes adultlike by the end of the 3rd week.[16]

Flexor and extensor dominance of the vertebral musculature, owing to an imbalance of the nervous innervation to them, is not highly consistent among kittens. Flexor dominance is present in most kittens from birth into adolescence (Fig. 9–1). After about the 1st month the curled up posture may modify so that the neck is extended, but the rest of the body position is similar to what it had been. Extensor dominance is much more variable. Starting as early as day 1, this activated vertebral extensor stage also can last into adolescence (Fig. 9–2). Kittens initially may exhibit extensor dominance and then, within a few seconds, progress into a more prolonged flexor dominant stage. This dual sequence is especially noticeable between days 15 and 40. Other kittens show neither dominance at birth, and still others exhibit a great deal of squirming when suspended from the neck.

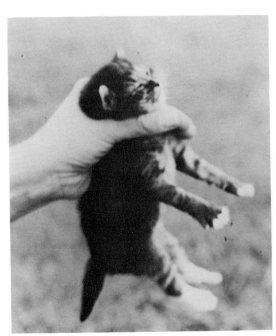

FIGURE 9–1. A 14-day-old kitten exhibiting flexor dominance.

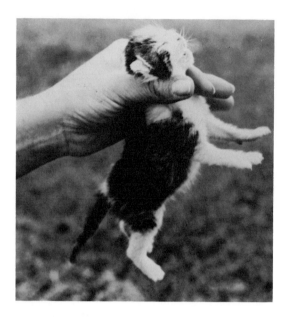

FIGURE 9–2. A 7-day-old kitten exhibiting extensor dominance.

Nonvisual placing of a limb onto a surface in response to its touching the edge of the surface consistently occurs for the thoracic limbs first, sometime during the first 5 days of life (mean is 2.3 days). (See Fig. 2–11.) Development of nonvisual placing of the pelvic limbs is much less uniform, and initially may appear during the first 12 days (mean is 3.6 days), although not consistently until sometime during the first 19 days (mean is 11.3 days).

When a young kitten is suspended by the ventral midline while still in a normal dorsoventral relation, the Landau reflex may be activated. In this reflex the forelimbs and hindlimbs are extended in response to the positioning. Although the reflex can last up to 19 days, the mean ending age is 6.8 days.

The forelimb crossed-extensor reflex is acquired by some individuals before birth. For others, this reflex and the hindlimb crossed-extensor reflex may appear up to the 3rd day of life (mean is 1.4 days), although either or both may never develop (Fig. 9–3). The crossed-extensor reflex ends between days 2 and 17 (mean is 8.1 days).

Body support by the limbs develops in four stages shortly after birth. In the first stage, when the kitten is held by the lumbar and pelvic areas and lowered to a table, its forelimbs start to support weight between 1 and 10 days of age (mean is 3.5 days). Direct forelimb support of the body weight, the second stage, also appears during the first 10 days, but the mean is 5.7 days (Fig. 9–4). Pelvic limb support, the third stage, begins to be demonstrated during the first 16 days (mean is 14.3 days)

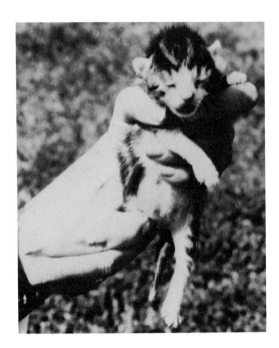

FIGURE 9-3. The crossed-extensor reflex of the pelvic limbs in a 7-day-old kitten.

when the kitten is suspended by the thorax and the pelvic limbs are allowed to touch the table (Fig. 9–5). Finally, the ability to completely elevate the body off the ground by the additional strength in the hindlimbs begins between days 5 and 25 (mean is 10.0 days).

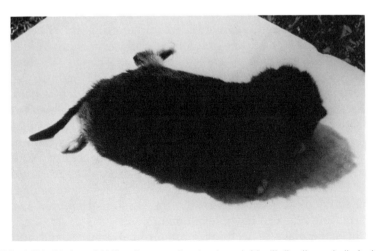

FIGURE 9-4. This 14-day-old kitten is supporting body weight with the thoracic limbs but not yet with the pelvic limbs.

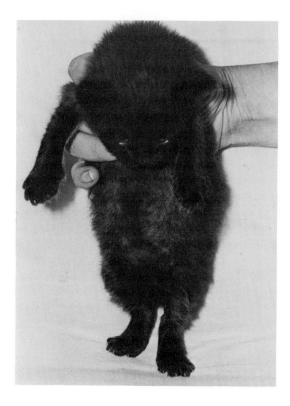

FIGURE 9–5. The pelvic limbs are supporting weight when this 2-week-old kitten is lowered to a solid surface.

Walking and Other Later Movements

Locomotor functions continue to mature, so that by 20 days the kitten is sitting, and it is unsteadily walking in another day or two. With early body support and standing, or with infant handling, the process can be speeded up, so that the kitten actually is walking at about 15 days.

Once walking has begun, several behaviors change. The avoidance reaction progresses from a primitive stage, in which the kitten vocalizes and squirms, to one more typical of an adult, in which it backs away from the stimulus. This latter type of avoidance appears about the 25th day.[72] Kittens actively approach specific people and littermates as early as 18 days of age, especially if the earlier experience has been enriched by handling, and they become good followers, a necessity, so that they can undergo visual learning from the queen's examples.[19, 66] Running first appears toward the end of the 3rd week, and is accompanied by the onset of active play. Shortly thereafter the kitten has matured enough for the air-righting reflex to have developed.[11]

Within a few days of walking, normally between 23 and 40 days of age (mean is 31 days), the kitten starts climbing, usually in an attempt to escape from the nesting box. At first these escapes are brief, but within

5 days 68 per cent of the young one's time is spent out of the box.[59] By 8 weeks of age 82 per cent of the time is spent out, an increase that coincides with the time the kitten changes its orientation from the home area to the queen.[59, 62, 63] Once out of the box, the kitten's climbing attempts are made on other environmental obstacles. Success in climbing is related to another factor: controllability of the claws. During the first 2 weeks of life the young cat does not have the ability to retract its claws. Through a gradual process, control is gained over retractability, so that by 3 weeks the kitten has reasonable control over its distal phalanges.

Sensorimotor Coordination

The sense of vision plays a significant role in the development of certain aspects of locomotion. Kittens raised experimentally without being able to see their forelimbs are not able to place their feet accurately at a later age. In addition, batting at dangling objects, reaching for objects, or avoidance stepping is not successful for these individuals because the controlled placing response requires a certain amount of integration of the visual and motor systems.[30, 32] Kittens allowed to watch one paw but not the other are permanently unable to guide the unseen paw.[30, 31] Similar studies have been conducted under conditions of light deprivation. After a minimum of 4 weeks of darkness visual depth discrimination is affected. Minimal stimulation, such as 1 hour per day of exercise on a patterned surface, with exercise being the key factor, results in normal movement discrimination.[60, 79] Time to develop this ability in older kittens that have been deprived is somewhat similar to that required for visually normal neonates to acquire it after birth.[75] For the kitten that has visual stimulation but is experimentally never allowed to propel itself, with locomotion supplied by others, visually guided behavior is severely affected.[33] Therefore, both factors are necessary for sensorimotor coordination.

Weight Gains

In addition to developing locomotor skills, kittens are growing in size. A kitten will double in size each week, from a birth weight of 85 to 140 g, until the 8th week. This weight increase is significant not only because the youngster is growing larger, but also because it necessitates growing stronger at a much faster rate. Rapid cerebellar growth also is necessary, and any or all of these processes can be severely impaired by malnutrition.

ADULT MOVEMENTS

Adult patterns of movement can be described as alternative or in-phase locomotion.[55] In alternative gates (walk, amble, trot) the ipsilateral limbs strike at alternate halves of stride. In-phase gates (pace, gallop) are characterized by limbs on the same side of the body moving forward during the same part of the stride.

Walking

The walk is a four-beat gait, meaning that each of the cat's paws contacts the ground at a separate time during the stride. During any one phase of this gait at least two feet have ground contact. In a slow walk, such as the stalking walk, usually three and occasionally four feet have ground contact (Fig. 9–6). In the rapid walk two or three feet are on the ground at a time (Fig. 9–7). The walk also has been described as symmetric because the left limbs repeat the position of the right, one-half stride later. The forward speed is about 0.9 m/sec; a rapid walk almost doubles the rate.[21, 24]

Vertical and horizontal forces are associated with walking, with the vertical thrust fluctuating between a high of about 4000 g to a low of about 2600 g twice during each complete cycle. Of these amounts, 60 per cent of body weight load is carried by the thoracic limbs, primarily because the center of gravity is closer to them. At normal speed the maximal vertical thrust is realized during the three-foot support phase, whereas minimal thrust occurs when only two paws are on the ground. Individual horizontal forces are greater for the thoracic limbs than for the pelvic limb counterparts. Both the period of forward propulsion and that of negative, retarding propulsion, when the forelimb is being returned to a cranial position, provide greater calculated values than corresponding values for the pelvic limbs. Because of the vertical thrust of the forelimbs, the net longitudinal force is a small forward impulse, much less than for the hindlimbs.[24, 53] In forward movement the primary function of the thoracic limbs is to produce the upward acceleration of the body, whereas that of the pelvic limbs is for forward progress. Neural and electromyographic aspects of locomotion also have been studied.[13, 86, 87]

Cats often submit and almost appear to enjoy going for walks on lead. However, they usually prefer to choose the course. Resistance may be shown by the cat when it and its owner do not want to go in the same direction.

Ambling

Another four-beat gait used by the cat has been referred to by a number of terms, including the amble, slow pace, running walk, and walk. The footfall pattern is the same as for the walk, but the timing of limb placement differs (Figs. 9–8 and 9–9). At this gait the cat has the appearance of moving the limbs on one side of the body forward at almost the same time. Whether the cat uses the walk, amble, or a sequence somewhat in between is an individual factor.

Trotting

For traveling long distances at fair speed the trot most frequently is used. This two-beat gait is less tiring than other gaits because there is less body movement over the center of gravity. An added feature, as a result of steadying the shift of gravity, is that the gait provides more stability of footing. To achieve this symmetric gait, the contralateral forefeet and hindfeet are on the ground simultaneously. At normal or fast speeds one pair of contralateral paws propels the body forward, leaving a brief suspended interval when no limbs are supporting the body (Fig. 9–10). The alternate pair of limbs then lands and pushes off to complete the cycle. At a slow rate of speed the suspension stage does not occur because the third and fourth paws contact the ground before the first and second leave it (Fig. 9–11).

Pacing

Another two-beat gait of fair speed, the pace, is not frequently used by cats. Except that ipsilateral limbs move forward and back as a unit, the ground contact and suspension phases are the same as those described for the trot (Figs. 9–12 and 9–13).

Galloping

When speed is needed to chase prey or escape enemies, the gallop is used. This four-beat, asymmetric gait has several variations, depending on the speed needed and on the individual performing it. At a slow rate (a gait that also is called a "canter"), there is at least one paw on the ground at all times or as many as three during certain phases (Fig. 9–14). As the caudal paws touch the ground, the foot contacting the ground last is positioned in advance of the other. The same positioning occurs when the cranial paws land. The foot that lands last and ahead of its counterpart may be termed the lead foot, and if these were the right forelimb and the right hindlimb, the cat could be said to have the right lead in front and the right lead behind.

When its speed increases the cat has a suspension phase after the push with the pelvic limbs (Fig. 9–15). At great speed a second suspension phase occurs after the push by the thoracic limbs (Fig. 9–16). About 80 per cent of a stride is spent in extended flight, almost 20 per cent in forelimb ground contact, and a minimal amount in ground time for the pelvic limbs.[21]At faster speeds the cat leads with opposite feet, fore and rear, to allow for overreaching as a result of the great amount of flexion in its back. The supple spine can increase the speed and length of each stride by several inches. If the vertebral column extends just before the last foot leaves the ground, before the suspended phase, and does not flex until the next foot touches the ground, the effect is that of adding several inches to the length of the animal and, thus, adding length to its stride. If the extension occurs after the cat is airborne, the effect on its stride and speed is nullified.[36] Faster speeds require more energy to obtain the suspension phase, and therefore seldom are maintained for prolonged distances.

A very short, fast chase has been termed "dashing," and is thought to use the half-bound variation of the gallop (Fig. 9–17).[12, 21] At this gait the cat pushes off with both hind feet at the same time, although they usually are not positioned adjacent to each other. When landing on the forepaws the cat has a timing sequence that is the same as for the gallop; one limb lands first and is caudal to the second.

Climbing

A general concept associated with cats is that they climb trees. Some individual cats, notably Siamese, spend a considerable amount of time on tall objects, including ceiling beams, roofs, and people, as well as trees, but prefer to find these new or odd places themselves. Thus climbing is an important part of the cat's locomotor behavior. Cats that like to climb people often learn this behavior as a kitten from owners who do not discourage it or, in some cases, actually encourage this "cute" kitten behavior. For the adult animal, climbing may represent an attempt to get close to the person's face, as in the facial approach of social greeting, or it may be an attempt to get to a higher location, especially if the shoulder or head is the final destination. The limb movement in climbing follows the same sequence as that used for walking: It is a four-beat rhythm. If the cat is in a hurry, a form of gallop pattern is used. The presence of claws is not required for climbing all objects, although claws are used if they are present. The removal of these ungual processes may necessitate a feline relearning experience.

Climbing down is difficult, and a kitten needs time to perfect the technique. At first the kitten backs down, but later it learns to come down head first in a rather haphazard manner. On reaching a certain height it jumps the remainder of the distance. Unless the cat is in a state of shock, it eventually will come down from any object it climbs if given enough time and motivation. In most cases the owner's lack of time and patience results in attempts to "rescue" the cat, rather than there being a real need by the animal.

Air-righting

Cats have the ability to alter their position in midair so that they can land feet first after a fall. Air-righting develops over a period of time and is seen first as a head rotation, shortly followed by the beginning of a rotation of the trunk. The reflex appears between 21 and 30 days of age (mean is 23.5 days), with complete righting abilities being perfected between 33 and 48 days (mean is 40 days).[8, 11, 81] Deaf cats develop this reflex because their vestibular apparatus seldom is defective. Sight is required to perfect the righting reflex, the development of which correlates with that of visual acuity; once righting abilities are perfected, blindfolding the cat does not greatly hinder the process.

A cat that is dropped with its feet higher than its body responds by turning so that it will land on its feet. The basic occurrences that result in this air-righting begin when the vertebral column flexes so that the cranial half of the body is about at a right angle from the initial starting position (Fig. 9–18). The thoracic limbs are held close to the body, and the pelvic limbs and tail are held away from the trunk (Fig. 9–19). The cranial half is then rotated 180 degrees about its axis while this motion is offset by a 5-degree counterrotation of the caudal body (Fig. 9–20). The thoracic limbs now are extended and vertical, and the pelvic limbs retain their relation with the caudal part of the body, although they are

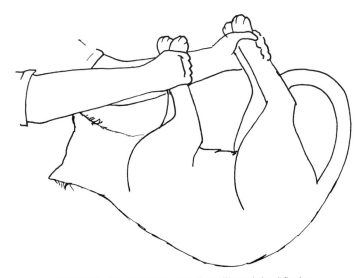

FIGURE 9–18. Air-righting begins with vertebral flexion.

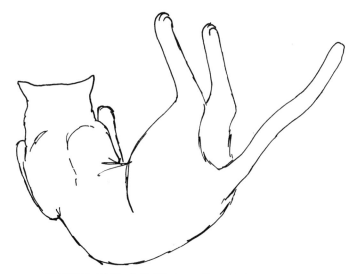

FIGURE 9–19. The initial limb positions during air-righting.

slightly flexed (Fig. 9–21). Then the caudal body rotates to line up with the front of the body (Fig. 9–22). Sometimes cats overrotate the caudal body by as much as 30 degrees, but a counterrotation by the tail and other body muscles usually corrects this problem rapidly. The original flexion of the vertebral column is maintained during the turn so that when landing, the back is arched with the four limbs extended (Fig. 9–23).[40, 54]

When falling, a cat can turn in a distance equal to that of its standing

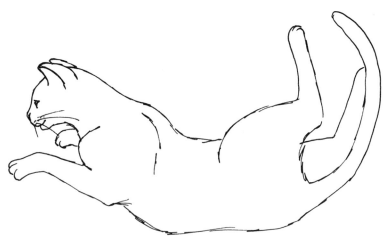

FIGURE 9–20. Cranial body rotation during air-righting.

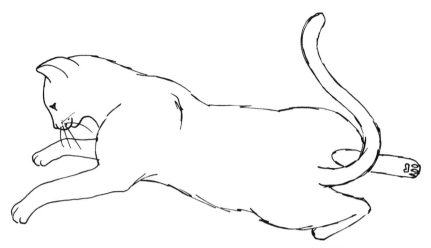

FIGURE 9–21. Changes in limb positions during air-righting.

height and in a time span between 0.125 and 0.5 second.[40, 54] Because it takes 0.4 second to fall 5 ft, most cats are capable of making the turn.[40, 70]

Many remarkable falls have been survived by cats, some even without physical damage. The free-fall record was 129 ft, or 11 stories, by a London cat in 1965.[92] Later reports have taken into account the surface landed on, and survival records for those have been established. When the landing is a hard surface, 18 stories have been the maximal distance survived; 20 stories are the maximum for shrubbery; and 28 stories for a

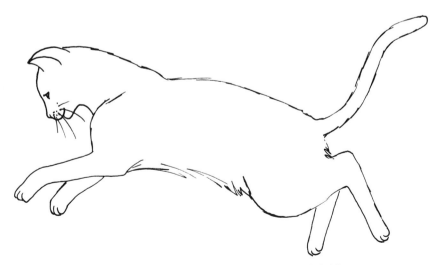

FIGURE 9–22. Caudal body rotation during air-righting.

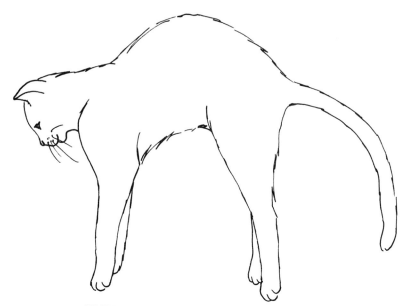

FIGURE 9–23. The landing posture after air-righting.

canopy or awning.[61] When falling, a cat reaches a terminal velocity approaching 40 mph in 60 ft.[54] Theoretically, then, if a cat can survive a fall of 60 ft, it should be able to withstand a fall from any height.

Most cats have an excellent sense of balance, but when they do slip from a precarious perch or fall out of an unexpectedly open window, medical reports of the "high-rise syndrome" reflect the cat's unique righting behavior. Of all traumatic occurrences to cats, 13.9 per cent are the result of a fall. Of these reported injuries, 31 per cent to 57 per cent occur to the head, usually the mandible, 31 per cent to 68 per cent occur to the thorax, and 39 per cent to 43 per cent occur to the limbs.[48, 88]

To show the air-righting reflex, the cat must be dropped so that its limbs are in about the same horizontal plane. When dropped with the cranial or caudal end first, the cat cannot correct its position until one pair of limbs touches the ground (Fig. 9–24).[54]

Jumping

Several behavioral series participated in by cats involve a leaping start from a standing position. Whether a cat is jumping down from a tree, jumping onto a windowsill, or starting after fleeing prey, its basic starting position is the same. The body weight initially is shifted over the hindlimbs, which are situated so that one is slightly in front of the other. Rapid extension of these limbs provides the propulsion for the cat's

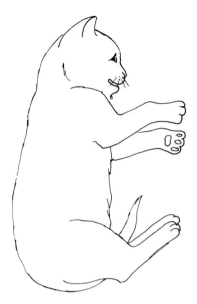

FIGURE 9–24. The air-righting reflex does not correct a position if the limbs are not in the same horizontal plane.

spring and is a modified form of the half-bound gallop gait. (See Fig. 9–17.) The animal lands on its forelimbs, one at a time, with the second foot landing forward of the first. The amount of energy necessary for the initial propulsion is significantly greater than that required for the other gaits, and the force of the support provided by each limb in turn is four to five times greater than that developed during walking.[21] This amount of power must be generated because the weight supported by each limb in turn is about four times the body weight.[21]

The distances jumped by a cat depend on a number of factors, including the physical ability of the individual as well as the distance to the goal; if conditions are right, a maximal leap would cover about 170 cm (5.5 ft).[21]

Swimming

Like most mammals, cats are natural swimmers, although it usually is not a favored behavior. The Turkish cat is a breed exception to this dislike for swimming. The limb movements, which are used to provide slow forward progress, commonly are referred to as the "dog paddle," the same combination of movements used in walking. This four-beat, symmetric pattern also is used by the dog, but the posture differs slightly, in that the cat keeps more of its back and tail out of the water.

Retrieving

The queen brings prey home for the young to use in practicing their hunting skills, and when the mouse escapes the young, the queen catches it and brings it back for her offspring. This is the most common and natural form of retrieving that is done by cats. For other individuals, live prey is repeatedly released only to be recaptured and dragged back. Members of the Kuiat breed, as well as a few other individuals, have an innate retrieving ability: They will catch a ball or other toy and bring it back for the owner to throw again.

Digging

The digging of soil by cats is well known as being part of the eliminative behavior pattern. Cats are capable of earth-raking relatively loose dirt only because their claws are retractable and not available to break the ground initially. The toes must do all the work of loosening and moving the dirt. This is the primary reason cats do not dig into rodent burrows after their prey as other animals do.

Paw Dominance

Felis catus shows a paw dominance similar to the right- and left-handedness observable in humans. Right forepaw usage is preferred by 20 per cent of the cats, and another 38.3 per cent favor the left side for manipulatory tasks.[10, 82] The remaining 41.7 per cent are ambidextrous. Preferences are determined by the sensorimotor cerebral cortex and can be modified only slightly by environmental factors, such as convenience for reaching something.[82, 83]

Limb-flicking

Cats respond to foreign material on their feet by lifting the paw and rapidly shaking it outward from the body. If more than one limb is involved, the cat alternately shakes each paw, repeating the cycle as often as necessary to rid the foot of the substance. Cats that have been dosed with d-lysergic acid diethylamide (LSD) spontaneously exhibit limb-flicking behavior.[38]

Bipedal Standing

A cat is capable of standing on its hindlimbs for relatively long periods. This posture frequently is displayed when the cat is begging or searching for food (Fig. 9–25). The cat is an exception with this behavior because the posture is considered uncommon for predatory animals; their long, slender limbs do not readily adapt to bipedal balance.[12]

Unusual Patterns of Locomotion

Otherwise normal cats occasionally are observed to show episodes of slow-motion movement. The events described are of varying duration and may include a period of apparently normal sleep. Walking movements are less than half as fast as normal, as are eating and grooming motions. Even urination has been observed at this slow speed.

Another unusual pattern observed in cats is a sudden aversion to a particular carpet, such that the cat will do almost anything to avoid walking on it. In seeking the reason for this behavior, several aversive causative situations must be considered. Chemicals used in rug cleaning may be physically irritating or leave an offensive odor. A traumatic event associated with laying a new carpet and even the odor of a new carpet are other factors for consideration. Sometimes an adequate history is difficult to obtain, but at other times the history may not provide any clues to the cause of the problem.

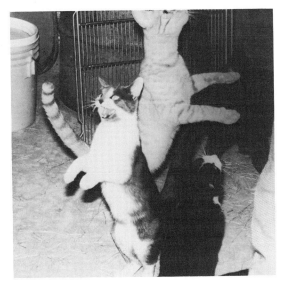

FIGURE 9–25. Bipedal posture used to request food.

RESTING BEHAVIORS

The resting stage of cat activity varies from sitting to sleeping, with several associated postures in between.

Sitting

In a sitting posture the thoracic limbs are positioned much like those of a normal standing cat, with the angulation of each joint remaining about the same. In contrast, the major joints of the pelvic limbs are flexed to lower the caudal portion of the body until the skin covering the ischiatic tuberosities contacts the ground. The tail may be directed caudally, especially when the sit is of short duration (Fig. 9–26 left), or the tail may be wrapped around the paws during a less transient period (Fig. 9–26 right).

Lying Down

Resting often is equated with the lying positions, and although that usually is true, it does not necessarily have to be. To lie down, the cat can lower either the sternum or the pelvis to the ground first; to rise, the cat can raise either end first or both ends at one time, as is most frequently done when springing after prey or stretching. If resting on a windowsill, the cat may slide head first off its perch to the ground.

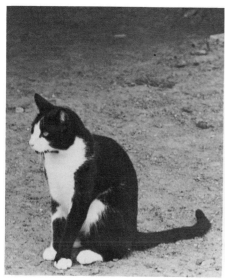 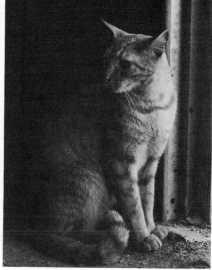

FIGURE 9–26. Common sitting postures of the cat.

There are three basic body postures associated with lying. Sternal recumbency is the first, and with it the forepaws may be pointed forward, usually with the tail directed caudally (Fig. 9–27 top). Another, more common version of sternal recumbency has the forepaws rotated and flexed so that they are tucked back under the cat (Fig. 9–27 bottom). In this situation the tail usually is curled around the cat's body and across its paws. This posture should be considered when treating ear mites. Unless the cat's whole body is treated initially, the mites can survive on other body areas and return to the ears when the treatment has been discontinued. Transfer of this parasite to the tail while the cat is lying

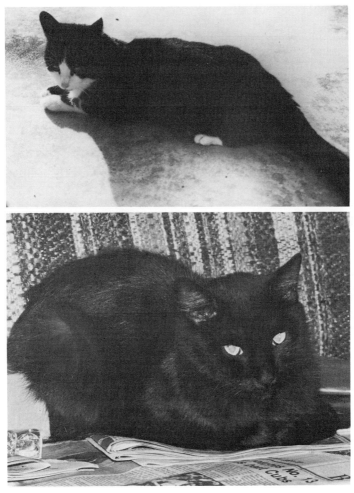

FIGURE 9–27. Sternally recumbent lying postures.

in this curled position is a frequent occurrence in individuals whose ears alone are treated.

The second lying posture is complete lateral recumbency (Fig. 9–28). Either side may contact the ground, and the cat may be stretched out or curled into a ball with the paws folded around one another. In the former case the tail also is outstretched; in the latter case the tail is curved around the body. The cooler the environmental temperature, the more tightly curled is the posture, so that the cat's head and paws are tucked under its body and enclosed by its tail.[7] Both of these are the postures associated with true sleep.

The third of the general postures associated with lying is a combination of cranial sternal recumbency and caudal lateral recumbency (Fig. 9–29). This position frequently is used by cats and is often associated with a "quiet alert" conscious phase.[85]

Preferences for sleeping places change periodically, but they often involve areas that are warm, quiet, and elevated. For a cat to accept a bed, it is best to encourage an area's use by providing warmth with a lamp or hot-water bottle.[6] An enclosed sleeping compartment also may be beneficial, especially for nervous or upset individuals.

Sleeping

The phenomenon known as sleep is not a state of the absence of activity, as has been described, but an active process. It begins with the

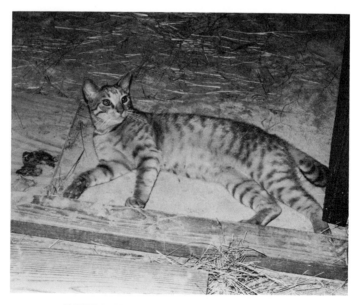

FIGURE 9–28. Laterally recumbent lying posture.

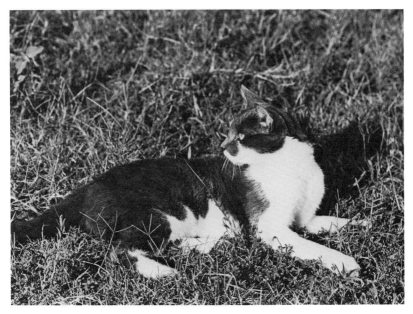

FIGURE 9–29. Combination of sternally and laterally recumbent lying postures.

neural initiation of a search for a place to sleep. Special posturing for sleep is part of this appetitive portion.[14, 57] The two consummatory phases of sleep are behaviorally evident at birth but cannot be differentiated by electroencephalographic means until the kitten is 2 to 3 weeks of age.[20] Until that time about 50 per cent of the kitten's day is spent sleeping, but only the deep phase is evident electronically.[1, 28] The amount of sleeping done by kittens is inversely proportional to the amount of play participation. Adult cats kept in controlled lighting sleep 10 hours per day.[37] Older cats have increased sleep bout fragmentation and show significantly less rapid-eye-movement (REM) sleep.[3]

Slow-wave (light) sleep usually occurs when the cat is in either a sternally recumbent posture with its forepaws tucked under and its tail wrapped around its body or the curled-up form of lateral recumbency. For both positions some muscle tone must be maintained for balance and head posture.[28, 41] There is a low-voltage, synchronized, slow cortical activity.[17, 42] Physiologic conditions also reflect this slowed state with breathing rates that are decreased and steady, and the eyes exhibit myosis of the pupils, stillness of the extrinsic muscles, and protrusion of the third eyelid.[42] Most sleep states of the cat are slow-wave in nature, taking up between 9 and 12 hours, about 40 per cent to 50 per cent of each day. Because the nocturnal activity patterns of cats are not observed, the relative amount of slow-wave sleep may appear to be greater than it actually is. Afternoon naps are easily observed, but hunting in the dark of night is not. Sleep studies indicate that modern cats are phasic throughout the day and night, thus not being truly nocturnal. More than half of the active time is during daylight and more than three-fourths of the sleep is during dark hours.[73] There also is evidence to support the idea that when deprived of slow-wave sleep, a cat can neurally compensate for this deficit during conscious minor activity.[15]

Within 10 to 30 minutes after falling asleep a cat may progress into paradoxical sleep, a deeper stage.[41, 42] Electroencephalographic recordings show desynchronization of the high-voltage cortical activity, some of which resembles normal wake patterns.[4] Although neck and general body muscle tone is lax, periodic movement of various parts can be observed. Digital flexion, twitching of the ears, irregular breathing, movement of vibrissae, flicking of the tongue, twitching of the tail, and sudden pupillary dilatation frequently occur. Rapid eye movements of 8 to 30 at a time are responsible for the other name for paradoxical sleep, REM sleep.[41] Lasting for 6 to 7 minutes, REM sleep usually alternates with 20 to 30 minutes of slow-wave sleep, but it takes up about 15 per cent of a 24-hour period.[28, 41, 56, 64, 71, 74] This represents about one-fourth of the total sleep time.[34] The phase of paradoxical sleep is known to be the time when dreaming occurs in human sleep, and although it may never be known whether animals do in fact dream, there is no reason to assume that they do not.[28, 29, 34, 56] The body movements that accompany REM sleep do not necessarily indicate the subject of the dream.[29]

Cats that are forced to remain awake for prolonged periods become increasingly irritable, even to the point of illness, but effects of sleeplessness on learning are not conclusively defined.[77] Deprivation of paradoxical sleep is the most significant aspect of this prolonged wakefulness because when allowed to sleep, the cat increases the amount of the REM phase until its deficit has been made up.[41, 51] Not until that time will the accelerated heart rate return to normal.[41] Fasting, use of antihistamines, and increased external stimulation all decrease sleep episodes, but the opposite is true for added food intake and quiet.

Awakening

Cats usually awaken from a slow-wave phase of sleep because the arousal threshold for REM sleep is 300 times greater than that needed for slow-wave sleep.[42] Cats that are sleeping on the lap of a person while being petted may awaken in a somewhat disoriented state and react to being "caught" by clawing. It is not until they have jumped free that full consciousness brings back the reality of the situation. When awaking naturally, most cats exhibit stretching behavior, usually of the thoracic limbs first. In addition, scratching nearby objects may serve as an action that in itself is a form of stretching.[25] (See Fig. 3–15.)

Reflexive Immobility

A young kitten is carried from place to place by the queen's holding the dorsum of its neck. (See Fig. 6–9.) This results in a partial flexor dominant position and passivity, which function to keep the kitten from struggling and to keep its tail out of the way so the queen will not step on it. Humans can successfully use the same method to immobilize adult cats, although its effectiveness decreases with the age of the cat. This reflexive posture, which also might be responsible for passivity during the male's mating neck grip, may be initiated by a number of factors.[27] External stimuli, such as visual, auditory, and tactile factors, as well as internal stimuli, such as emotional, visceral, and proprioceptive factors, bring about reflexive immobility.[45]

THE BRAIN AND LOCOMOTION

The cerebellum has long been recognized for functioning in motor coordination as a regulator, not an initiator. The functions of maintenance of equilibrium and body posture also are performed by this neural area. Degeneration or hypoplasia of the cerebellum does not become obvious until the kitten is at least 4 weeks of age because normal ambulation does not stabilize until then. Malnutrition of kittens from the prenatal period to as late as 6 weeks after birth significantly and permanently affects the cerebellum and, thus, motor coordination.[26, 68, 69]

Visually directed forelimb placement, although regulated by the cerebellum, probably is under fine control by the caudal sigmoid gyrus.[22] The frontal lobes also are known to affect motor abilities, particularly placing. Vertigo can be associated with motion sickness, labyrinthitis, cerebellar lesions, proprioception problems, and drug intoxication, including salicylates and streptomycin.[58, 65, 67]

The reticular activating system of the brainstem maintains consciousness, and is opposed by other central areas collectively called the "forebrain inhibitory system."[9] The thalamus of the brain is associated with sleep because stimulation of that region produces this homeostatic response, possibly by way of the thalamocortical radiations.[39, 57] Thalamic connections with the hypothalamus regulate the sleep-wake cycle, with destruction of the hypothalamus producing an abnormal amount of sleepiness. Conversely, stimulation of these areas results in hyperactivity and increased locomotion. The hypothalamic association with somatomotor responses, such as circling, rolling over, limb extension, claw extension, and head movements, can be demonstrated by stimulation soon after a kitten's birth.[46] The hippocampus has been experimentally shown to facilitate REM sleep, and the rostral raphe nuclei provide the major control of slow-wave sleep and the capacity of the brain to shift to sleep patterns.[1, 43, 44] Pontine activity stimulates the medullary inhibitory center, which then inhibits spinal cord motor neurons from initiating muscle contractions.[56] Stimulation of or damage to the forebrain system's pontine formations also is associated with disruptions in normal sleep-wake rhythms.[2, 9, 52]

Specific cerebral cortical areas regulate movement of certain body areas by the time the kitten is 47 days old.[84]

Locomotion is motivated by homeostatic drives, which are associated with rest and sleep and elicited by internal stimuli, as well as by nonhomeostatic drives caused by external stimuli, such as movement to escape a dog's approach. A combination of homeostatic and nonhomeostatic drives also can be effective, such as the prey-catching behavior of a cat that is initiated by both hunger and the squeak of a mouse.[57]

LOCOMOTIVE BEHAVIOR PROBLEMS

Most problems associated with locomotion are related to lameness, but because these are of minor significance in a feline practice and because these are traditionally covered in other subjects of veterinary medicine, this chapter does not discuss lameness.

Narcolepsy

Narcolepsy is an uncommon neurologic condition in the cat that results in sudden, recurring episodes of sleep. The condition can occur at any time, and thus could be potentially dangerous to the animal. Treatment of the narcolepsy with dextroamphetamine (1.25 mg P.O. as needed) has been successful.[47]

Other Sleep Disorders

With the exception of narcolepsy, sleep disorders are not well understood in domestic animals. Seizurelike activity during REM sleep has been reported in an otherwise healthy cat.[35]

Stereotyped Pacing

Animals that are in chronically frustrating situations, such as being confined in small cagelike environments or not getting enough exercise or environmental enrichment, frequently develop a behavioral vice called "stereotyped pacing." Although normally associated with zoo animals, stereotyped behavior patterns can be developed by cats, too, and are characteristic for each individual, regardless of the cause. Two basic patterns have been described in cats. The first involves the movement of the head and neck in a continuous lateral to-and-fro motion.[18, 80] The animal may have enough momentum to cause weight-shifting over the appropriate forepaw at the same time. The second stereotyped behavior is that the cat stands at a particular location, usually near the cage door, and sniffs.[80] Certain drugs potentiate these behaviors in cats known to have already acquired them.[80] Affected cats may be increasingly irritable to environmental stimuli, striking out at minor changes, such as new people feeding them or cleaning their cages. Neutering has been the most successful control because of its calming effect on the animal.[5] Progestin drugs for tomcats and neutered females and tranquilizers have been used successfully, but in all cases it is highly desirable to change the exercise plan for the cat. This can readily be accomplished by providing movable toys or another cat if space and social natures permit.

Overactivity

Overactivity as a problem can have a number of causes.[78] In young cats play behaviors may involve a lot of running, especially in sporadic bouts. The channeling of this energy into a play bout before bedtime can allow the owners a night without the kitten bouncing over them. Hyperthyroidism is a common clinical entity that causes young-acting geriatric cats, so owners need to be warned that the animal's activity may decrease after treatment. The feline hyperesthesia syndrome is manifested by overactivity and is discussed in Chapter 10.

CASE PRESENTATION

CASE 9–1. Two-and-one-half-year-old domestic shorthair neutered male. The cat had jumped on the kitchen counter ever since the owners got it 3 months ago. They had tried beating it and yelling at it. The owners believed that the cat was hungry all the time and fed it twice daily.

Diagnosis. Normal behavior of jumping onto high structures.

Treatment. The cat probably learned to get food by jumping onto counters at its previous home, so it was important not to leave food out on the counters. Access was controlled so that the cat could be punished with a squirt gun. The jumping decreased in incidence but continued to occur occasionally.

REFERENCES

1. Adrien, J.: Lesion of the anterior raphe nuclei in the newborn kitten and the effects on sleep. Brain Res. 103:579, 1976.
2. Bard, P., and Macht, M. B.: The behavior of chronically decerebrate cats. In Wolstenholme, G. E. W., and O'Connor, C. M., ed.: Neurological Basis of Behavior. Boston: Little, Brown & Co., 1952.
3. Bowersox, S. S., Baker, T. L., and Dement, W. C.: Sleep-wakefulness patterns in the aged cat. Electroencephalogr. Clin. Neurophysiol. 58:240, 1984.
4. Brooks, D. C., and Gershon, M. D.: Eye movement potentials in the oculomotor and visual systems of the cat: A comparison of reserpine induced waves with those present during wakefulness and rapid eye movement sleep. Brain Res. 27:223, 1971.
5. Brunner, F.: The application of behavior studies in small animal practice. In Fox, M. W., ed.: Abnormal Behavior in Animals. Philadelphia: W. B. Saunders Co., 1968.
6. Bryant, D.: The Care and Handling of Cats. New York: Ives Washburn, 1944.
7. Burton, M.: The Sixth Sense of Animals. New York: Taplinger Publishing Co., 1973.
8. Carmichael, L.: The genetic development of the kitten's capacity to right itself in the air when falling. J. Genet. Psychol. 44:453, 1934.
9. Clemente, C. D.: Forebrain mechanisms related to internal inhibition and sleep. Cond. Reflex. 3:145, 1968.
10. Cloe, J.: Paw preference in cats related to hand preference in animals and man. J. Comp. Physiol. Psychol. 48:137, 1955.
11. Cruickshank, R. M.: Animal infancy. In Carmichael, L., ed.: Manual of Child Psychology. New York: John Wiley & Sons, 1946.
12. Dagg, A. I.: Gaits in mammals. Mammal. Rev. 3:135, 1973.
13. English, A. W.: Interlimb coordination during stepping in the cat: An electromyographic analysis. J. Neurophysiol. 42:229, 1979.
14. Ewer, R. F.: Ethology of Mammals. London: Paul Elek, Ltd., 1968.
15. Ferguson, J., and Dement, W.: The effect of variations in total sleep time on the occurrence of rapid eye movement sleep in cats. Electroencephalogr. Clin. Neurophysiol. 22:2, 1967.
16. Fish, M. W., and Windle, W. F.: The effect of rotatory stimulation on the movements of the head and eyes in newborn and young kittens. J. Comp. Neurol. 54:103, 1932.
17. Foulkes, D.: Dream reports from different stages of sleep. J. Abnorm. Soc. Psychol. 65:14, July 1962.
18. Fox, M. W.: New information on feline behavior. Mod. Vet Pract. 56:50, Apr. 1965.
19. Fox, M. W.: Understanding Your Cat. New York: Coward, McCann & Geoghegan, 1974.
20. Fox, M. W.: The behavior of cats. In Hafez, E. S. E., ed.: The Behavior of Domestic Animals. 3rd ed. Baltimore: Williams & Wilkins Co., 1975.
21. Gambaryan, P. P.: How Mammals Run. New York: John Wiley & Sons, 1974.
22. Glassman, R. B.: Cutaneous discrimination and motor control following somatosensory cortical ablation. Physiol. Behav. 5:1009, 1970.
23. Gottlieb, G.: Ontogenesis of sensory function in birds and mammals. In Tobach, E., Aronson, L. R., and Shaw, E., ed.: The Biopsychology of Development. New York: Academic Press, 1971.
24. Gray, J.: Animal Locomotion. New York: W. W. Norton & Co., 1968.
25. Hart, B. L.: Behavioral aspects of scratching in cats. Fel. Pract. 2:6, Mar.- Apr. 1972.
26. Hart, B. L.: Behavior of the litter runt. Fel. Pract. 4:14, Sept. 1974.
27. Hart, B. L.: Handling and restraint of the cat. Fel. Pract. 5:10, Mar.-Apr. 1975.
28. Hart, B. L.: Sleeping behavior. Fel. Pract. 7:8, July 1977.
29. Hart, B. L.: The client asks you: A quiz on feline behavior. Fel. Pract. 8:10, Mar. 1978.
30. Hein, A.: Prerequisite for development of visually guided reaching in the kitten. Brain Res. 71:259, 1974.
31. Hein, A., and Diamond, R. M.: Locomotory space as a prerequisite for acquiring visually guided reaching in kittens. J. Comp. Physiol Psychol. 8:394, 1972.
32. Hein, A., and Held, R.: Dissociation of the visual placing response into elicited and guided components. Science 158:390, 1967.
33. Held, R., and Hein, A.: Movement-produced stimulation in the development of visually guided behavior. J. Comp. Physiol. Psychol. 56:872, 1963.

34. Hendricks, J. C., and Morrison, A. R.: Normal and abnormal sleep in mammals. J. Am. Vet. Med. Assoc. 178:121, 1981.
35. Hendricks, J. C., Morrison, A. R., Farnbach, G. L., et al.: A disorder of rapid eye movement sleep in a cat. J. Am. Vet. Med. Assoc. 178:55, 1981.
36. Hildebrand, M.: How animals run. Sci. Am. 202:148, 1960.
37. Houpt, K. A., and Wolski, T. R.: Domestic Animal Behavior for Veterinarians and Animal Scientists. Ames: Iowa State University Press, 1982.
38. Jacobs, B. L., Trulson, M. E., and Stern, W. C.: An animal behavior model for studying the actions of LSD and related hallucinogens. Science 194:741, 1976.
39. Jenkins, T. W.: Functional Mammalian Neuroanatomy. Philadelphia: Lea & Febiger, 1972.
40. Johnson, L. N.: Design of the master hunter. Cat Fancy 16:23, Dec. 1973.
41. Jouvet, M.: The states of sleep. Sci. Am. 216:62, 1967.
42. Jouvet, M.: Neurophysiology of the states of sleep. Physiol. Rev. 47:117, 1967.
43. Kim, C., Choi, H., Kim, C. C., et al.: Effect of hippocampectomy on sleep patterns in cats. Electroencephalogr. Clin. Neurophysiol. 38:235, 1975.
44. Kim, C., Choi, H., Kim, J. K., et al.: Sleep pattern of hippocampectomized cat. Brain Res. 29:223, 1971.
45. Klemm, W. R.: Neurophysiologic studies of the immobility reflex ("animal hypnosis"). Neurosci. Res. 4:165, 1971.
46. Kling, A., Kovach, J. K., and Tucker, T. J.: The behavior of cats. In Hafez, E. S. E., ed.: The Behavior of Domestic Animals. 2nd ed. Baltimore: Williams & Wilkins Co., 1969.
47. Knecht, C. D., Oliver, J. E., Redding, R., et al.: Narcolepsy in a dog and a cat. J. Am. Vet. Med. Assoc. 162:1052, 1973.
48. Kolata, R. J., Kraut, N. H., and Johnston, D. E.: Patterns of trauma in urban dogs and cats: A study of 1,000 cases. J. Am. Vet. Med. Assoc. 164:499, 1974.
49. Langworthy, O. R.: Histological development of cerebral motor areas in young kittens correlated with their physiological reaction to electrical stimulation. Contrib. Embryol. 19:177, 1927.
50. Langworthy, O. R.: A correlated study of the development of reflex activity in fetal and young kittens and the myelinization of tracts in the nervous system. Contrib. Embryol. 20:127, 1929.
51. Lucas, E. A.: Effects of five to seven days of sleep deprivation produced by electrical stimulation of the midbrain reticular formation. Exp. Neurol. 49:554, 1975.
52. Mancia, M.: Electrophysiological and behavioral changes owing to splitting of the brain-stem in cats. Electroencephalogr. Clin. Neururophysiol. 27:487, 1969.
53. Manter, J. T.: The dynamics of quadrupedal walking. J. Exp. Biol. 15:522, 1938.
54. McDonald, D.: How does a cat fall on its feet? New Scientist 7:1647, 1960.
55. Miller, S., Van Der Burg, J., and Van Der Meché, F. G. A.: Locomotion in the cat: Basic programmes of movement. Brain Res. 91:239, 1975.
56. Morrison, A. R.: A window on the sleeping brain. Sci. Am. 248:94, 1983.
57. Moruzzi, G.: Sleep and instinctive behavior. Arch. Ital. Biol. 107:175, 1969.
58. Pierce, J. H.: Disturbed equilibrium in small animals. Mod. Vet. Pract. 49:32, Oct. 1968.
59. Rheingold, H. L., and Eckerman, C. O.: Familiar social and nonsocial stimuli and the kitten's response to a strange environment. Dev. Psychobiol. 4:71, 1971.
60. Riesen, A. H., and Aarons, L.: Visual movement and intensity discrimination in cats after early deprivation of pattern vision. J. Comp. Physiol. Psychol. 52:142, 1959.
61. Robinson, G. W.: The high risk trauma syndrome in cats. Fel. Pract. 6:40, 1976.
62. Rosenblatt, J. S.: Suckling and home orientation in the kitten: A comparative developmental study. In Tobach, E., Aronson, L. R., and Shaw, E., ed.: The Biopsychology of Development. New York: Academic Press, 1971.
63. Rosenblatt, J. S.: Learning in newborn kittens. Sci. Am. 227:18, 1972.
64. Ruckebusch, Y., and Gaujoux, L.: Sleep patterns of the laboratory cat. Electroencephalogr. Clin. Neurophysiol. 41:483, 1976.
65. Schmidt, J. P.: Psychosomatics in veterinary medicine. In Fox, M. W., ed.: Abnormal Behavior in Animals. Philadelphia: W. B. Saunders Co., 1968.
66. Schneirla, T. C., Rosenblatt, J. S., and Tobach, E.: Maternal behavior in the cat. In Rheingold, H. L., ed.: Maternal Behavior in Mammals. New York: John Wiley & Sons, 1963.

67. Shimazu, H., and Precht, W.: Tonic and kinetic responses of cat's vestibular neurons to horizontal angular acceleration. J. Neurophysiol. 28:991, 1965.
68. Smith, B. A., and Jansen, G. R.: Early undernutrition and subsequent behavior patterns in cat. J. Nutr. 103:xxix, 1973.
69. Smith, B. A., and Jansen, G. R.: Behavior and brain composition of offspring of underfed cats. Fed. Proc. 36:1108, 1977.
70. Smith, R. C.: The Complete Cat Book. New York: Walker & Co., 1963.
71. Sterman, M. B., Knauss, T., Lehmann, D., and Clemente, C. D.: Circadian sleep and waking patterns in the laboratory cat. Electroencephalogr. Clin. Neurophysiol. 19:509, 1965.
72. Tilney, F., and Casamajor, L.: Myelinogeny as applied to the study of behavior. Arch. Neurol. Psychiatry 12:1, 1924.
73. Turner, D. C., and Meister, O.: Hunting behaviour of the domestic cat. In Turner, D. C., and Bateson, P., eds.: The Domestic Cat: The Biology of Its Behaviour. New York: Cambridge University Press, 1988.
74. Ulrsin, R.: Sleep stage relations within the sleep cycles of the cat. Brain Res. 20:91, 1970.
75. Van Hof-van Duin, J.: Development of visuomotor behavior in normal and dark reared cats. Brain Res. 104:233, 1976.
76. Villablanca, J. R., and Olmstead, C. E.: Neurological development of kittens. Dev. Psychobiol. 12:101, 1979.
77. Vogel, G. W.: A review of REM sleep deprivation. Arch. Gen. Psychiatry 32:749, 1975.
78. Voith, V. L., and Marder, A. R.: Feline behavioral disorders. In Morgan, R., ed.: Handbook of Small Animal Practice. New York: Churchill Livingstone, 1988.
79. Walk, R. D.: The study of visual depth and distance perception in animals. In Lehrman, D. S., Hinde, R. A., and Shaw, E., eds.: Advances in the Study of Behavior. Vol. 1. New York: Academic Press, 1965.
80. Wallach, M. B., and Gershon, S.: The induction and antagonism of central nervous system stimulant-induced stereotyped behavior in the cat. Eur. J. Pharmacol. 18:22, Apr. 1972.
81. Warkentin, J., and Carmichael, L.: A study of the development of the air righting reflex in cats and rabbits. J. Genet. Psychol. 55:67, 1939.
82. Warren, J. M., Abplanalp, J. M., and Warren, H. B.: The development of handedness in cats and rhesus monkeys. In Stevenson, H. W., Hess, E. H., and Rheingold, H. L., eds.: Early Behavior, Comparative and Developmental Approaches. New York: John Wiley & Sons, 1967.
83. Warren, J. M., Cornwell, P. R., Webster, W. G., and Pubols, B. H.: Unilateral cortical lesions and paw preferences in cats. J. Comp. Physiol. Psychol. 81:410, 1972.
84. Weed, L. H., and Lanworthy, O. R.: Physiological study of cortical motor areas in young kittens and in adult cats. Contrib. Embryol. 17:89, 1926.
85. West, M.: Social play in the domestic cat. Am. Zool. 14:427, 1974.
86. Wetzel, M. C.: Independently controlled EMG responses in treadmill locomotion by cats. Am. J. Phys. Med. 60:292, 1981.
87. Wetzel, M. C.: Operant control and cat locomotion. Am. J. Phys. Med. 61:11, Feb. 1982.
88. Whitney, W. O., and Mehlhaff, C. J.: High-rise syndrome in cats. J. Am. Vet. Med. Assoc. 191:1399, 1987.
89. Windle, W. F., and Fish, M. W.: The development of the vestibular righting reflex in the cat. J. Comp. Neurol. 54:85, 1932.
90. Windle, W. F., and Griffin, A. M.: Observations on embryonic and fetal movements of the cat. J. Comp. Neurol. 52:149, 1931.
91. Windle, W. F., O'Donnell, J. E., and Glasshagle, E. E.: The early development of spontaneous and reflex behavior in cat embryos and fetuses. Physiol. Zool. 6:521, 1932.
92. Wood, G. L.: Animal Facts and Feats. Garden City, NY: Doubleday & Co., 1972.

ADDITIONAL READING

Alstermark, B., and Wessberg, J. Timing of postural adjustment in relation to forelimb target-reaching in cats. Acta Physiol. Scand. 125:337, 1985.

Anand, B. K. Nervous regulation of food intake. Physiol. Rev. 41:677, 1961.

Beadle, M. The Cat: History, Biology, and Behavior. New York: Simon & Schuster, 1977.

Beaver, B. V. Reflex development in the kitten. Appl. Anim. Ethol. 4:93, 1978.

Beyer, C., Almanza, J., De La Torre, L., and Guznán-Flores, C. Brain stem multi-unit activity during "relaxation" behavior in the female cat. Brain Res. 29:213, 1971.

Bogen, J. E., Suzuki, M., and Campbell, B. Paw contact playing in the hypothalamic cat given caffeine. J. Neurobiol. 6:125, 1975.

Camuti, L. J. Cat ahoy! Fel. Pract. 4:50, May-June 1974.

DeLahunta, A. Veterinary Neuroanatomy and Clinical Neurology. Philadelphia: W. B. Saunders Co., 1977.

Dowd, P. J. Effects of congenital feline cerebellar hypoplasia on developmental behavior and the vestibular system. J. Psychol. 62:89, 1966.

Ewer, R. F. The Carnivores. Ithaca, NY: Cornell University Press, 1973.

Hall, V. E., and Pierce, G. N. Litter size, birth weight and growth to weaning in the cat. Anat. Rec. 60:111, 1934.

Hart, B. L. Behavioral aspects of selecting a new cat. Fel. Pract. 6:8, Sept. 1976.

Hart, B. L., and Voith, V. L. Sexual behavior and breeding problems in cats. Fel. Pract. 7:9, Jan. 1977.

Hemmer, H. Gestation period and postnatal development in fields. In Eaton, R. L., ed. The World's Cats. 3rd ed. Seattle: Carnivore Research Institute, 1976.

Kemp, I. R., and Kaada, B. R. The relation of hippocampal theta activity to arousal, attentive behavior and somato-motor movements in unrestrained cats. Brain Res. 95:323, 1975.

Kilham, L., Margolis, G., and Colby, E. D. Cerebellar ataxia and its congenital transmission in cats by feline panleukopenia virus. J. Am. Vet. Med. Assoc. 158:888, 1971.

Koepke, J. E., and Pribram, K. H. Effect of milk on the maintenance of sucking behavior in kittens from birth to six months. J. Comp. Physiol. Psychol. 75:363, 1971.

Konrad, K. W., and Bagshaw, M. Effect of novel stimuli on cats reared in a restricted environment. J. Comp. Physiol. Psychol. 70:157, 1970.

Langworthy, O. R.: Behavior disturbances related to the decomposition of reflex activity caused by cerebral injury: An experimental study of the cat. J. Neuropathol. Exp. Neurol. 3:87, 1944.

Lockard, D. E., Traher, L. M., and Wetzel, M. C.: Reinforcement influences upon topography of treadmill locomotion by cats. Physiol. Behav. 16:141, 1976.

Meier, G. W. Infantile handling and development in Siamese kittens. J. Comp. Physiol. Psychol. 54:284, 1961.

Munson, J. B. Multi-unit activity with eye movements during fast-wave sleep in cats. Exp. Neurol. 37:446, 1972.

Prinz, P. A. N. Pharmacological alterations of patterns of sleep and wakefulness in the cat. Diss. Abstr. Int. 30:3794B, 1969.

Scott, P. P. Diet and other factors affecting the development of young felids. In Eaton, R. L., ed. The World's Cats. 3rd ed. Seattle: Carnivore Research Institute, 1976.

Skoglund, S. On the postnatal development of postural mechanisms as revealed by electromyography and myography in decerebrate kittens. Acta Physiol. Scand. 49:299, 1960.

Suzuki, J., and Cohen, B. Integration of semicircular canal activity. J. Neurophysiol. 29:981, 1966.

Warkentin, J., and Smith, K. U. The development of visual acuity in the cat. J. Genet. Psychol. 50:371, 1937.

Weigel, I. Small cats and clouded leopards. In Grzimek, H. C. B., ed.: Grzimek's Animal Life Encyclopedia. Vol. 12. New York: Van Nostrand Reinhold Co., 1975.

Widdowson, E. M. Food, growth and development in the suckling period. In Graham-Jones, O., ed.: Canine and Feline Nutritional Requirements. New York: Pergamon Press, 1965.

Wilson, M., Warren, J. M., and Abbott, L. Infantile stimulation, activity and learning by cats. Child Dev. 36:843, 1965.

Worden, A. N. Abnormal behavior in the dog and cat. Vet. Rec. 71:966, 1959.

10

Feline Grooming Behavior

The various grooming behaviors are important to a normal, healthy cat. Not only does the lack of these behaviors indicate depression or ill health, but also the potential for ectoparasite infestation and accompanying secondary conditions greatly increases.

GROOMING FUNCTIONS

Newborn kittens depend on the dam for grooming, especially during the first few days of life. Her licking not only conditions their coats but also stimulates urination and defecation until the young can move to a special area to eliminate. This reflex control of eliminations keeps both the nest and the kittens clean. As motor skills mature, the kittens begin self-grooming, but it is incomplete and awkward at first.

As the cat matures, grooming becomes increasingly significant until 30 per cent to 50 per cent of the awake time is spent performing some type of this behavior.[11] Variations do exist, probably as a result of early experience, genetic factors, and hair coat, with long hair needing more attention.

Grooming serves several purposes, with the most important probably being maintenance of healthy skin. Body hygiene is apparently learned early because kittens that are not well cared for develop into unkempt adults more frequently than those with normal histories. Although hair is shed by normal cats year round, losses are heaviest in the spring and when the cat is ill or staying in dry indoor heat. The hair coat between the eye and ear normally is thinner than on other parts of the body, but during shedding it may almost disappear, so that Siamese cats can almost lose their masks.[5] Removal of loose hair is necessary to keep the coat unmatted and minimize ectoparasite infestations. Grooming also removes parasites and dander. In hot weather as much as a third of the cat's evaporative-cooling loss can be achieved by licking the skin and hair.[11] Another function of grooming is to relieve tension, as may occur preceding a thunderstorm, after a reprimand from the owner, or after an encounter with a very aggressive cat.[10]

GROOMING PATTERNS

Each type of grooming has an appetitive and a consummatory phase. The former phase is made up of the orienting components that direct the animal's attention to the affected body surface. The consummatory phase completes the response and consists of the lick, bite, or scratch.[28] Normal tactile stimulation results in either grooming of the region or, more frequently, no response.[28]

Oral Grooming

The cat grooms much of its body with its tongue or teeth. Licking as a form of grooming usually appears near the beginning of the kitten's 2nd week with attempts at licking the forepaw. Within a few days the kitten is licking the rest of its body. The caudally directed, well-developed lingual papillae are particularly suited for this form of grooming.

After eating a cat spends considerable time grooming by licking, particularly around the oral area. In addition, direct licking is useful from the caudal to the midcervical area (Fig. 10–1). The cat can assume some unusual positions to reach various areas (Fig. 10–2). The anogenital area is groomed after mating as well as during normal grooming periods.

The incisors are useful for pulling burrs and tangles out of the hair coat and frequently are used to clean between the toes. This type of grooming is most effective for the body caudal to the neck (see Fig. 10–1).

Feline oral grooming, particularly by licking, may someday prove to be a useful tool in evaluating the environment.[17] The cat's metabolic concentrations of pollutants gathered by grooming could serve as sentinels of public health.

Paw Grooming

Areas that cannot be groomed directly by the mouth are cared for by using either fore paws or hind paws (Fig. 10–1). Because the head and neck are so difficult to care for, problems are more numerous in these areas.[11] The common form of grooming that follows eating, which is

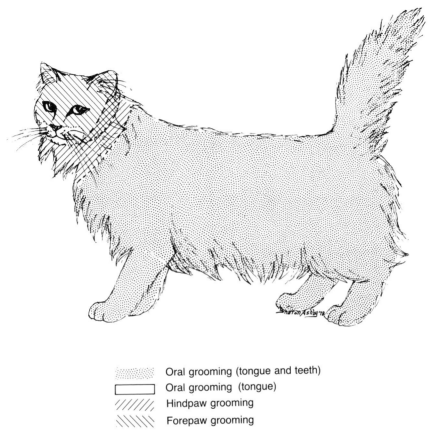

```
[dotted]    Oral grooming (tongue and teeth)
[  ]        Oral grooming (tongue)
//////      Hindpaw grooming
\\\\\\      Forepaw grooming
```

FIGURE 10–1. Areas groomed in various manners by the cat.

second only to licking, is use of the fore paw as a washing tool. The paw is licked several times (Fig. 10–3) and then its medial side is wiped across the neck, the back of the head and ears, and, finally, the face (Fig. 10–4). The head and neck often are moved to accommodate this action. After every few swipes the cat again licks its paw. The young kitten usually begins this fore paw–washing behavior before it is 4 weeks of age.

Scratching various parts of the body with the hind paw in grooming begins about 18 days after birth. (See Appendix D.) As in paw-washing, the areas most frequently scratched are those that cannot be licked, particularly the neck and auricular areas (see Fig. 10–1).

The cat conditions its claws by scratching favorite objects, usually near its sleeping quarters, or by chewing off the frayed and worn parts. (See Fig. 3–15.) Scratching usually grooms the thoracic claws, whereas claws on the pelvic limbs are primarily cared for by the teeth.

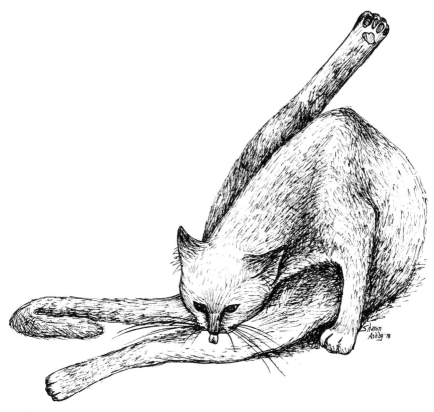

FIGURE 10–2. Cats can assume some unusual positions during grooming sessions.

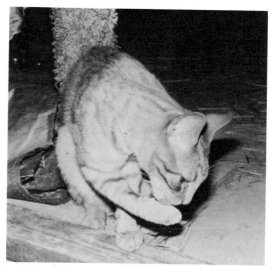

FIGURE 10–3. The licking of the forepaw before using it as a washing tool.

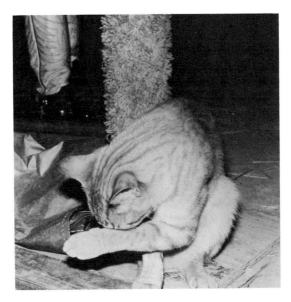

FIGURE 10–4. The forepaw is used to groom facial areas.

Mutual Grooming

Ancestors of the cat were not social animals and so did not have social behavior patterns. Only after human interaction did the cat evolve social behaviors in grooming. When two cats are together by mutual agreement, it is common for one to lick the other. This type of mutual, or social, grooming most frequently involves the head and neck, the most difficult places to care for (Fig. 10–5). Cats have been known to chew off another's tactile hairs during a mutual-grooming session.[5] Beginning at a few weeks of age, social behavior tends to reach a peak when the kitten is between 5 weeks and 4 months.[31] After that time the frequency of the mutual-grooming sessions decreases.

Mutual grooming can be extended to humans by licking them and accepting their petting, especially on the cranial regions. Most cats patiently accept a prolonged session of caressing, probably because they have no built-in mechanism to limit it.[9] In nature, one cat spends only a limited amount of time grooming another cat, which becomes almost immobile. Humans often extend this grooming session well beyond the normal length of time, and the cat accommodates them by not moving.

Displacement Grooming

On a number of occasions a cat suddenly starts grooming for a brief duration as a displacement activity. When a cat is in a conflict or a

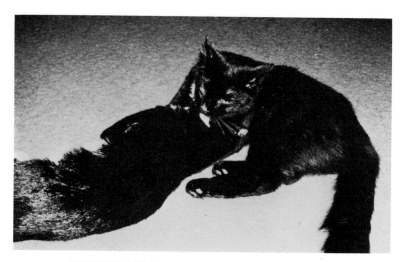

FIGURE 10–5. Mutual grooming of one cat by another.

stressful situation, it may appear ready to react but instead suddenly stops and performs an act that is out of context with the situation at hand, such as licking a paw and rubbing it across its face. Presumedly, this behavior reduces anxiety. A queen with kittens may increase her grooming of the young or of her own perineal and mammary regions during stress, and a cat, if reprimanded frequently, may react by walking a distance away and then grooming. Cats that roll over and accidentally slide off a table or chair also respond with a grooming session, usually after glancing around the room.

NEUROENDOCRINE AND GROOMING RELATIONSHIPS

Central controls of grooming behavior are not completely understood but are related to the pontine area of the brain and may be the same as for locomotion.[7] When lesions are created in this location, a dissociation develops between the appetitive and consummatory phases of grooming.[19, 25] This abnormality is exhibited as an immediate response to a tactile stimulus that is independent of the appetitive component. Thus, although the response is appropriate, the orientation may be poorly directed. For example, touching the ear might produce midair scratching movements.[28] Similar abortive grooming has been observed with frontal neocortical lesions.[14, 24–26] In both cases tryptophan hydroxylase levels of the rostral colliculi decrease, indicating a relation between this area of the mesencephalon and grooming behavior.[24, 26]

Thyroid hormones and glucocorticoids play a role in central control of grooming behavior, although the exact mechanism is uncertain. Thyroidectomized cats show the same enzyme changes in the rostral colliculi mentioned above, but the relation between these two situations is not understood.[28]

Hallucinogenic drugs can produce dissociated grooming. The body is properly positioned, but licking, biting, or scratching either does not occur or is poorly directed.[13]

Circadian rhythms are difficult to identify, but studies of fragmented grooming behaviors have provided evidence that such cycles exist in the cat. Body temperature, caloric intake, and abnormal grooming activity fluctuate in 3- to 4-month periods, peaking in October or November and in June, and ebbing between February and May and in August.[18, 20, 25–28]

Hormone levels affect hair coat. Castrated males show a significant tendency toward longer hair.[22] Queening, extended lactation, or both may result in hair loss, producing a thinner or shorter coat.

GROOMING BEHAVIOR PROBLEMS

Nongrooming Behavior

Stressful conditions that are emotionally upsetting to a cat can result in cessation of grooming behaviors.[10, 15] (See Fig. 4–7.) Certainly disease can be a causal factor, but so can such things as overcrowding or a new dog in the house. The security of a box or paper sack may be all that is needed.

Excessive Grooming Behavior

Nervousness, boredom, and desire for human contact can be expressed with forms of excessive grooming, particularly by Siamese and Abyssinian cats.[11] In these situations licking most frequently is the used type of grooming, and the caudal half of the body, particularly the medial thigh and ventral abdomen, most frequently is involved. Affected areas usually have well-defined borders, normal skin, and almost no hair within the area. In extreme cases self-mutilation can result, and queens may overgroom their kittens to the point of mutilation.[10] Tail-chasing and excessive scratching of the head are other forms of this behavior. When stress is a contributing factor, treatment ideally involves removal of the cause.[32] This could include treating fleas or other causes of pruritus, minimizing visualization of stray cats, or decreasing environmental disturbances. These may need to be supplemented with a secluded area, progestins, which have a calming effect, and/or tranquilizers, especially the antianxiety tranquilizers such as diazepam (1 to 2 mg P.O. b.i.d.), amitriptyline hydrochloride (5 to 10 mg P.O. s.i.d.), and chlorpheniramine maleate (2 to 4 mg P.O. b.i.d.).[30] The affection-craving individual should be placed on a strict routine that includes rewarding the grooming behavior only with inattention.

Excessive grooming may indicate involvement of the central nervous system, probably in a number of ways. Direct stimulation of the ventral hippocampus can produce reactions with emotional manifestations, including restlessness, vocalizations, body postures of fear and retreat, and excessive perineal licking.[8] There also is a connection between grooming and several forms of epilepsy, an understanding of which is useful in combining several diagnoses and treatments into a more common grouping.[8] Excessive groomers, especially tail-biters or mutilators, have been treated with varying success with repository corticosteroids, progestins, and antiepileptic medications. A combination of drugs often is most successful, particularly when using corticosteroids and progestins; feline leukemia apparently plays a role in the pathologic behavior of some of these cats because diagnostically positive individuals have a much lower success rate for treatment.[3, 23]

The feline hyperesthesia syndrome (rolling skin syndrome, feline neurodermatitis) is another behavioral abnormality. It is exhibited by a cat suddenly rising with vertical tail and with the skin over the dorsum appearing to roll.[2, 32] Then the cat howls and dashes away. This cutaneous muscle movement may represent a form of epilepsy because it usually responds to antiepileptics and occasionally to progestins or steroids as well.[1, 4, 15, 16, 29] A similar startle reaction is seen with pontine and certain rostral hypothalamic lesions.[12]

A secondary problem in excessive grooming is the formation of hairballs. Because most of the hair that pulls loose during grooming sticks to the papillae of the tongue, it eventually is swallowed. If enough is ingested and not lost by normal vomition or defecation, anorexia and generalized depression result.[11]

Hair Loss

Generalized hair loss and alopecia can occur in cats that are under severe emotional stress, especially nervous individuals and purebred animals.[6, 21] In contrast, localized hair loss caudal to the ears or along the lumbar spine, possibly accompanied by ulceration, is due to the vigorous scratching of this area by the hind feet. This hair loss is indicative of an *Otodectes cynotis* or flea infestation.

Skin Problems

In addition to dermatoses resulting from nongrooming, allergens, and bacteria, the cat can suffer from psychic eczema.[21] Affected individuals frequently lick excessively, producing skin trauma, until they are hospitalized, where new surroundings distract them. Lesions of cutaneous lymphedema or lymphedemic dermatitis are characteristic.

CASE PRESENTATIONS

CASE 10–1. Four-year-old domestic shorthair female. The cat was a tail mutilator. The owner thought that the cat became frightened when it saw its tail and then attacked. Once the cat began chewing, it did not seem to be able to stop. The problem occurred at least three times in 5 days.

Medical Workup. The physical examination, laboratory data, and electroencephalogram were normal. The cat was reported feline leukemia negative.

Diagnosis. Excessive grooming, probably caused by epilepsy (as seen by episodes of sudden fear).

Treatment. The condition is fairly well controlled with phenobarbital (1/8 gr t.i.d.).

CASE 10–2. Two-year-old Burmese neutered female. About 2 weeks before presentation the cat started licking its fore paws. The licking progressed to the mammary area and to the tail. While licking, the cat seemed unaware of its surroundings but suddenly stopped the behavior. It would lick a hand if it got in the way. The cat had previously been reported feline leukemia negative.

Medical Workup. The physical examination and laboratory data were within normal limits. A second feline leukemia report was positive.

Diagnosis. Excessive grooming, possibly related to feline leukemia.

Treatment. Medroxyprogesterone acetate (50 mg I.M.) and methylprednisolone acetate (10 mg I.M.) stopped the licking within a week, but the cat began running and jumping onto high objects and calling as if hurting. Antiepileptics did not help.

CASE 10–3. Three-and-one-half-year-old domestic shorthair female. The cat had daily occurrences of cutaneous muscle twitches, at which time it also cried out and raced around the apartment. This behavior occurred for about 1 year. During each attack, the animal apparently was oblivious to anything going on around it.

Diagnosis. Feline hyperesthesia syndrome (rolling skin syndrome).

Treatment. Phenobarbital (1/8 gr P.O. t.i.d.) eliminated the problem within 3 days. During a vacation period when the cat was not medicated for 2 weeks, the syndrome recurred within 2 days but was brought under control shortly after treatment was resumed.

CASE 10–4. Twelve-year-old domestic shorthair neutered female. The cat was described as very fearful, and 3 years ago spent most of the year hiding in dark corners. In the past 2 years the cat has started to spend more time in the room but also has been licking its abdomen, inner thighs, and sides excessively. The problem started about the time the owner moved to town to go to college.

Diagnosis. Psychogenic alopecia.

Treatment. Getting the cat on a rigid schedule, including interactions with the owner, helped to control the degree of excessive grooming.

CASE 10–5. Four-and-one-half-year-old Burmese neutered female. The cat had started licking its abdomen, forearm, and elbow about 1½ years before being presented. The problem seemed to end during the winter but recurred the next spring. The cat was quite attached to the owner and could be described as very nervous. The owner later mentioned that outdoor cats had actually torn the window screens where this cat normally spends its day. Because the owners are moving soon, they were thinking of getting a kitten to be with this cat while they are gone.

Medical Workup. Other than alopecia on the abdomen and right forearm, the cat appeared to be physically healthy. The blood counts and chemistry panel were within normal limits. A dermatology workup with antigen testing also was normal.

Diagnosis. Psychogenic alopecia with a seasonal incidence probably related to the roaming cats during their mating season.

Treatment. The owners were told to keep the cat away from the area where it could see other cats and to confine it to a small room that had the owners' odors when they did move. They were told that getting a kitten was not advisable. The response was good, particularly by several months after the move.

CASE 10–6. Six-year-old domestic shorthair neutered female. The cat had a long history of not liking people other than the husband and wife owners. There is an 8-month-old son in the family who is now crawling. Within the past 6 months the cat started licking its abdomen, and in the last month she occasionally defecated on the dining room carpet.

Diagnosis. Psychogenic alopecia and housesoiling by defecation related to the presence of the baby.

Treatment. The owners tried to confine the cat away from the child, but the situation became more difficult as the baby started walking. The cat eventually was placed in a new home.

CASE 10–7. Ten-year-old Siamese neutered female. Two weeks before presentation the owner of this cat passed away and the cat was taken home by the married son. Since arriving the cat had spent its entire time under the bed. It stopped grooming, eliminated only when no one was at home, and would not eat.

Diagnosis. Stress-related nongrooming and anorexia nervosa.

Treatment. The cat was started on megestrol acetate (5 mg P.O.) and within 3 days had started eating. The drug dose gradually was reduced. Within 10 days the cat was considered to be normal again.

CASE 10–8. Three-year-old Siamese neutered female. When the wife started back to work in the middle of April, the owners noticed that the cat was getting bald on the dorsal midline. They brought the cat in for the problem about 1 month later.

Diagnosis. Psychogenic alopecia.

Treatment. The owners put the cat on diazepam (2 mg P.O.) for 2 weeks and started on a schedule of attention so that it was interacted with at specific times. It was given a rag with the owners' scent on which it normally slept during the day. This helped some, but the problem got worse again about 3 months later, when the man, a teacher, returned to work.

Also see case 2–8.

REFERENCES

1. Alterman, H. P., Hart, B. L., Mosier, J. E., and Parker, A. J.: Use of primidone in cats questioned. Fel. Pract. 7:4, Nov. 1977.
2. Beaver, B. V.: Disorders of behavior. In Sherding, R. G., ed.: The Cat: Diseases and Clinical Management. New York: Churchill Livingstone, 1989.
3. Beaver, B. V.: Feline behavioral problems other than housesoiling. J. Am. Anim. Hospital. Assoc. 25:465, 1989.
4. Blum, S. R.: Aggressive behavior. Fel. Pract. 9:9, Mar.-Apr. 1979.
5. Bryant, D.: The Care and Handling of Cats. New York: Ives Washburn, 1944.
6. Chertok, L., and Fontaine, M.: Psychosomatics in veterinary medicine. J. Psychosom. Res. 7:229, 1963.
7. Deliagina, T. G., Orlovsky, G. N., and Perret, C.: Efferent activity during fictitious scratch reflex in the cat. J. Neurophysiol. 45:595, 1981.
8. Dhume, R. A., Gogate, M. G., deMascarenhas, J. F., and Sharma, K. N.: Functional dissociation within hippocampus: Correlates of visceral and behavioral patterns induced on stimulation of ventral hippocampus in cats. Indian J. Med. Res. 64:33, 1976.
9. Ewer, R. F.: Ethology of Mammals. London: Paul Elek, Ltd., 1968.
10. Fox, M. W.: Understanding Your Cat. New York: Coward, McCann & Geoghegan, 1974.
11. Hart, B. L.: The role of grooming activity. Fel. Pract. 6:14, July 1976.
12. Hart, B. L.: Sleeping behavior. Fel. Pract. 7:8, July 1977.
13. Jacobs, B. L., Trulson, M. E., and Stern, W. C.: An animal behavior model for studying the actions of LSD and related hallucinogens. Science 194:741, 1976.
14. Langworthy, O. R.: Behavioral disturbances related to the decomposition of reflex activity caused by cerebral injury: An experimental study of the cat. J. Neuropathol. Exp. Neurol. 3:87, 1944.
15. Mosier, J. E.: Common medical and behavioral problems in cats. Mod. Vet. Pract. 56:699, 1975.
16. Parker, A.: Feline hyperesthesia syndrome. Virg. Vet. Notes 19:2, Jan.-Feb. 1986.

17. Priester, W. A.: Cats are pollution sentinels. J. Am. Vet. Med. Assoc. 160:341, 1972.
18. Randall, W. L., and Parsons, V.: The concomitancy in the rhythms of caloric intake and behavior in cats: A replication. Psychon. Sci. 15:35, 1969.
19. Randall, W. L., and Parsons, V.: Thyroidectomy produces abnormal grooming behavior in cats. Psychon. Sci. 21:268, 1970.
20. Rogers, W., Parsons, V., and Randall, W.: Comsummatory grooming fragments: A model for periodic behaviors. Psychon. Sci. 23:375, 1971.
21. Schmidt, J. P.: Psychosomatics in veterinary medicine. In Fox, M. W., ed.: Abnormal Behavior in Animals. Philadelphia: W. B. Saunders Co., 1968.
22. Searle, A. G.: Gene frequencies in London's cats. J. Genet. 49:214, 1949.
23. Stein, B.: Personal communication, 1977.
24. Trulson, M. E.: Role of superior colliculus serotonin in the grooming behavior of cats. Neuropharmacology 15:91, 1976.
25. Trulson, M. E.: Biological bases for the integration of appetitive and consummatory grooming behaviors in the cat: A review. Pharmacol. Biochem. Behav. 4:329, 1976.
26. Trulson, M. E., Nicolay, J., and Randall, W.: Abnormalities in grooming behavior and tryptophan hydroxylase activity in the superior colliculi in cats with pontile and frontal neocortical lesions. Pharmacol. Biochem. Behav. 3:87, 1975.
27. Trulson, M. E., and Randall, W.: 5-Hydroxytryptamine metabolism, superior colliculus, and grooming behavior in cats with pontile lesions. J. Comp. Physiol. Psychol. 85:1, Oct. 1973.
28. Trulson, M. E., and Randall, W.: Similarities in the physiological bases of an abnormal grooming behavior in thyroidectomized cats and in cats with lesions of the central nervous system. J. Comp. Physiol. Psychol. 90:917, 1976.
29. Tuttle, J. L., and Parker, A. J.: Diagnosing, treating feline hyperesthesia syndrome. D.V.M. 11:72, Feb. 1980.
30. Voith, V. L., and Marder, A. R.: Feline behavioral disorders. In Morgan, R., ed.: Handbook of Small Animal Practice. New York: Churchill Livingstone, 1988.
31. West, M.: Social play in the domestic cat. Am. Zool. 14:427, 1974.
32. Young, M. S., and Manning, T. O.: Psychogenic dermatoses. Derm. Reports 3:1, 1984.

ADDITIONAL READING

Beadle, M. The Cat: History, Biology, and Behavior. New York: Simon & Schuster, 1977.
Beaver, B. V. G. Feline behavioral problems. Vet. Clin. North Am. 6:333, 1976.
Blacklock, G. A. A cat's purr. . . On purpose? Cat Fancy 16:20, Aug. 1973.
Boudreau, J. C., and Tsuchitani, C. Sensory Neurophysiology. New York: Van Nostrand Reinhold Co., 1973.
Fox, M. W. New information on feline behavior. Mod. Vet. Pract. 56:50, Apr. 1965.
Fox, M. W. Aggression: Its adaptive and maladaptive significance in man and animals. In Fox, M. W., ed. Abnormal Behavior in Animals. Philadelphia: W. B. Saunders Co., 1968.
Hart, B. L. Behavioral aspects of scratching in cats. Fel. Pract. 2:6, Apr. 1972.
Hart, B. L. Social interactions between cats and their owners. Fel. Pract. 6:6, Jan. 1976.
Hart, B. L. Aggression in cats. Fel. Pract. 7:22, Mar. 1977.
Kling, A., Kovach, J. K., and Tucker, T. J. The behavior of cats. In Hafez, E. S. E., ed. The Behavior of Domestic Animals. 2nd ed. Baltimore: Williams & Wilkins Co., 1969.
Randall, W., and Parsons, V. Rhythmic dysfunctions in 11-hydroxycorticoid excretion after midbrain lesions and their relationship to an abnormal grooming behavior in cats. J. Interdiscipl. Cycle Res. 3:3, Mar. 1972.
Randall, W., Trulson, M., and Parsons, V. Role of thyroid hormones in an abnormal grooming behavior in thyroidectomized cats and cats with pontile lesions. J. Comp. Physiol. Psychol. 90:231, 1976.
Tilney, F., and Casamajor, L. Myelinogeny as applied to the study of behavior. Arch. Neurol. Psychiatry 12:1, July 1924.

APPENDIX A

Phonetics of Feline Vocalization*

Murmur patterns
1. Grunt
2. Purr   ['hrn-rhn-'hrn-rhn . . .]
   a. Greeting (request)   ['mhrn]
3. Call   ['ə mhrn]
4. Acknowledgement   ['mhrŋ]

Vowel patterns
1. Demand   ['mhrn-a':ou]
   a. Whisper   ['mhrn-ɛ̃']
   b. Begging demand   ['mhrn-a:ou]
2. Bewilderment   ['maou:?]
   a. Worry   ['mæ ou:?]
3. Complaint   ['mhŋ-a:ou]
4. Mating cry (mild form)   ['mhrn-a:ou]
5. Anger wail   [wa:ou:]

Strained intensity patterns
1. Growl   [grrr . . .]
2. Snarl   ['æ:o]
3. Hiss   ['sss . . .]
   a. Spit   [fft!]
4. Mating cry (intense form)   ['ø-ø':ə]
5. Scream   [æ!]
6. Refusal   ['æᶻ'æᶻ'æ]

KEY: [a] as in father, [æ as in cat, [ɛ] as in get, [ə] as in momma,
    [o] as in go, [ø] as in French eux, [u] as in pool, [f] as in fan,
    [g] as in gone, [h] as in hunt, [m] as in mouse, [n] as in kitten,
    [ŋ] as in sung, [r] as in rat, [t] as in cat, [s] as in see,
    [:] indicates prolongation, [~] indicates nasalization, ['] indicates
    stress-accent, ['] indicates inhalation, [?] indicates rising inflec-
    tion, [ᶻ] indicates wavering or discontinuity, [!] indicates abrupt,
    stress-accent ending.

*Data from Moelk, M.: Vocalizing in the house cat; a phonetic and functional study. Am. J. Psychol. 57:184-205, 1944.

APPENDIX B

Sensory Response Development

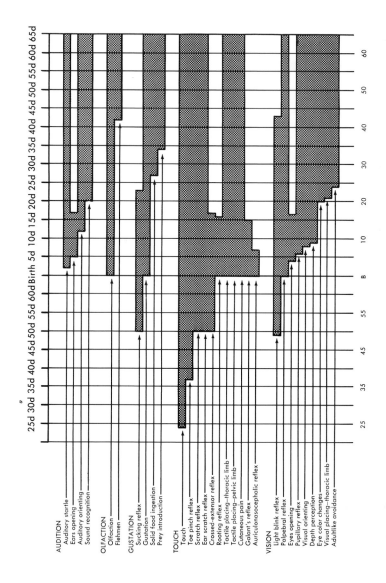

APPENDIX C

Motor Response Development

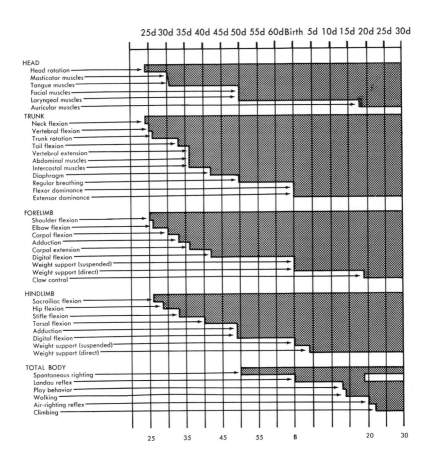

APPENDIX D

Miscellaneous Response Development

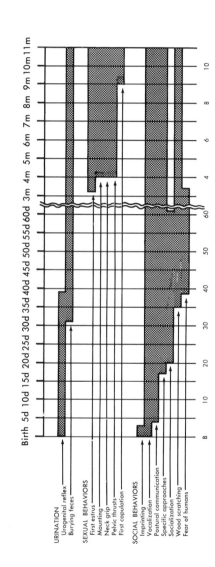

Index

271